6- 10-
263639

AF324225

MENTAL RETARDATION RESEARCH ADVANCES

MENTAL RETARDATION RESEARCH ADVANCES

ELIZABETH B. HEINZ
EDITOR

Nova Biomedical Books
New York

Copyright © 2007 by Nova Science Publishers, Inc.

All rights reserved. No part of this book may be reproduced, stored in a retrieval system or transmitted in any form or by any means: electronic, electrostatic, magnetic, tape, mechanical photocopying, recording or otherwise without the written permission of the Publisher.

For permission to use material from this book please contact us:
Telephone 631-231-7269; Fax 631-231-8175
Web Site: http://www.novapublishers.com

NOTICE TO THE READER

The Publisher has taken reasonable care in the preparation of this book, but makes no expressed or implied warranty of any kind and assumes no responsibility for any errors or omissions. No liability is assumed for incidental or consequential damages in connection with or arising out of information contained in this book. The Publisher shall not be liable for any special, consequential, or exemplary damages resulting, in whole or in part, from the readers' use of, or reliance upon, this material.

Independent verification should be sought for any data, advice or recommendations contained in this book. In addition, no responsibility is assumed by the publisher for any injury and/or damage to persons or property arising from any methods, products, instructions, ideas or otherwise contained in this publication.

This publication is designed to provide accurate and authoritative information with regard to the subject matter covered herein. It is sold with the clear understanding that the Publisher is not engaged in rendering legal or any other professional services. If legal or any other expert assistance is required, the services of a competent person should be sought. FROM A DECLARATION OF PARTICIPANTS JOINTLY ADOPTED BY A COMMITTEE OF THE AMERICAN BAR ASSOCIATION AND A COMMITTEE OF PUBLISHERS.

Library of Congress Cataloging-in-Publication Data

Mental retardation research advances / Elizabeth B. Heinz (editor).
    p. ; cm.
Includes bibliographical references.
ISBN-13: 978-1-60021-658-9 (hardcover)
ISBN-10: 1-60021-658-7 (hardcover)
1. Mental retardation. 2. Mental retardation. I. Heinz, Elizabeth B.
[DNLM: 1. Mental Retardation. WM 300 M55345 2007]
RC570.M4224 2007
616.85'880072--dc22

2007010567

Published by Nova Science Publishers, Inc. ✦ New York

Contents

Preface   **vii**

Chapter I   Simple Reaction Times and Timing of Unimanual and Bimanual Serial Actions in Adolescents with Mental Retardation, Autism, and Down Syndrome   **1**
Nobuyuki Inui

Chapter II   Regular Exercise as a Healthy Strategy to Reduce Oxidative Stress in Adolescents with Down Syndrome   **35**
F.J. Ordonez and M.Rosety-Rodriguez

Chapter III   Stress and Quality of Life in Families of People with Intellectual Disabilities   **45**
Verri Annapia, Cremante Anna, Kaltchewa Dimitrina and Ronchi Guido

Chapter IV   Supporting Families of Children with Down Syndrome: What the Literature Teaches Us   **59**
Judy O. Berry and River J. Smith

Chapter V   Distractor Interference Effects and Identification of Safe and Dangerous Road-Crossing Sites by Children with and without Mental Retardation   **75**
A. Alevriadou and G. Grouios

Chapter VI   Neurotrophic Factors in the Pathogenesis of Mental Retardation in Children   **89**
Raili Riikonen

Chapter VII   Mental Retardation and Mental Illness: An Overview   **105**
Alka S. Ahuja and Srinivas Reddy

Chapter VIII   Challenging Symmetry on Mental Retardation:
Evidence from Williams Syndrome   **147**
Andreia Santos, Duncan Milne,
Delphine Rosset and Christine Deruelle

Chapter IX   Access to Childhood and Adolescent Mental Health
Services for Young People with Mental Retardation   **175**
Renato Donfrancesco and Dario Calderoni

Chapter X   Information Technology for People with Mental Retardation   **185**
Cecilia Li-Tsang and Nichael Wong

Index   **197**

Preface

Mental retardation is a term for a pattern of persistently slow learning of basic motor and language skills ("milestones") during childhood, and a significantly below-normal global intellectual capacity as an adult. One common criterion for diagnosis of mental retardation is a tested intelligence quotient (IQ) of 70 or below. This book presents leading-edge research from around the world.

Chapter I - A large body of study has yielded longer and more variable simple reaction times for mentally retarded participants than for normal participants. Scientists have assumed that the slowness of mentally retarded individuals has been associated with central and peripheral processing components as well as structural alterations within the central nervous system. The present review showed experimental evidence for simple reaction times and timing of unimanual and bimanual serial actions of adolescents with mental retardation, autism, and Down syndrome. First, this review showed that adolescents with mental retardation, autism, and Down syndrome had slower and more variable simple reaction time than did unafflicted participants. The autistic adolescents had further faster simple reaction time than ones with Down syndrome. Second, on a task of tracking a serial light stimulation, the review showed that while mentally retarded adolescents had faster reaction time than normal those, the autistic adolescents had faster anticipatory reaction times than did those in the other three groups. To the contrary, adolescents with Down syndrome had remarkably slower and more variable reaction times than did those with non-Down syndrome mental retardation. Third, on a bimanual finger-tapping task of a 3:2 polyrhythm, the author revealed that because strong negative correlations between-hand taps were observed for adolescents with mental retardation, and their slow-hand movements were further subordinate to the movements of the fast hand, they adopted a hierarchical integrated organization. These findings thus allow for a speculation about the control of timing and force in serial movements: the output chunking can be regarded as a developmental milestone for the control in serial movements.

Chapter II - In recent years it has been claimed trisomic cells are more sensitive to oxidative stress. This fact is of particular interest since oxidative stress has been proposed as a pathogenic mechanism of atherosclerosis, cell aging and neurodegeneration in individuals with Down syndrome.

In general population it has been recently published regular exercise may increase antioxidant system. However, far less information is available on handicapped populations such as Down syndrome.

For the reasons already mentioned the authors designed a research project to assess the influence of a 12-week training program on redox metabolism in adolescents with Down syndrome in order to determine its capacity to attenuate their increased oxidative damage.

Thirty-one male adolescents with Down syndrome (16.3 ± 1.1 years) performed a 12-week training program, 3 sessions/week, consisting of warm up (15 min) followed by a main part (20-35 min [increasing 5 minutes each three weeks]) at a work intensity of 60-75% of peak heart rate according to the equation HRmax=194.5-[0.56 age] (increasing 5% each three weeks) and by a cool-down period (10 min). No one of them suffered acute medical problems at that moment and had not taken part in any physical activity program in the last six months. Written informed consent was obtained from all their parents.

Blood samples were collected from an antecubital vein while participants 72-hours before the beggining of the program and after its ending. Lysed erythrocytes were prepared by putting cells through three freeze-thaw cycles in dry ice and by the addition of five volumes of ice-cold distilled water. After centrifugation, supernatant was frozen at -20 °C until analysis.

Main outcome measurements included the assessment of lipoperoxidation -in terms of MDA content- and protein oxidation -in terms of carbonyl group content-. Antioxidant enzymes such as superoxide dismutase (SOD) glutathione peroxidase (GPX), glutathione reductase (GR), catalase (CAT) and glucose-6-phophate-dehydrogenase (G6PDH) were also assessed.

When compared to baseline values, lipoperoxidation and protein oxidation were significantly reduced. It may be explained, at least in part, since the activity of antioxidants enzymes such as glutathione persoxidase (GPX), glutathione reductase (GR) and glucose-6-phophate-dehydrogenase (G6PDH) were significantly increased after the training period.

Consquently it may be concluded regular exercise improved redox metabolism in adolescents with Down syndrome. Further studies on other handicapped populations are highly required.

Chapter III - This paper reports the results of study into stress and quality of life in the parents of people with intellectual disability. Recent studies have shown that families caring for disabled members report significantly greater stress compared with families who are not providing such care. It is also known that as stress increases, the quality of life decreases.

The Questionnaire on Resources and Stress (QRS-F) (Friedrich, 1983), which is considered a general measure of adaptation and coping, was used to measure the impact of caring for a disabled person on other family members. It contains four subscales as: parent and family problems (I); pessimism (II); child characteristics (III); physical incapacitation (IV). Quality of life was measured using the Comprehensive Quality of Life Scale (Cummins, 1997).

The sample was composed by parents (55 mothers, 47 fathers) of disabled subjects with mild to severe intellectual disability (39 males, 26 females) and a control group (10 mothers and 10 fathers) caring for not-disabled family members (5 females and 5 males). It was found that stress was correlated with parental and familiar problems and a pessimistic attitude towards the situation. No differences were found between mothers and fathers although there was a tendency for mothers to give greater importance to such familiar and parental problems. Parents of male family members experience greater stress and this was more marked in the disabled sample. Moreover the relationship between stress, familiar problems and pessimistic attitudes increases with age of the family member.

Chapter IV - Down syndrome affects 1 in 800 children. These children are frequently served in early intervention programs and these first services provide a bridge for continuation of programs over the child's life course. It is well documented that these programs effectively provide needed services and help children make developmental progress. Less is known about the efficacy of support services for parents, although this is clearly a population at risk for stress. This chapter reviews research on services that parents receive, including information, emotional support, tangible help and direct psychological intervention, the effectiveness of these supports, and the importance of family resilience.

Chapter V - This study provides some reasoning to support the notion that individuals with mental retardation are less likely to actively inhibit response tendencies to irrelevant information in their visual field. Inherent in this idea is the notion that selective attention processes operate differently for subjects with and without mental retardation. Selection by individuals with mental retardation only involve facilitatory processes directed at the target stimulus, whereas selection by individuals without mental retardation involve both facilitatory processes directed toward the target and inhibitory processes directed against irrelevant information. The aim of the present study was to test the suppression of irrelevant information in a non-laboratory context (testing road crossing abilities of children with and without mental retardation). The sample of the study consisted of 104 young individuals. The participants were further subdivided into four groups (n=26 per group) matched on mean mental age, using the Raven's Colored Progressive Matrices: two groups with children with mental retardation (Group A and Group B) and two groups with children without mental retardation (Group C and Group D). Group A and Group C were matched on mental age at 5.6 yr.; Group B and Group D were matched on mental age at 8.0 yr. Ability to identify safe and dangerous road–crossing sites was assessed using computer presentations. The task featured the image of a child standing at the edge of a road facing towards the road. Two tasks were designed using a number of road-crossing sites in each one: recognition task without irrelevant information (i.e., distracting visual stimuli were removed from the scene, allowing the participant to focus on the road site) and recognition task with irrelevant information (i.e., distracting visual stimuli were included in the scene, obscuring the participant to focus on the road site). Every participant was asked to select the "safe" and "unsafe" (dangerous) road-crossing sites. Results demonstrated statistically significant differences between Groups A and C and Groups B and D in task conditions, especially in those in which irrelevant information was involved. Conclusions were drawn concerning the empirical and theoretical benefits for psychology and education, which arise from the study of safety road education in children with mental retardation.

Chapter VI - This study provides some reasoning to support the notion that individuals with mental retardation are less likely to actively inhibit response tendencies to irrelevant information in their visual field. Inherent in this idea is the notion that selective attention processes operate differently for subjects with and without mental retardation. Selection by individuals with mental retardation only involve facilitatory processes directed at the target stimulus, whereas selection by individuals without mental retardation involve both facilitatory processes directed toward the target and inhibitory processes directed against irrelevant information. The aim of the present study was to test the suppression of irrelevant information in a non-laboratory context (testing road crossing abilities of children with and without mental retardation). The sample of the study consisted of 104 young individuals. The participants were further subdivided into four groups (n=26 per group) matched on mean mental age, using the Raven's Colored Progressive Matrices: two groups with children with mental retardation (Group A and Group B) and two groups with children without mental retardation (Group C and Group D). Group A and Group C were matched on mental age at 5.6 yr.; Group B and Group D were matched on mental age at 8.0 yr. Ability to identify safe and dangerous road–crossing sites was assessed using computer presentations. The task featured the image of a child standing at the edge of a road facing towards the road. Two tasks were designed using a number of road-crossing sites in each one: recognition task without irrelevant information (i.e., distracting visual stimuli were removed from the scene, allowing the participant to focus on the road site) and recognition task with irrelevant information (i.e., distracting visual stimuli were included in the scene, obscuring the participant to focus on the road site). Every participant was asked to select the "safe" and "unsafe" (dangerous) road-crossing sites. Results demonstrated statistically significant differences between Groups A and C and Groups B and D in task conditions, especially in those in which irrelevant information was involved. Conclusions were drawn concerning the empirical and theoretical benefits for psychology and education, which arise from the study of safety road education in children with mental retardation.

Chapter VII - There have been significant advances in our understanding of the pathophysiology of mental retardation in the last decade. This has been associated with a sociocultural change in conscience regarding people with mental retardation and carer support ushering a revolution in ethics of care. This chapter aims to review the current understanding of the concept of mental retardation, etiological understanding of intelligence and its impairment, assessment methods and management strategies for associated mental health disorders and disabilities. Mental retardation is identified clinically as a developmental disorder. Research in etiology of mental retardation has identified biological, environmental and psychological factors capable of producing deficits in intellectual function. The co-occurrence of psychiatric illness with mental retardation has been well established, and people with mental retardation are more likely to suffer from ill mental health (including behavioural disorders, personality disorders, autistic-spectrum disorders and attention- deficit hyperactivity disorder). These conditions are often underdiagnosed due to issues such as " diagnostic overshadowing", the tendency by which clinicians tend to overlook additional psychiatric diagnosis once a diagnosis of mental retardation is made; or "masking" in which the clinical characteristics of a mental disorder are masked by a cognitive, language or speech deficit. People with mental retardation share many mental health needs with the general population. The concept of 'normalisation', individual rights and respect for the wishes of individuals with mental retardation has complemented the deinstitutionalised community care, career support and psychopharmacological advances in psychiatry. However, due to a variety of reasons their care has to be specifically tailored to meet these needs.

Chapter VIII - This paper examines the notion of symmetry on mental retardation (MR). Of the more than 1000 known genetic causes of MR, here we focus on Williams syndrome (WS) because it is characterized by an outstanding juxtaposition of deficits and preservations. Despite mild to moderate MR, WS is thought to present strengths in most social cognitive domains and in particular in face processing. Along this paper we will review studies on face and facial-emotion processing in WS. Several researchers have claimed for a link between "intact" face-processing skills and gregarious social behaviour. However, to date, this hypothesis remains unclear. Recent findings of our group showed that individuals with WS are able to decode emotions expressed in human, but not in non-human faces. This striking dissociation challenges the notion of symmetry on MR and suggests domain-specific rather than subaverage general cognitive functioning in WS. Findings are interpreted in light of a developmental rather than modular approach of cognition.

Chapter X - The development of the information and communication technology (ICT) has made a huge revolution of human's lifestyle in the past few decades. A lot of daily chores could be performed by just pressing a few icons on the computer at home such as paying bills, booking of appointments etc. However, people with mental retardation were often deprived of the opportunities to learn ICT skills. This has created a digital divide among people with mental retardation to get into the ICT world. It is believed that through systematic training and special assistive device (e.g. software programme) designed for people with mental retardation, they can get into the ICT world. The digital barrier could thus be removed. Previous studies have been focused on "Identification of barriers for people with mental retardation to the ICT world", "Training of people with mental retardation in learning various ICT skills" and "Enhancement of people with mental retardation to use ICT skills in vocational and leisure perspectives".

This chapter will carefully describe how people with mental retardation manage to get into the ICT world through systematic training and societal support.

In: Mental Retardation Research Advances
Editor: Elizabeth B. Heinz, pp. 1-33

ISBN: 978-1-60021-658-9
© 2007 Nova Science Publishers, Inc.

Chapter I

Simple Reaction Times and Timing of Unimanual and Bimanual Serial Actions in Adolescents with Mental Retardation, Autism, and Down Syndrome

Nobuyuki Inui[*]
Department of Human Motor Control, Faculty of Health and Living Science
Naruto University of Education, Takashima, Naruto-cho, Naruto-shi 772-8502, Japan

Abstract

A large body of study has yielded longer and more variable simple reaction times for mentally retarded participants than for normal participants. Scientists have assumed that the slowness of mentally retarded individuals has been associated with central and peripheral processing components as well as structural alterations within the central nervous system. The present review showed experimental evidence for simple reaction times and timing of unimanual and bimanual serial actions of adolescents with mental retardation, autism, and Down syndrome. First, this review showed that adolescents with mental retardation, autism, and Down syndrome had slower and more variable simple reaction time than did unafflicted participants. The autistic adolescents had further faster simple reaction time than ones with Down syndrome. Second, on a task of tracking a serial light stimulation, the review showed that while mentally retarded adolescents had faster reaction time than normal those, the autistic adolescents had faster anticipatory reaction times than did those in the other three groups. To the contrary, adolescents with Down syndrome had remarkably slower and more variable reaction times than did those with non-Down syndrome mental retardation. Third, on a bimanual finger-tapping task of a 3:2 polyrhythm, the author revealed that because strong negative correlations between-hand taps were observed for adolescents with mental retardation, and their slow-hand

---

[*] Nobuyuki Inui: Tel: (+81) 88-687-6517; Fax: (+81) 88-687-6028; E-mail: inui@naruto-u.ac.jp

movements were further subordinate to the movements of the fast hand, they adopted a hierarchical integrated organization. These findings thus allow for a speculation about the control of timing and force in serial movements: the output chunking can be regarded as a developmental milestone for the control in serial movements.

1. Simple Reaction Times

From an information-processing perspective, simple reaction time has been reported frequently in the research of motor performance for individuals with mental retardation (Baumeister and Kellas, 1968; Berkson, 1960a; Karrer, 1986). Many studies have yielded longer and more variable simple reaction time for mentally retarded participants than for normal participants. The slowness of mentally retarded individuals is thought to be primarily due to problems in information-processing in the central nervous system, such as the difficulty of the storage and ordering of information (Karrer, 1986).

Berkson (1960b) also reported simple reaction times in participants with Down syndrome to be considerably longer than those of severely subnormal and subnormal participants. A substantial number of studies have reported longer and more variable simple reaction time for participants with Down syndrome than for mentally retarded participants without Down syndrome, indicating that increases in simple reaction time for the participants with Down syndrome varied from 25 % to greater than 300 % (for review, Anson, 1992).

Although little research on reaction time for autistic individuals was reported until recently (for example, Courchesne et al., 1994a), Inui et al. (1995) examined differences among individuals of mental retardation, autism, and Down syndrome for simple reaction time to understand their differences for a information-processing of perceptual-motor skills.

Their data were obtained from four groups. Three contrasting groups consisted of 7 mentally retarded females and males (IQ: 60-72), 8 autistic males (IQ: 42-65), and 3 males with Down syndrome (IQ: impossible to measure), all students of a high school for handicapped children attached to the university. Their chronological ages ranged from 16 to 18 years. The control group consisted of 10 normal male undergraduate students. Their chronological ages ranged from 20 to 24 years.

Figure 1 showed experimental setup. Participants were seated directly in front of a vertical panel consisting of six stimulation lights. The stimuli were six luminous diodes covered with red lens caps and mounted three cm apart on a vertical display board. Six touch switches were placed beneath the lights. Stimulus presentation was controlled by a personal computer. The responses were also recorded by the computer.

In a simple reaction time task, participants were instructed to respond as fast as possible to a light flash by touching a touch switch on twenty trials. Although the stimulation interval was always 100 ms, the interstimulus interval from 300 ms to 1500 ms was randomly presented.

Figure 2 showed means and standard deviations of simple reaction times for the four groups. The control participants had significantly faster and less variable simple reaction times than all three contrasting groups. Also, the autistic group had significantly faster simple reaction time than the Down syndrome group. Although the mentally retarded group had somewhat faster simple reaction times than the Down syndrome group, the difference between groups was not statistically significant. Similarly, the autistic group had somewhat faster simple reaction time than the mentally retarded group, but the difference between groups was not statistically significant.

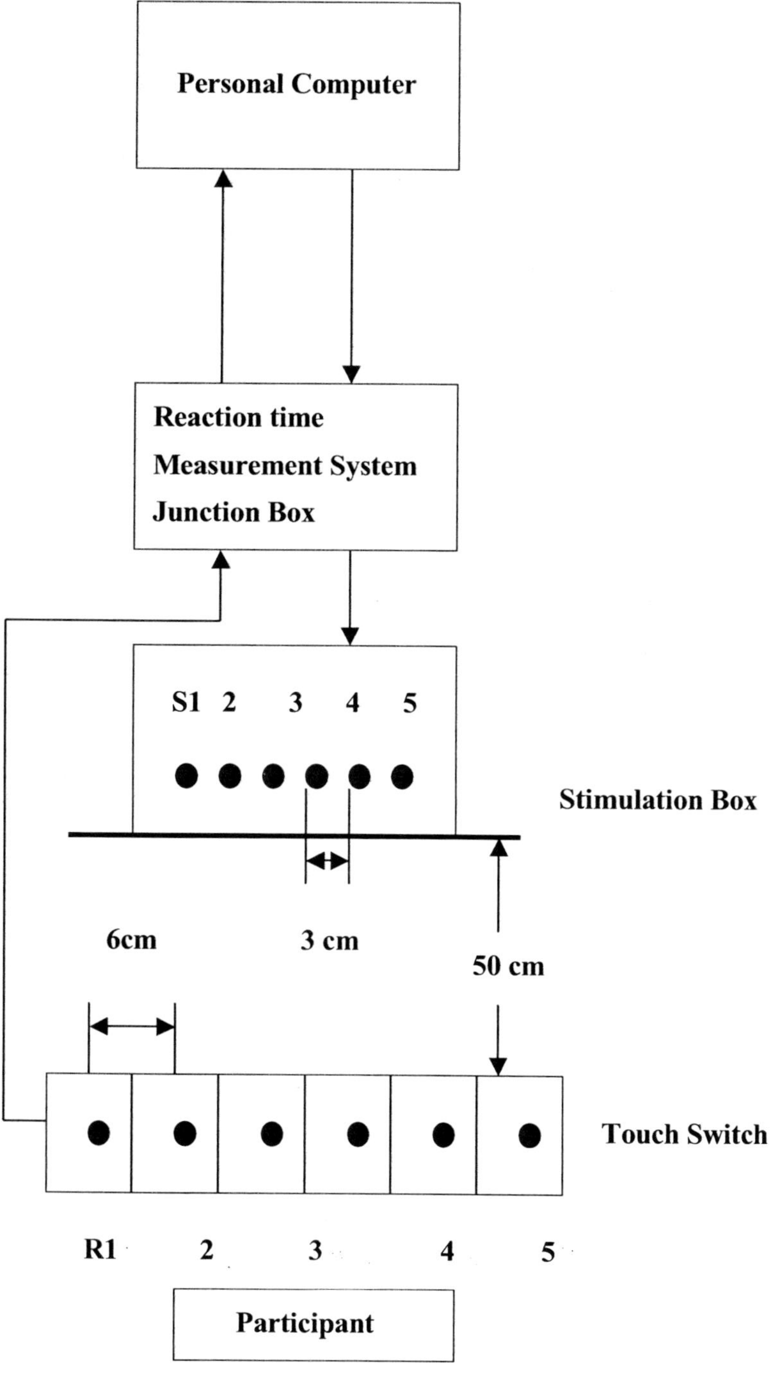

Figure 1. Experimental setup (Modified from Inui et al., 1995).

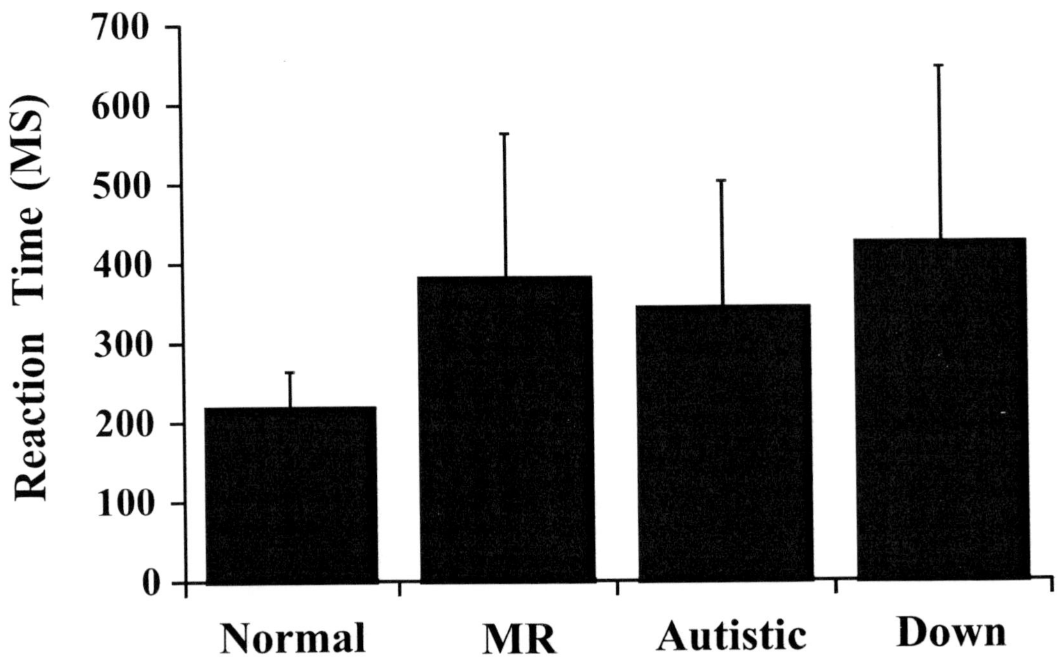

Figure 2. Mean Simple Reaction Times (ms) and Standard Deviations for Four Groups (Modified from Inui et al., 1995). Abbreviations. MR: mental retarded.

These results indicated that the adolescents with mental retardation, autism, and Down syndrome had significantly slower and more variable simple reaction time than did normal participants. Also, the autistic adolescents had significantly faster simple reaction time than adolescents with Down syndrome.

The results were thus consistent with many previous reports (Anson, 1992; Baumeister and Kellas, 1968; Berkson, 1960a; Karrer, 1986). On the other hand, although simple reaction time for autistic individuals was not reported until recently, Inui et al. (1995) found that autistic adolescents had faster simple reaction time than adolescents with Down syndrome.

Such differences in simple reaction time have often been associated with central and peripheral processing components (Davis et al., 1991; Inui et al., 1995; Un and Erbahceci, 2000) as well as structural alterations within the central nervous system (LeClair et al., 1993; Saccuzzo and Michael, 1984). Although this mechanism was examined by using electromyogram (EMG)-reaction time, some studies reported that individuals with mental retardation were longer for both premotor and motor times than normal those (for individuals with mental retardation and Down syndrom, Davis et al., 1991; for individuals with mental retardation, Horvat et al., 2003). Premotor time is the first component of reaction time and is the "silent" interval of time between stimulus and muscular activity. Premotor time is regarded as central processes involved in a motor response. Premtor time was operationally defined as the period between the onset of the stimulus and the beginning of muscle activity. Motor time is the second component of reaction time and defined as the period from the initial change in EMG to the actual beginning of the observable movement (Schmidt, 1988).

On the other hand, there are a few excellent reviews of relationship between reaction time and muscle activity for individuals with Down syndrome (Anson, 1992; Anson and Mawston, 2000; Simon et al., 2003). In spite of frequent observations of slow simple reaction time in individuals with Down syndrome, a satisfactory explanation remains elusive. As for slow reaction time of persons with Down syndrome, Simon et al. (2003) pointed out in their review that three possible factors included hypotonia, differences in central and peripheral processing, and differences in the ordering of limb segments during initiation of goal-directed upper limb movements.

Hypotonia refers to the absence or markedly reduced levels of electrical activity in a muscle. Hypotonia, the muscle appears as floppy or lacks tone, has frequently been observed for individuals with Down syndrome, in particular, for infants with Down syndrome (Simon et al., 2003). Although Anwar and Hermelin (1979) linked hypotonia to slow reaction time, recent studies suggest no relationship between hypotonia and reaction time. For example, Shumway-Cook and Woollacott (1985) reported that normal stretch reflex was observed by young individuals with Down syndrome. Investigation of changes in joint stiffness further showed no presence and influence of hypotonia in Down syndrome (Davis and Kelso, 1982; Davis and Sinning, 1987).

Mean fractionated reaction time (simple reaction time, premotor time, and motor time) has shown that although for individuals with Down syndrome simple reaction time is longer, the delay are greater in both central and peripheral components of simple reaction time. Mawston and Anson (1994) reported that within the central component, the increased delay (increase in premotor time) is not associated with slower nerve conduction velocity, which has been reported to be normal. However, when attention to performing the task of simple reaction time at hand was observed, there was a substantial difference between the performances of the normal group and the Down syndrome group. From recorded videotape, attention was crudely measured by counting the number of times participants glanced away from the target during the movement preparation interval. The movement preparation interval was the period between the verbally presented command and an imperative auditory stimulus. The number of off-task glances per second was computed as an indicator of inattention. Whereas the normal group maintained to focus attention on the target in 99 per cent of trials, the score for the Down syndrome group was 24 per cent on task. For the participants with Down syndrome, fluctuation in attention may have produced to increase both variability and delay in central processing (Simon et al., 2003).

Although simple reaction time is usually measured at the tip of index finger and at the elbow, Anson and his colleagues measured reaction time at different anatomical points on the upper limb segments to examine the order of limb segment displacement during movement initiation (Simon et al., 2003). Reaction times measured at elbow and index finger from two switches showed that whereas a proximal-to-distal pattern of segment activation associated with movement initiation was observed by normal participants, a distal-to-proximal pattern was observed by participants with Down syndrome (Figure 3). This was kinematically revealed in reaction times being faster at the index finger than at the elbow for the participants with Down syndrome. This observation was further physiologically supported by premotor times that indicated extensor indicis muscle was activated before anterior deltoid.

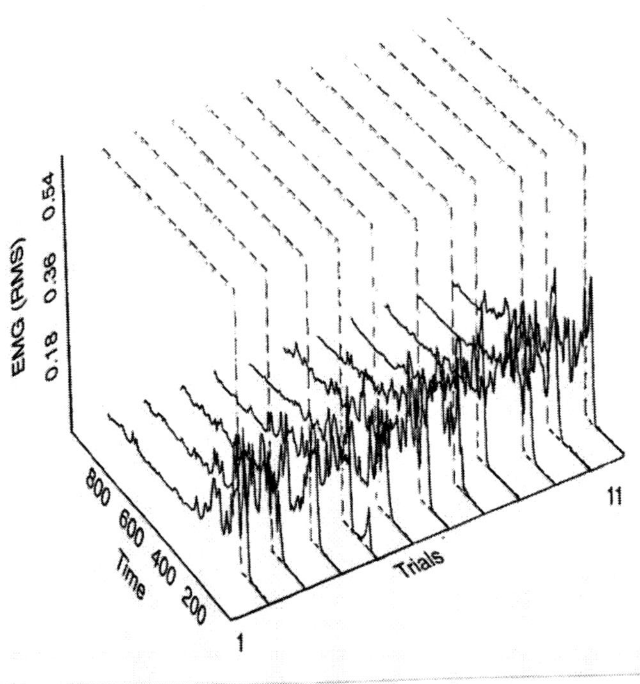

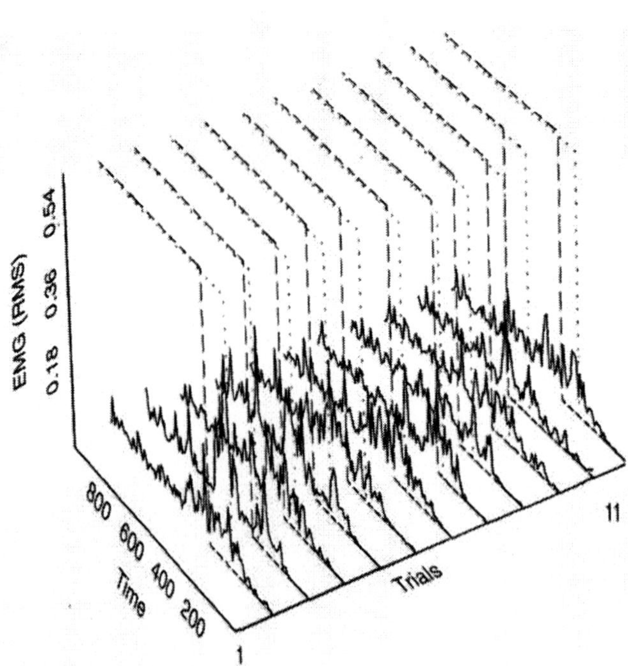

Figure 3. Simple reaction times (elbow = dashed; finger = dotted) and electromyogram (root mean square) for 11 trials for one normal participant (top) and one with Down syndrome (bottom) showing consistent trial-to-trial performance in the pattern of distal muscle activation (extensor indicis) (Modified from Anson and Mawston, 2000).

From the perspective of practice for individuals with Down syndrome, on the other hands, a substantial number of studies have reported no effect of practice on tasks of tracking, tapping, reaction time, and the control of grip force in a lifting movement (Anson, 1992). Kerr and Blais (1987), however, found after 2400 responses, practice improved performance on reaction time without effecting changes in movement time. Kerr and Blais (1988) consequently pointed out that a minimum of 100 responses or trials and not less than 400 were required to assess effects in reaction time and movement time tasks. From studies of the non-Down syndrome mentally retarded persons, Hoover et al. (1981) further reported that the mentally retarded had task-component specific effects of practice. Participants reacted from a switch and reached to a target in the experimental task of Hoover et al. When the participants were instructed to focus on the reaction time component, it improved, and movement time similarly improved when focused on the component of movement speed. Anson (1992) thus pointed out that the equivocal effect of practice for persons with Down syndrome was perhaps associated with the difficulty of determining whether some parts of the neuromuscular system were more suitable for practice effects than others.

2. Serial Reaction Times

Motor planning and programming have been often discussed in the motor control of mentally retarded individuals. However, little study of serial reaction time, wherein decision-making was more than simple reaction time, has been reported for mentally retarded individuals. Inui et al. (1995) therefore examined serial information processing dependent motor control in adolescents with mental retardation, Down syndrome, and autism by using a task of tracking a serial light stimulation.

The same experimental set-up (Figure 1) and participants as the study of simple reaction time was used in this study. In a task of tracking a serial light stimulation, participants were instructed to execute switch responses corresponding to light onsets during trials. The serial pattern which participants tracked on twenty trials was 123456. The stimulus interval (100 ms) and interstimulus interval (500 ms) were always constant during trials.

Figure 4 showed means and standard deviations of serial reaction times and serial anticipatory reaction times corresponding to each serial position for the four groups. The mentally retarded group had significantly faster serial reaction time than the control group. The autistic group had markedly mean anticipatory reaction times, and this group thus had faster anticipatory reaction time than all other three groups. To the contrary, the Down syndrome group had marked slow mean reaction times, and this group thus had slower reaction time than all other three groups.

To examine individual variations of reaction times and anticipatory reaction times, Figure 5 showed plots of all 120 responses during each trial for a typical example of four groups. A single normal participant (A) responded with six movements, in which this participant pressed a series of keys (1, 2, 3, 4, 5, and 6), as a chunk. The other participants of the control group also responded with six movements in chunk. A single mentally retarded adolescent (B) also responded with movements as a chunk, as exhibited by the normal participnat, until the 12th trial. However, she did not produce this movement-output chunking after the 13th trial. Although four other participants executed this movement-output chunking, two participants did not make this response.

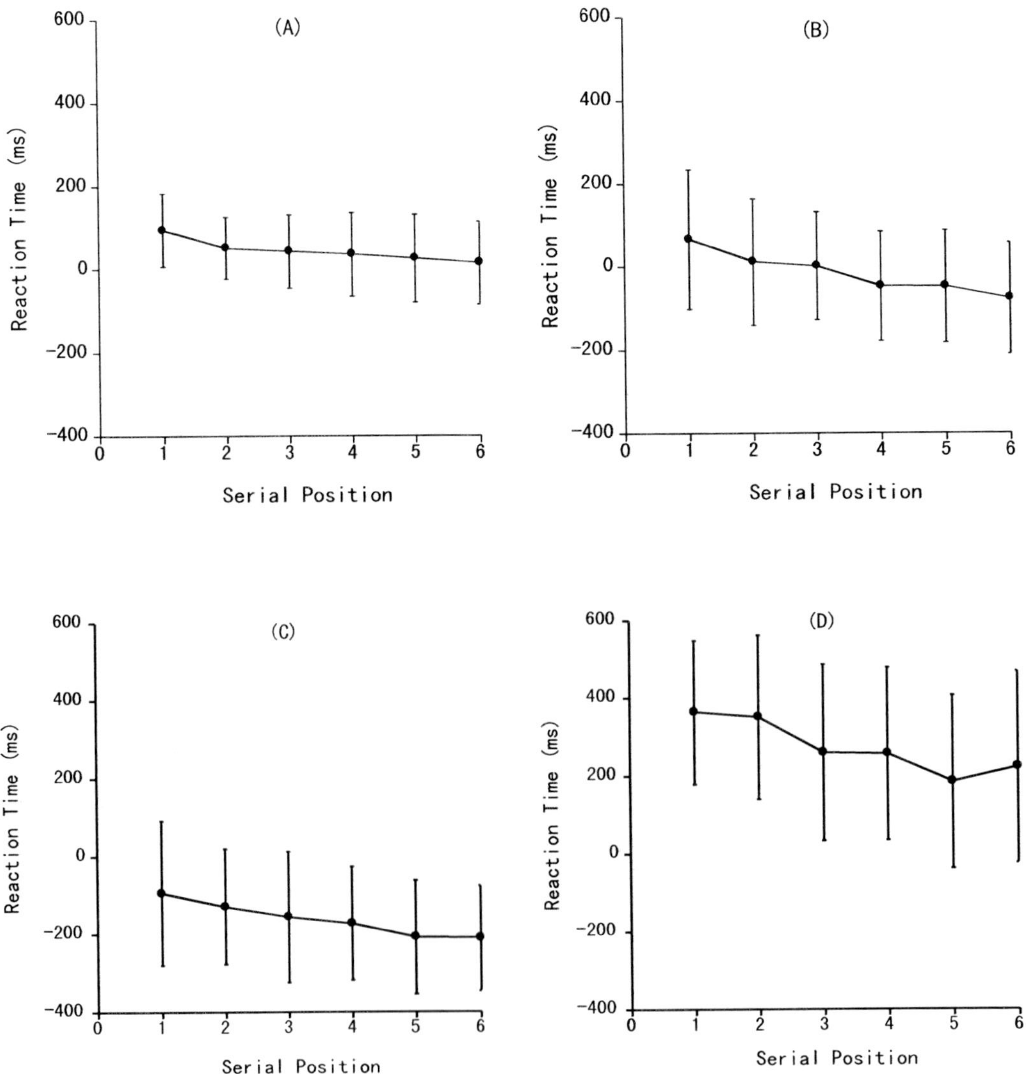

Figure 4. Mean reaction times (ms), mean anticipatory reaction times (ms), and standard deviations for four groups in a task of tracking a serial pattern (Modified from Inui et al., 1995). Figures show means and standard deviations of undergraduate students (A), and adolescents with mental retardation (B), with autism (C), and with Down syndrome (D).

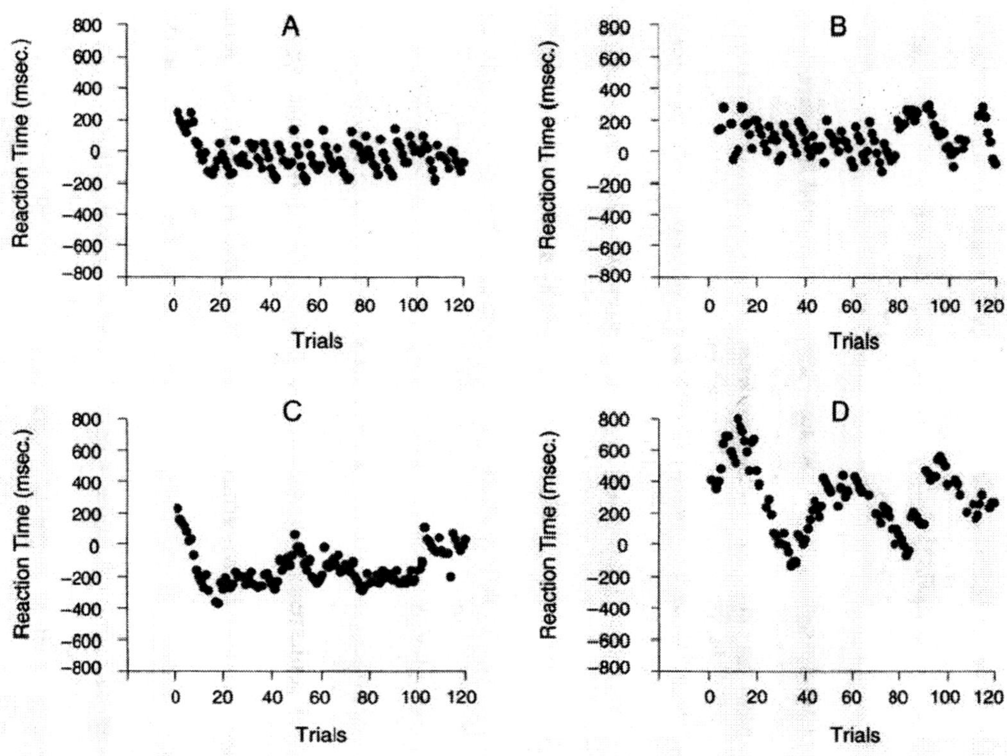

Figure 5. Reaction times and anticipatory reaction times for individuals of four groups in a task of a tracking serial pattern (Inui et al., 1995). Figures show 120 responses of an undergraduate student (A), and an adolescent with mental retardation (B), with autism (C), and with Down syndrome (D).

Although an adolescent with autism was unable to produce the similar clear movement-output chunking as both normal and mentally retarded adolescents, adolescents with autism made the unclear movement-output chunking. A few autistic adolescents often made a stereotyped movement during trials. Adolescents with Down syndrome, on the other hand, did not produce the movement-output chunking. They had more variable reaction times than did participants of the other three groups.

In a task of tracking a serial light stimulation, mentally retarded adolescents had significantly faster reaction time than normal participnats. Kondo (1978) also found that the mentally retarded adolescents had minimal simple reaction time under the conditions in which the cue stimuli were presented regular in a spatial order.

Kondo (1978) examined information processing during the warning intervals of simple reaction time task performed by mentally retarded adolescents. His data were obtained from two groups. The contrasting group consisted of 12 mentally retarded females and males (IQ: 46-78). Their chronological ages ranged from 13 to 15 years. The control group consisted of 12 normal females and males. Their chronological ages ranged from 12 to 15 years. Stimulation panel was placed in front of participants. Seven cue stimulation lights on the panel were arranged over an arcing course. The warning stimulation light was put above the cue stimulation light. The response stimulation light was put below the cue stimulation lights.

The cue stimuli were consisted of a combination of both the modes of the temporal presentation (regular vs. irregular) and the spatial presentation (regular vs. irregular), introducing during the warning interval. The responses were recorded by the digital counter.

Kondo's analysis (1978) showed that although there was little reaction time difference among the four experimental conditions for normal participants, the spatial regularity was more effective than the temporal regularity for mentally retarded those. Adolescents with mental retardation had the fastest simple reaction time under the conditions in which the cue stimuli were presented regular in a spatial order. The experiment of Inui et al. (1995) also regularly presented a series of six stimuli in a similar spatial order to Kondo's experimental set-up. Mentally retarded adolescents for both the experiments are thus thought to have a preparatory state for response to serial stimulation.

Adolescents with Down syndrome had slower and more variable serial reaction time than mentally retarded adolescents without Down syndrome, as exhibited in the simple reaction time. As for the cause of these slowness and variation for adolescents with Down syndrome, they are thought to be unable to form and utilize motor program (Anwar, 1983; Frith and Frith, 1974; Kerr and Blais, 1987). Individuals with Down syndrome are perhaps more likely to be dependent on feedback at all stages of responding (Anson, 1992).

On the other hand, little research on reaction time for autistic individuals has been reported. This study indicated that autistic adolescents had markedly faster reaction times and serial anticipatory reaction times than those with mental retardation and Down syndrome. Autistic adolescents were perhaps chunking together the whole series of responses and were unable to coordinate the timing of individual responses with individual stimuli, as in normal participants, in a task of tracking a serial stimulation. Autistic adolescents did not thus control a visually-initiated movement, but executed a self-pacing movement.

Kanner (1943) first described a patient with autism, noting that his arousal, attention, and sensory responsiveness were severely impaired. In the neurobiological theory of autism, Rimland (1964) first hypothesized that the dysfunction of reticular activating system underlay the characteristic social and cognitive deficits in this disorder. As the first neuropathological evidence of autism, Williams et al. (1980) found Purkinje neuron loss throughout the cerebellum of a single patient. Because the Purkinje neuron is an exclusive output cell from the cerebellar cortex, the neuron plays an important role on cerebellar function. The finding of Williams et al. (1980) then led Courchesne et al. (1988) to the finding of hypoplasia of cerebellar vermal lobules VI and VII and hemispheres in the great majority of patients with autism. These cerebellar area receive information from visual and auditory systems.

The cerebellum has been known to have neuroanatomical connections with the reticular activating system and attentional systems (Nieuwenhuys et al., 1988), and to have a modulatory effect on sensory responsiveness (Crispino and Bullock, 1984). The cerebellum also has neuroanatomical rich connections with brainsten, thalamic, and parietal systems implicated in shifting attention in studies of individuals with focal lesions (Posner and Petersen, 1990). Thus, substantial decrease in the Purkinje neuron of the cerebellar cortex could be of great significance in explaining attention, arousal, and sensory dysfunction in autism.

Courchesne et al. (1994a) therefore hypothesized (1) that the cerebellum might play an important role in the coordination of attention as well as in motor control and (2) that cerebellar maldevelopment in children with autism asks them unable to adjust their mental focus of attention to follow the rapidly changing verbal, gestural, postural, tactile, and facial cues that signal changes in a stream of social information (for review see Courchesne et al., 1994b).

Courchesne et al. (1994a) asked participants to perform two experimental tasks: focus attention task and shift attention task in which visual and auditory stimuli were randomly intermixed and rapidly presented. Visual stimuli were red and green squares presented on a video monitor. Auditory stimuli were presented over headphones. All visual and auditory stimuli were 50 ms in duration, and interstimulus intervals varied between 450 and 1,450 ms. Twenty-five percent of all stimuli were target stimuli to which participants were required to respond by pressing a button.

The focus attention task tested the participant's ability to continuously maintain a focus of attention and to detect rare target stimuli in one sensory modality while ignoring all stimuli in the other modality. This served as a control for the shift attention task. The focus attention task consisted of two conditions: a visual focus attention condition and an auditory focus attention condition. The hit and false data in the task were analyzed at five intervals of elapsed time immediately following the onset of the last correctly detected target: 0.4-2.5 s, 2.5-4.5 s, 4.5-6.5 s, 6.5-10.5 s, and 10.5-30.0 s. The focus attention task thus contains both factors of simple and selective reaction times.

The shift attention task asked participants to alternate attention between visual and auditory stimuli as signaled by the appearance of the rare target stimuli. Correct detection of a target in the attended modality served to signal the participants to disengage their attention to stimuli in the current modality and to move and reengage their focus of attention as rapidly as possible to stimuli in the other modality in order to detect the very next target appearing in that modality. The hit and false data in the task were analyzed at the same five intervals of elapsed time immediately following the onset of each correctly detected target, as the focus attention task. The shift attention task thus contains both factors of selective and serial reaction times.

Courchesne et al. (1994a) reported two findings. First, autistic patients had shorter reaction times than either the patients with cerebellar lesions or the younger normal controls in the focus attention task. Second, autistic patients and patients with acquired cerebellar lesions had substantially longer reaction times in the shift attention task.

Figure 6 showed the index of the speed of shifting and detecting targets as the percentage difference in reaction time. The percentage was computed as follows: the different between the reaction time to the short cue-to-target delay (0.4-2.5-s interval) and the reaction time to the long cue-to-target delay (2.5-4.5-s interval) divided by the latter reaction time. In the shift task, then, the more positive the percentage difference score, the poorer the ability to rapidly shift and detect targets. On this score, autistic patients and patients with acquired cerebellar lesions had substantially longer reaction times than the normal participants. In the focus task, the more positive the percentage difference score, the poorer the ability to detect two rapid targets in a row while keeping a single constant focus of attention. On this score, autistic patients had shorter reaction times than either the patients with cerebellar lesions or the younger normal participants. These findings indicated that cerebellar malvdevelopment in persons with autism perhaps produced an inability to execute rapid attention shifts, and consequently impaired social and cognitive development.

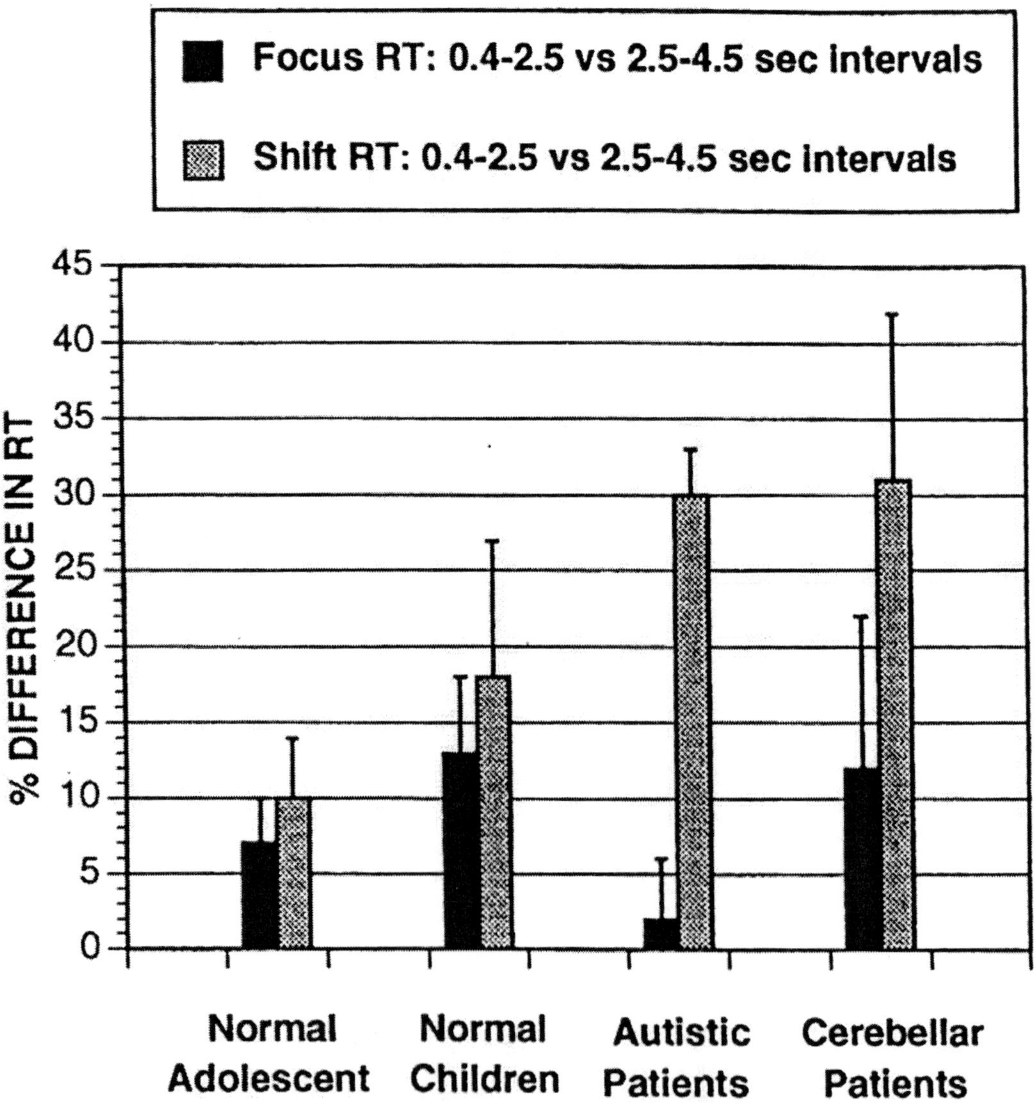

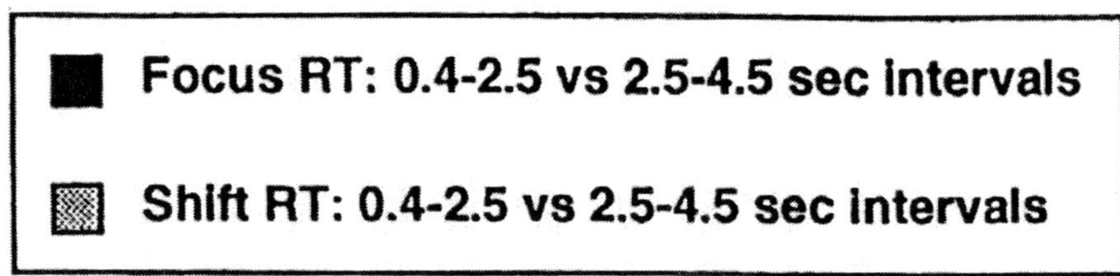

Figure 6. Percentages of difference in reaction time (RT) at the two time intervals in the two tasks for four groups (Courchesne et al., 1994). The index of speed of shifting and detecting targets is shown as the percentage difference and was computed as follows: the difference between the RT to the short cue-to-target delay (0.4-2.5 s interval) and the RT to the long cue-to-target delay (2.5-4.5 s interval) divided by the latter RT.

3. Effects of Practice on Serial Reaction Times of Adolescents with Autism

On a task of tracking a serial light stimulation, Inui et al. (1995) showed that while mentally retarded adolescents had faster reaction time than normal those, the autistic adolescents had faster anticipatory reaction times than did those in the other three groups. To the contrary, adolescents with Down syndrome had markedly slower and more variable reaction times than did those with non-Down syndrome mental retardation.

The motor organization seems to be different among these types of participants. On the six keystrokes on the tracking task, whereas adolescents with mental retardation and autism responded with six movements as a chunk, those with Down syndrome did not produce this movement-output chunking.

Adolescents with Down syndrome have been reported to have no practice effect (Anson, 1992), but autistic adolescents have not yet been studied about this effect. Inui and Suzuki (1998) therefore examined effects of practice on timing of serial reactions of adolescents with autism by using a task of tracking a serial light stimulation.

Data were obtained from two groups. The contrasting group was seven adolescents with autism. They consisted of three male and two female students (16-18 yrs, IQ: 36-57) of a high school for handicapped children and two male students (15 yrs, IQ: 41 and 68) of a similar junior high school attached to the university. The control group consisted of five normal male and female high school students (16-18 yrs) and five normal male and female junior high school students (15 yrs). The same experimental set-up as the study of Inui et al. (1995) was used in this study (figure 1).

Simple reaction times were measured by the same procedure as the study of Inui et al. (1995). As a task of serial reactions, participants were instructed to tap touch switches corresponding to light onsets on each of the six diodes. Fifty trials were given and serial reaction times corresponding to light onsets on the six diodes were measured. The serial pattern of switches was 123456 for all 50 trials. The stimulus duration (100 ms) and interstimulus interval (800 ms) were always constant during trials. Prior to beginning each experimental trial, each participant performed a few practice trials. All participants practiced the same experimental task of serial reactions for four days.

Adolescents with autism were first compared with the control for simple reaction times served as a baseline for serial reaction times. The analysis showed that adolescents with autism (M=387.70 ms., SD=184.30) had a significantly slower and more variable mean simple reaction time than the control group (M=228.99 ms., SD=58.10). This result was consistent with the previous study of Inui et al. (1995).

Figure 7 showed percentages of trials consisting of reaction times, of anticipatory reaction times, and of both reaction times and anticipatory reaction times for four days for both groups in the serial reaction time. Normal participants' trials mainly consisted of both reaction times and anticipatory reaction times. Autistic adolescents' trials, on the other hand, mostly consisted of anticipatory reaction times. Error and omission responses did not reach low percentage of 5 across all participants.

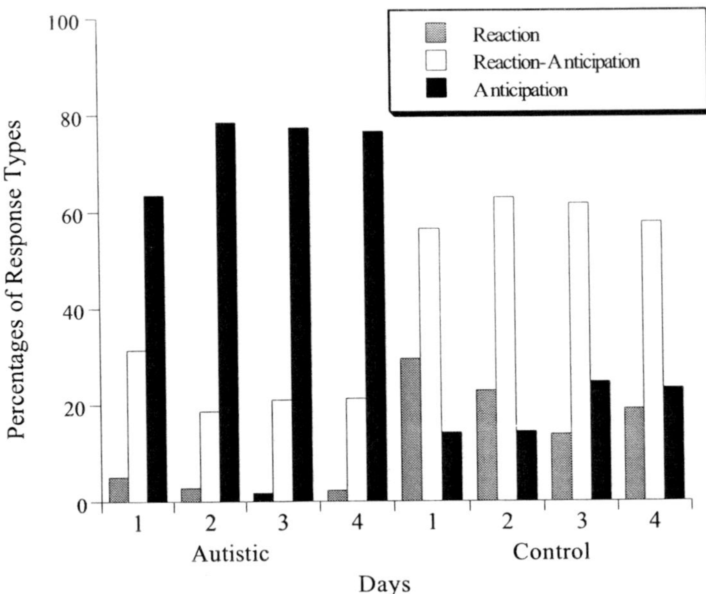

Figure 7. Percentages of trials consisting of reaction times (RT), of anticipatory reaction times (anticipatory RT), and of both reaction times (RT + anticipatory RT) over four days for both groups in a task of a tracking serial pattern (Inui and Suzuki, 1998). A "RT" trial is when all six responses on a trial are more than 0 ms. An "anticipatory RT" trial is when all six responses on a trial are less than 0 ms. A "RT+anticipatory RT" trial, on the other hand, consists of both reaction times and anticipatory reaction times.

Table 1. Means (ms) and standard deviations of reaction times corresponding to serial position within the sequences for both groups in a task of a tracking serial pattern for four days (Inui and Suzuki, 1998).

Group	n	Day	RT (msec)	Serial Position					
				1	2	3	4	5	6
Control	10	1	M	215.97	178.36	168.35	158.27	161.41	144.83
			SD	81.68	60.56	67.40	69.87	83.73	75.35
		2	M	138.26	115.51	106.12	103.11	102.73	91.12
			SD	77.98	63.73	60.43	57.00	51.39	56.76
		3	M	124.68	107.90	95.56	99.16	87.13	85.35
			SD	54.86	54.71	55.59	51.79	50.94	48.30
		4	M	115.44	106.01	99.37	85.52	82.40	77.84
			SD	64.23	57.17	53.29	49.17	54.80	52.42
Autistic	7	1	M	566.78	520.28	446.17	431.67	395.50	320.72
			SD	401.14	347.37	313.26	338.93	320.58	316.80
		2	M	347.80	389.60	304.70	70.00	269.40	204.40
			SD	428.40	462.77	360.69	356.41	326.22	243.55
		3	M	685.83	778.00	617.67	452.00	372.83	284.50
			SD	615.49	645.97	507.72	422.46	287.44	212.77
		4	M	14.75	94.50	90.25	81.25	58.63	58.50
			SD	140.43	56.55	70.57	51.25	68.88	38.80

Table 1 showed means and standard deviations of reaction times corresponding to serial position within the sequences for both groups in the serial reaction time. The first day had significantly slower reaction times for the control group than the other days. The second day had also significantly slower reaction times for the control group than the fourth day. Effects of practice on timing of serial reactions were thus found for mean reaction times of the control group.

For reaction times of adolescents with autism, although the means of the first day were not different from those of the second and third days, the fourth day were significantly faster for the means than the first and third days. Effects of practice on timing of serial reactions were thus found for mean reaction times of adolescents with autism.

Table 2 showed means and standard deviations for anticipatory reaction times corresponding to serial position within the sequences for both groups in the serial reaction time. The analysis indicated the control group did not have significantly faster anticipatory reaction times on the first day than the fourth day, but did with respect to the second and third days. What the magnitude of anticipation becomes smaller is the effects of practice on the anticipatory reaction time. So that effects of practice on timing of serial reactions were found for mean anticipatory reaction times of the control group.

Table 2. Means (ms) and standard deviations of anticipatory reaction times corresponding to serial position within the sequences for both groups in a task of a tracking serial pattern for four days (Inui and Suzuki, 1998)

Group	n	Day	Anticipatory RT (msec)	Serial Position					
				1	2	3	4	5	6
Control	10	1	M	-62.23	-107.20	-127.09	-129.49	-121.57	-120.89
			SD	35.19	60.43	72.04	67.09	66.10	71.46
		2	M	-57.31	-67.03	-79.75	-84.32	-87.56	-87.10
			SD	46.26	44.14	49.01	48.54	58.61	115.94
		3	M	-60.33	-76.45	-86.13	-94.13	-108.11	-100.48
			SD	42.98	48.73	57.96	61.51	67.62	61.04
		4	M	-77.57	-89.04	-96.31	-98.24	-120.26	-109.04
			SD	56.94	57.11	58.52	59.60	68.19	85.51
Autistic	7	1	M	-196.41	-370.87	-325.97	-335.78	-366.99	-363.05
			SD	151.25	343.16	266.34	218.23	245.35	239.77
		2	M	-232.92	-294.92	-333.73	-340.61	-358.17	-353.44
			SD	126.84	158.05	194.63	191.79	206.88	187.23
		3	M	-221.65	-289.74	-314.67	-336.14	-342.64	-355.39
			SD	126.14	139.66	135.42	156.94	177.58	203.78
		4	M	-248.98	-325.84	-354.35	-382.70	-400.70	-415.96
			SD	187.96	163.64	168.74	202.52	205.74	235.80

The first day was not different from the other three days for mean anticipatory reaction times of adolescents with autism. However, the fourth day had significantly faster anticipatory reaction times for adolescents with autism than the second and third days. Thus, because mean anticipatory reaction times of adolescents with autism did not approach 0 ms, effects of practice on timing of serial reactions were not found for them.

In order to examine individual variations of serial reaction times and anticipatory reaction times, figure 8 showed plots of all 300 responses on the first and fourth days for three typical examples. Although reaction times and anticipatory reaction times for control participants (Figure 8, A and B) were distributed around 0 ms, the first day was not different from the fourth day for both reaction times. There was no practice effect over the four days as a result.

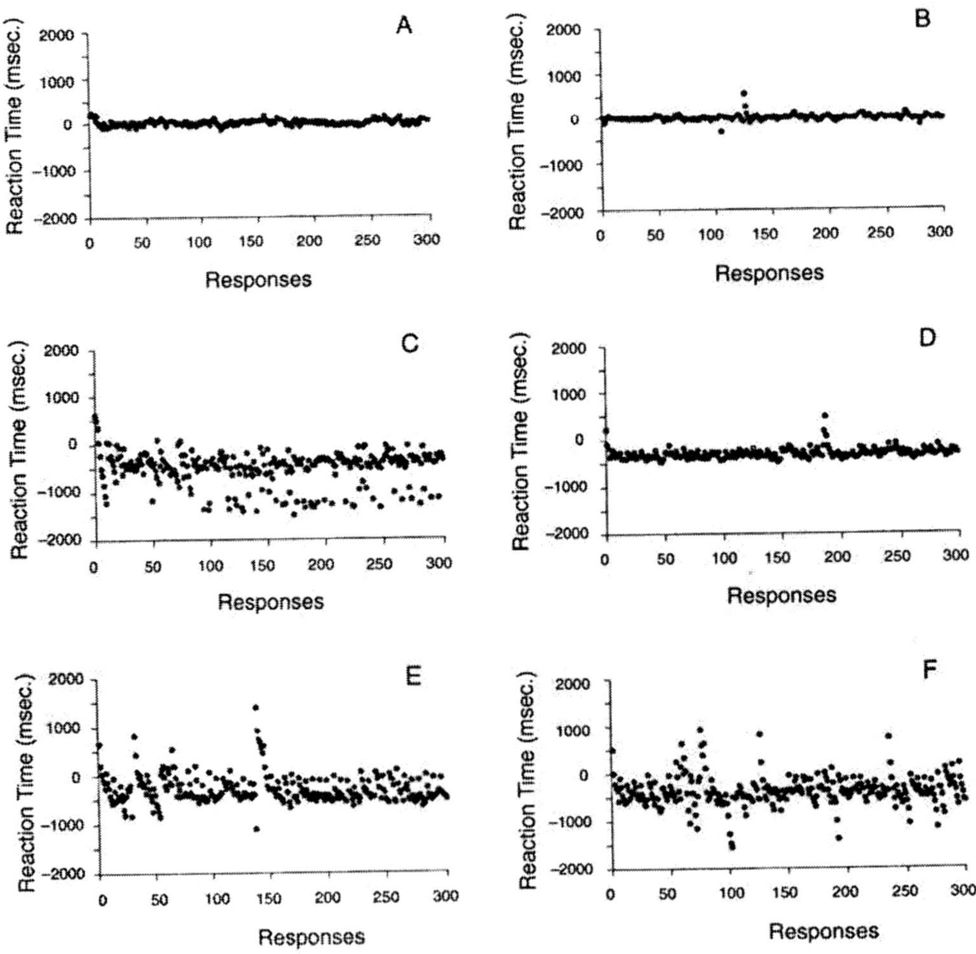

Figure 8. Reaction times and anticipatory reaction times for individuals of three typical examples on the first (A, C, and E) and fourth (B, D, and F) days in a task of a tracking serial pattern (Inui and Suzuki, 1998). Figures show 300 responses of a single control participant (A and B), an autistic participant having practice effect (C and D), and an autistic participant showing no practice effect (E and F).

Although reaction times and anticipatory reaction times for an autistic participant (figure 8, C and D) were largely distributed from -500 ms to 0 ms, the fourth day had slower and less variable both reaction times than the first day with practice. Four of seven participants with autism similarly had practice effects on timing of serial reactions. However, there was no practice effect over the four days for the other three participants with autism (figure 8, E and F).

The results for mean simple and anticipatory reaction time of autistic adolescents were consistent with Inui et al. (1995). These results indicate that although mean anticipatory reaction times of adolescents with autism did not approach to 0 ms with practice, practice effects on the timing of mean reaction times were found. From individual variations of reaction times and anticipatory reaction times, four of seven participants with autism had effects of practice on timing of serial reactions.

Normal adolescents respond with six movements as a chunk and are able to coordinate the timing of individual responses with individual stimuli. In contrast, autistic adolescents appear to chunk together the whole series of responses and are unable to coordinate the timing of individual responses with individual stimuli. Thus, although Hermelin and O'Connor (1970) suggested that children with autism had marked difficulties in the serial information-processing required in perceptual-motor tasks, we believe that autistic adolescents are able to process the information serially because practice effects are found in their timing of serial reactions and make movement-output chunking. The data indicate that autistic adolescents can form and use motor programs with practice.

Courchesne et al. (1994a) reported in their study of autistic patients that there was a persistent and profound impairment in the patients' ability to accurately and rapidly shift attention despite repeated training and experience. The experiment of Inui and his colleagues (1995, 1998) required responding to a series of six stimuli presented regularly in spatial order, so the participants' inability to shift attention accurately and rapidly may contribute to the inability to coordinate the timing of individual responses with individual stimuli for autistic participants.

Courchesne et al. (1994a) further reported that autistic and cerebellar patients' responses to a correctly detected target were not impaired as long as there was no requirement to shift attention. They suggested that the inability to shift attention accurately and rapidly in these patients was not due to problems with motor control. Inui and his colleagues (1995, 1998) indicated that autistic participants were unable to coordinate the timing of individual responses with individual stimuli, but made movement-output chunking and formed and used motor programs with practice. These findings thus suggests the inability to coordinate the timing of individual responses with individual stimuli for autistic participants appears not to be due problems with motor control but with perceptual processing.

4. Timing of Bimanual Alternating Finger Tapping Movement

Bimanual motor coordination is of direct interest in the context of athletics, dancing, the performance of some musical instruments, and the operation of machines. Studies on such coordination are further useful for the education and therapy of individuals with mental retardation.

The author first refers to the information-processing approach to two-hand simultaneous tapping of Helmuth and Ivry (1996) and Vorberg and Hambuch (1978, 1984). They asked participants to tap simultaneously with one or two hands. Their analysis showed less variability in timing with two hands than with one hand, suggesting that the effect was due to combining the output of two separate timing systems by application of the Wing and Kristofferson model (1973). Wing et al (1989) further examined repetitive tapping with alternate hands, involving antiphase movements of the two hands. They found that at the fastest response rate (100 ms), adjacent between-hand intervals exhibited correlations more negative than the limit of minus one-half predicted by the Wing-Kristofferson model. The correlation for the alternate-hand tapping at longer tapping intervals (200 and 400 ms) were also more negative than single-hand tapping.

To date, the slowness in simple reaction times for individuals with mental retardation, autism, or Down syndrome is a persistent and robust finding in this line of research. However, as already stated, little research has been reported on their serial reactions or movements from an information-processing perspective. Moreover, their ability to coordinate bimanual movements has seldom been studied.

From a cognitive perspective, Inui and Asama (2003a, b) are therefore to examine the timing control of bimanual rhythmic finger-tapping sequences in adolescents with mental retardation, autism, or Down syndrome. To examine serial information processing in bimanual movements, the authors examined repetitive finger tapping with alternate hands as an easy bimanual movement. In other words, by examining serial information processing during repetitive finger tapping with alternate hands, the authors documented that the single-timer model (Wing and Kristofferson, 1973) was incapable of doing but two coupled Wing-Kristofferson timing systems with left and right clock (two coupled-timer model) could.

Participants were 9 male adolescents with mental retardation (IQ: 38-71), 5 with autism (IQ: 40-66), and 10 healthy individuals. The ages of the adolescents with mental retardation ranged from 13 to 16 years, with a mean of 14.5; those with autism ranged from 13 to 16 years, with a mean of 14.1; those of healthy adolescents ranged from 13 to 14 years, with a mean of 13.8. The adolescents with mental retardation or autism were recruited from a local school for handicapped children and healthy adolescents from a local junior high school. Although adolescents with Down syndrome participated in this experiment, they were not counted among participants because they were unable to meet the criteria in the recall trials.

Participants were seated facing two touch switches (figure 1). They alternately produced repetitive finger-tappings by an extension-flexion of the right and left arms at the elbow joint. While the three target intertap intervals of between-hand taps were 200 ms, 400 ms, and 800 ms, those of within-hand taps were 400 ms, 800 ms, and 1600 ms. In three practice trials, the participants were instructed to synchronize these hand taps on the touch switches with a computer-controlled metronome presented through a headphone for 30 s. These trials served to acquaint the participant with the tapping task. When they were unable to produce the three consecutive practice trials with an average deviation (obtained by averaging the absolute differences between the produced intertap interval and the target intertap interval) of 10% of the target intertap interval or less and a within-trial coefficient of variation (CV: obtained by dividing standard deviation by mean and multipling by 100) for target intertap interval of 30% or less, the practice trials were conducted two or three more times. They did not perform more than three additional practice trials so that fatigue effects in the hands and arms could be avoided. On the recall trial immediately after the practice trials, each participant spontaneously tapped once for 30 s. They were instructed to recall the intertap interval acquired during practice without feedback. If they were unable to produce accurate timing within the aforementioned criteria of average deviations and within-trial CVs in the practice trial, then the recall trial was conducted once again after practice trials had been repeated two or three times. If they were still unable to meet the criteria, they were eliminated. Then, they were not counted among participants. For both practice and recall trials, although no additional trial was taken by the normal participants, additional trials were taken by participants with mental retardation (6/9) or autism (5/5). The order of these three conditions presented to participants was randomly varied to avoid interaction effects.

Table 3 showed means and CVs for realized intertap intervals of within-hand taps in the recall trial (the self-pacing task, Inui and Asama, 2003a). To examine differences among groups and conditions, the analysis showed that normal adolescents approximately reproduced their taps with target intertap intervals under the three conditions. The analysis in the 800 ms condition showed that while the group with mental retardation used remarkably shorter intervals than the other two groups, the group with autism also used shorter intervals than the normal group. The analysis in the 400 ms condition showed that the group with autism used shorter intervals than the normal group, and in the 200 ms condition used shorter intervals than the other two groups. Thus, while the group with autism made faster tapping movements than the normal group over all three conditions, the group with mental retardation produced faster tapping movements than the other two groups only in the 800 ms condition.

Table 3. Means (M) and coefficients of variation (CV) for intertap interval of within-hand taps under three conditions in recall trials (Inui and Asama, 2003a). Abbreviations. MR: mental retardation, RH: right hand, LH: left hand

Group	n		Target intertap interval					
			200 ms		400 ms		800 ms	
			RH	LH	RH	LH	RH	LH
MR	8	M	416.35	416.65	778.01	777.63	1320.08	1320.42
		CV	14.50	14.77	8.19	8.20	10.53	10.45
Autism	5	M	345.12	342.90	742.70	743.10	1475.68	1475.36
		CV	20.53	21.00	5.93	5.86	7.38	7.65
Normal	10	M	394.49	395.10	787.19	786.67	1619.44	1615.25
		CV	8.29	8.98	4.34	4.25	5.50	5.39

Analysis of the CVs in the recall trial showed that while the group with mental retardation was more variable than the normal group over all conditions, the 200 ms condition had more variable realized intertap intervals than the other two conditions.

Table 4 showed means and CVs for realized intertap interval of within-hand taps in the practice trial (the synchronization task). Inui and Asama (2003b) examined differences among synchronization and self-pacing tasks and conditions for adolescents with mental retardation. Analysis of the means showed that there were significant main effects for task and condition. Whereas they produced longer intertap interval for the self-pacing task than for the synchonization task in the target interval of 200 ms, they produced shorter intertap interval for the self-pacing task than for the synchonization task in the target intervals of 400 and 800 ms. As a result, the interaction of task and condition was significant. For adolescents with autism, the analysis showed there were significant main effects for task and condition.

Although there was no difference between both the tasks in the target interval of 200 ms, they produced shorter intertap interval for the self-pacing task than for the synchonization task in the target intervals of 400 and 800 ms. The interaction of task and condition was consequently significant. For normal adolescents, the analysis showed there was no significant main effect for task but for condition. However, while there was no difference between both the tasks in the target intervals of 200 and 400 ms, they produced shorter intertap interval for the self-pacing task than for the synchonization task in the target interval of 800 ms. As a result, the interaction of task and condition was significant.

Table 4. Means (M) and coefficients of variation (CV) for intertap interval of within-hand taps under three conditions in practice trials (Inui and Asama, 2003b)

Group	n	Target intertap interval					
		200 msec		400 msec		800 msec	
		Right Hand	Left Hand	Right Hand	Left Hand	Right Hand	Left Hand
Mental Retardation	M	400.22	399.50	794.65	793.55	1579.35	1568.43
	CV	16.90	16.87	4.76	5.04	4.13	5.38
Normal	M	387.68	387.87	787.71	787.09	1661.24	1659.59
	CV	6.48	7.05	2.76	2.72	2.17	2.26

Analysis of the CVs showed that there were no significant main effect for task but for group and condition. However, while groups with mental retardation or autism had more variable intertap interval for synchonization task than for the self-pacing task in the target interval of 200 ms, all three groups had more variable intertap interval for the self-pacing task than for the synchonization task in the target intervals of 400 and 800 ms. As a result, the interaction of task and condition was significant.

All three groups thus made faster and variable movements for the self-pacing task than for the synchonization task in the longer target intervals. This suggests that whereas they were able to coordinate the timing of individual responses with individual stimuli in the synchonization task, they controlled the timing by a memory or the generation/setting of the incorrect timer rate in the self-pacing task.

To examine the single-timer model and two coupled-timer model with left and right clock in the bimanual alternate tapping, table 5 showed Pearson correlations between adjacent between-hand intertap intervals for each participant. At the shorter target intervals of 200 and 400 ms, the significant negative correlations were often observed for the groups with autism (5/10) and mental retardation (7/18). At the longer target interval of 800 ms, on the other hand, the rare significant positive correlations were unexpectedly observed (autism (1/5) and mental retardation (3/9)). Whereas at the longer target interval, the significant negative correlations were not realized for the normal group, the estimates at the shorter target intervals were observed (3/20). Thus, at the shorter target intervals adjacent between-hand intervals for some adolescents with autism and mental retardation and a few normal those exhibited correlations more negative than the limit of minus one-half predicted by the Wing-Kristofferson model. In addition, at the longer target interval the positive correlations for a few adolescents with autism and mental retardation suggest two separate Wing-Kristofferson timing systems in the bimanual alternate tapping.

Table 5. Pearson correlations between adjacent between-hand intertap intervals for each participant (Inui and Asama, 2003a). Abbreviations as in table 3

Paricipant		Target interval (ms)		
		200	400	800
Autism	Hi	-0.25	0.11	0.66**
	Ue	-0.41	-0.33	0.20
	Sa	-0.24	-0.45*	0.11
	Mo	-0.58**	-0.52*	-0.07
	Na	-0.62**	-0.58**	0.33
MR	Ic	-0.73	-0.38	0.53
	Ka	-0.27	0.15	0.43
	Nk	-0.37	-0.30	-0.13
	Ni	0.31	-0.11	-0.07
	Ok	-0.35	-0.23	0.84**
	Ki	-0.60**	-0.77**	0.28
	Nn	-0.38	-0.68**	0.59**
	Ha	-0.51*	-0.59**	0.01
	Hn	-0.67**	-0.48*	0.76**
Normal	Fu	0.27	0.01	-0.32
	Kn	0.08	0.22	0.24
	Ku	-0.26	-0.71**	-0.12
	Wa	-0.43	-0.24	0.08
	Mo	-0.71**	-0.32	0.16
	On	-0.25	-0.38	-0.06
	Ow	0.38	-0.22	-0.22
	Si	0.27	-0.60**	-0.29
	Ta	0.11	0.14	-0.07
	To	0.35	-0.16	-0.29

*p<0.05; ** p<0.01; df=18

Wing et al. (1989) examined repetitive tapping with alternate hands, finding that in the fastest alternate-hand condition (target interval 100 ms) adjacent to between-hand intervals exhibited correlations more negative than the limit of minus one-half predicted by the Wing-Kristofferson model (1973). They concluded that two coupled Wing-Kristofferson timing systems with left and right clock yielded negative correlations for adjacent between-hand intertap intervals of less than -0.5, which the single-timer model is incapable of doing. Similarly, Gentner (1983) and Shaffer (1978) earlier proposed that separation of left- and right-hand response streams combined with phase fluctuation would account for correlations of less than -0.5 observed between the hands in typing. Thus, they also concluded that the single-timer model might be spurious.

In the study of Inui and Asama (2003a), at the shorter target intervals of 200 and 400 ms the strong negative correlations were observed for adolescents with autism and mental retardation but not for normal adolescents. These results for adolescents with autism and mental retardation also suggested that this might be accounted for by two coupled Wing-Kristofferson timing systems with left and right clock intervals kept in appropriate relative phase by corrections involving the previously preceding produced intervals.

Normal adolescents, however, did not exhibit such strong negative correlations as those with autism and mental retardation. Wing et al. (1989) reported that for normal participants, negative correlations was greater in the target interval of 100 ms than in the target intervals of 200, 400, and 800 ms. Their results were consistent with the study of Inui and Asama (2003a). On the other hand, because the target intervals of 200 and 400 ms for adolescents with autism and mental retardation appear to correspond to the target interval of 100 ms for normal those, those with autism and mental retardation exhibited strong negative correlations at the target intervals of 200 and 400 ms.

5. Timing of Bimanual Polyrythmic Tapping Movement

Perhaps more than any other bimanual motor skill, bimanual coordination in polyrhythmic tapping tasks provides a focus for the current debate about the bimanual control of a coordinated skill. Because these skills have objective rhythmic structures, control models must take into account the need to produce specific rhythms rather than individually preferred rhythms. Current approaches to bimanual coordination in polyrhythmic tapping tasks follow the general distinctions between cognitive and dynamic systems approaches (for review, Wing and Beek, 2002).

In a cognitive approach, Jagacinski et al (1988) proposed two forms of motor organization in the production of polyrhythmic sequences (figure 9). One, an integrated organization, involves interleaving the timing of the two hands. The task then becomes a single sequence performed with two hands rather than two sequences performed by distinct hands. The other, a parallel organization, involves the use of separate timing mechanisms for the two hands so that each hand produces a separate sequence of responses. When such parallel organization is contrasted with the serial integrated organization in which a single timer is responsible for the between-hand intertap intervals, the pattern of covariances observed between intertap intervals disproves the parallel model (Jagacinski et al., 1988; Summers, Rosenbaum et al., 1993) even after extensive practice (Summers, Ford et al., 1993; Summers and Kennedy, 1992; Klapp et al, 1998). However, an experiment using highly skilled keyboard performance has recently produced evidence for parallel timing when the overall response rate is high (Krampe et al, 2000).

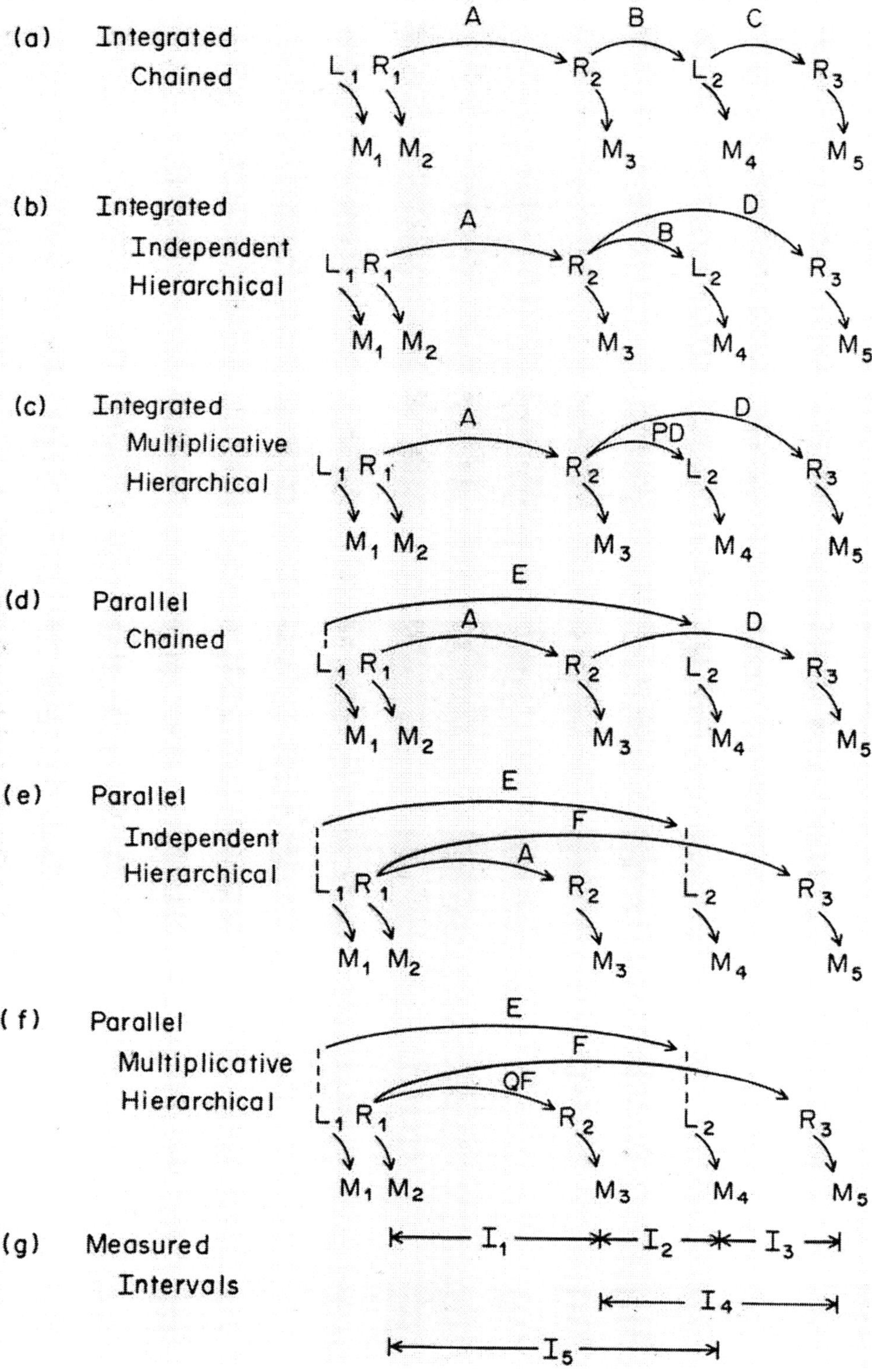

Figure 9. Six models of motor organization (Jagacinski et al., 1988). R1, L1, and so on, show internal events corresponding to tapping responses. A-F are internal timekeeper intervals. M1-M5 are motor delays. I1-I5 are observable intertap intervals.

To examine serial information processing in bimanual movements for adolescents with mental retardation, Inui and Asama (2003a) examined the bimanual task of a 3:2 polyrhythm as a complex bimanual movement. In other words, they examined the motor organization strategy adopted by participants in the bimanual task of a 3:2 polyrhythm requiring the concurrent production of two different isochronous sequences.

Participants were 6 male adolescents with mental retardation (IQ: 40-64) and 9 healthy those. The ages of the adolescents with mental retardation ranged from 17 to 18 years, with a mean of 17.8; those of healthy adolescents ranged from 18 to 19 years, with a mean of 18.4. All participants were right-handed. Handedness was tested using the Edinburgh handedness inventory (Oldfield, 1971). The adolescents with mental retardation were recruited from a local school for handicapped children, and healthy adolescents from a local college. To ensure that two conditions produced equivalent performance, whereas three adolescents with mental retardation and four undergraduate students were assigned to the task condition with the right hand taking the fast beat, the other participants were assigned to the task condition with the left hand taking the fast beat. Although 5 adolescents with autism participated in this experiment, they were not counted among participants because they were unable to meet the criteria in the recall trials.

Participants were seated facing two touch switches that were placed beneath each hand on a desk (figure 1). The responses were recorded by a personal computer through a junction box. The intertap intervals of each response were digitally measured.

The motor task required participants to tap out respectively a 3:2 polyrhythm on the two switches using the hands (Figure 10). Each cycle of the polyrhythm was initiated by a simultaneous right hand and left hand responses. Participants attempted to produce the polyrhythm with a cycle duration of 2100 ms. The fast hand was consequently to tap every 700 ms, and the slow hand every 1050 ms. The practice phase consisted of 10 trials, each trial continuing until the participant had produced 22 cycles of the polyrhythm. If participants were unable to produce the accurate timing within the aforementioned criteria of average deviations and within-trial CVs for the bimanual alternating finger-tapping, then the practice trials were conducted two or three more times. On the recall trial immediately after the end of the practice trials, each participant spontaneously tapped only 22 cycles of the polyrhythm. They were instructed to recall the intertap interval acquired during practice without feedback. If they were unable to produce the accurate timing with the aforementioned criteria of average deviations and within-trial CVs for the bimanual alternating finger-tapping, then the recall trial was conducted once again after practice trials had been repeated two or three times. If they were still unable to meet the criteria, they were eliminated. Then, they were not counted among participants. For both practice and recall trials, although no additional trial was taken by the normal participants, additional trials were taken by all participants with mental retardation.

The aim of this study was to determine the motor organizational strategies adopted by participants. One approach to this question is to examine mean proportions for fast hand and slow hand intervals. A parallel motor organization would be indicated by the maintenance of regular beats within each hand sequence. On the other hand, an integrated motor organization would be suggested by a departure from regularity in the intervals performed by one or both hands, as participants attempted to interlace the movements of the two hands.

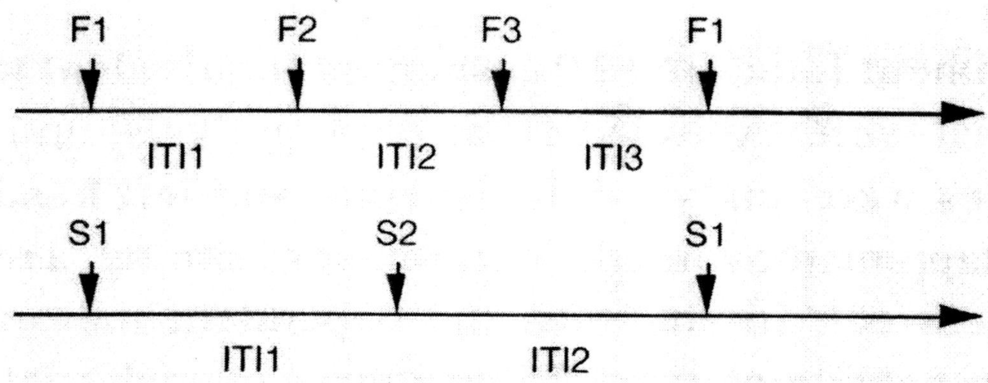
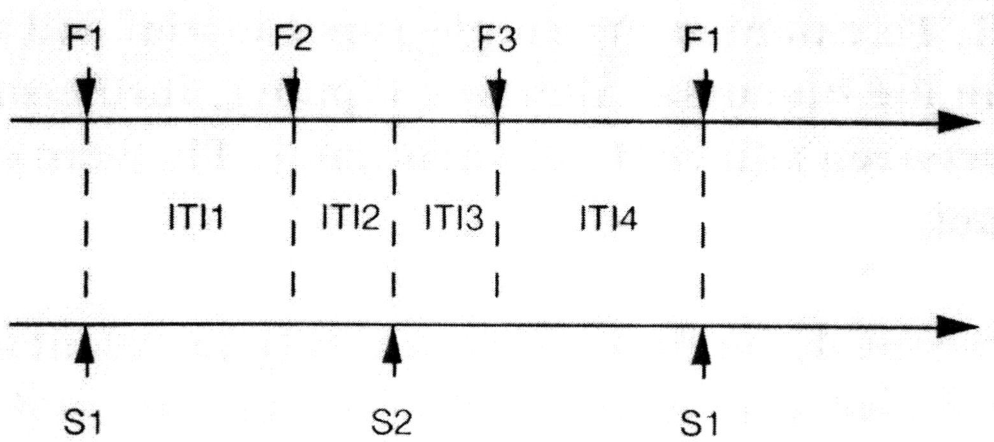

Figure 10. Schema of the temporal relationships between the two hands required for the 3:2 rhythm. Five within-hand intertap intervals (top) and four between-hand intertap intervals (bottom) are shown. Abbreviations. F: fast-hand tap, S: slow-hand tap, ITI: intertap interval.

Table 6 showed mean proportions for fast hand and slow hand intervals. Inui and Asama (2003a) examined the intertap intervals produced by converting each within-hand interval into a proportion of the total cycle duration to correct for tempo differences between participants, and then compared them to the required proportions. Both groups maintained a regular series of taps with both the fast and slow hands. Thus, because this study showed a regular series of taps with both the fast and slow hands exclusively in this stage, this suggested that both groups adopted the parallel motor organization.

Table 6. Mean proportions for fast-hand and slow-hand intervals (Inui and Asama, 2003a). Abbreviations as in Table 3 and Figure 10

Group	n	Fast hand			Slow hand	
		ITI1	ITI2	ITI3	ITI1	ITI2
MR	6	0.34	0.33	0.33	0.51	0.49
Normal	9	0.33	0.33	0.33	0.49	0.51

Table 7 showed means and CVs for realized intertap intervals of within-hand taps. Analysis of the means showed that the group with mental retardation used shorter intervals than the normal group. Thus, adolescents with mental retardation were unable to spontaneously reproduce the required target intertap intervals, but normal participants could. However, a similar tendency to adolescents with mental retardation has been reported in the production by skilled musicians of a 3:2 polyrhythm at similar slow (a cycle duration of 2,250 ms) rates (Summers, Rosenbaum et al., 1993). Rather it could indicate a memory problem or the generation/setting of the incorrect timer rate. Because the participants met the task requirements (table 6), realized intertap intervals performed by the slow hand were longer than realized intertap intervals performed by the fast hand. The interaction of group and serial position was not significant. Analysis of the CVs did not indicate any main effect and interaction.

Table 7. Means (M) and coefficients of variation (CV) for intertap interval of within-hand taps (Inui and Asama, 2003a). Abbreviations as in Table 3 and Figure 10

Group	n		Fast hand			Slow hand	
			ITI1	ITI2	ITI3	ITI1	ITI2
MR	6	M	644.82	636.04	626.19	971.04	936.02
		CV	7.43	6.54	9.51	7.51	9.26
Normal	9	M	707.08	703.94	706.80	1046.69	1071.13
		CV	8.84	8.47	10.35	8.45	9.29

Table 8 showed means and CVs for realized intertap intervals of between-hand taps. Analysis of the means showed that the group with mental retardation used shorter intervals than the normal group. This similar tendency to realized intertap intervals of within-hand taps could also indicate a memory problem or the generation/setting of the incorrect timer rate. Because the participants met the task requirements (Table 6), the intertap intervals 1 and 4 had longer intervals than the intervals 2 and 3. The interaction of group and serial position was not significant. Although analysis of the CVs for the normal group did not show any main effect or interaction, that for the group with mental retardation showed that the intertap intervals 2 and 3 had larger CVs than the intervals 1 and 4. In other words, the shorter intertap intervals were more variable than the longer intervals.

Table 8. Means (M) and coefficients of variation (CV) for intertap intervals of between-hand taps (Inui and Asama, 2003a). Abbreviations as in Table 3 and Figure 10

Group	n		ITI1	ITI2	ITI3	ITI4
MR	6	M	644.82	636.04	626.19	971.04
		CV	7.43	6.54	9.51	7.51
Normal	9	M	707.08	703.94	706.80	1046.69
		CV	8.84	8.47	10.35	8.45

Another approach to determine the motor organizational strategies adopted by participants is to examine correlations between adjacent intertap intervals of within-hand and between-hand taps. A parallel organization would be indicated by negative correlations between adjacent intertap intervals of within-hand taps. In contrast, an integrated organization would be suggested by negative correlations between adjacent intertap intervals of between-hand taps.

Table 9 showed Pearson correlations between adjacent within-hand intertap intervals for each participant. The correlations were scarcely observed in either group. Neither group thus adopted a parallel organization in the performance of a 3:2 polyrhythm. Table 10 showed Pearson correlations between adjacent between-hand intertap intervals for each participant. Although negative correlations between the intertap intervals 2 and 3 were observed for both groups, the correlations were observed more often and more strongly for the group with mental retardation (4/6) than for the normal group (3/9).

Table 9. Pearson correlations between adjacent within-hand intertap intervals for each participant (Inui and Asama, 2003a). "R" was attached to names of participants assigned to the task condition with the left hand taking the fast beat. Abbreviations as in Table 3 and Figure 10

Paricipant		Fast hand		Slow hand
		ITI1-2	ITI2-3	ITI1-2
MR	Ic	-0.02	0.01	-0.10
	Ka	0.25	0.24	0.04
	Nk	0.33	0.36	0.12
	Ni-R	-0.06	0.38	-0.16
	Ok-R	0.40	0.35	-0.33
	Ki-R	0.51*	0.34	0.35
Normal	Fu	-0.42	0.12	0.22
	Kn	0.71**	0.55*	0.53*
	Ku	0.31	0.30	-0.10
	Wa	0.27	0.40	0.50*
	Mo-R	0.15	0.48*	-0.15
	On-R	0.10	0.27	0.30
	Ow-R	-0.09	0.31	-0.24
	Si-R	0.22	-0.14	0.06
	Ta-R	-0.42	0.37	-0.36

*p<0.05; ** p<0.01; *df*=18

Table 10. Pearson correlations between adjacent between-hand intertap intervals for each participant (Inui and Asama, 2003a). "R" was attached to names of participants assigned to the task condition with the left hand taking the fast beat. Abbreviations as in Table 3 and Figure 10

Participant		ITI1-2	ITI2-3	ITI3-4
MR	Ic	0.11	-0.40	-0.10
	Ka	0.24	-0.68**	-0.37
	Nk	0.59**	-0.49*	0.21
	Ni-R	0.28	-0.60**	0.24
	Ok-R	0.67--	-0.76**	0.29
	Ki-R	0.23	-0.25	0.22
Normal	Fu	0.48*	0.19	0.52*
	Kn	0.63**	0.12	0.31
	Ku	0.48*	-0.47*	0.39
	Wa	-0.19	-0.44*	0.49*
	Mo-R	0.05	-0.54*	0.16
	On-R	-0.10	-0.39	0.26
	Ow-R	0.11	0.10	0.49*
	Si-R	-0.07	-0.01	-0.01
	Ta-R	-0.29	-0.06	-0.42

*p<0.05; ** p<0.01; df=18

From both approaches, whereas a few normal participants appeared to adopt the integrated organization, almost all participants with mental retardation adopted the organization. For participants with mental retardation, further, high negative correlations between the intertap intervals 2 and 3 of between-hand taps suggested that S2 of the slow hand taps did not influence F3 of the fast hand taps. The intertap intervals 2 and 3 of between-hand taps were more variable than the intervals 1 and 4 of between-hand taps (table 8), indicating that movements of the slow hand were subordinate to movements of the fast hand. They thus adopted the hierarchical integrated organization.

Summers, Rosenbaum et al. (1993) indicated that between-hand correlations increased with the complexity of polyrhythm (3:2 to 5:4) and the correlartions became more negative at the fast speed. Peters and Schwartz (1989) also reported strong negative Lag 1 autocorrelations between the intertap intervals 2 and 3 of between-hand taps in the performance of a 3:2 polyrhythm at the fast speed (target cycle durations 1086 ms and 1490.2 ms). These earlier results are similar to between-hand correlations in the performance of a 3:2 polyrhythm at the slow speed (target cycle duration 2100 ms) in the study of Inui and Asama (2003a) for normal participants. On the other hand, because a 3:2 polyrhythm for participants with mental retardation corresponds to more complex polyrhythms for normal participants, between-hand correlations in the performance of a 3:2 polyrhythm even at the slow speed were high negative for participants with mental retardation.

6. General Discussion

In a task of tracking a serial light stimulation, two components have been already observed for motor organization of unimanual serial reactions (Inui and Suzuki, 1998; Inui et al, 1995). Normal participants responded with six movements, in which these individuals pressed a series of keys 1, 2, 3, 4, 5, and 6, as a chunk and were able to coordinate the timing of individual responses with individual stimuli. However, although adolescents with mental retardation or autism appeared to chunk the whole series of responses, they were unable to coordinate the timing of individual responses with individual stimuli. To the contrary, adolescents with Down syndrome not only did not produce this movement-output chunking, but they were also unable to coordinate the timing of individual responses with individual stimuli. Thus, for motor organization of unimanual serial reactions, one component is to temporally chunk the whole series of reactions ("temporal component"), and another is to accurately coordinate the timing of individual responses with individual stimuli ("spatial component"). Similarly, when normal participants between 7 and 20 years old unimanually recalled the force pattern (300 g-300 g-300 g-100 g), adults and adolescents responded with four taps as a chunk, but younger children had difficulty with such chunking (Inui and Katsura, 2002). Adults and adolescents were further able to more accurately produce individual force magnitudes to match target magnitudes than younger children.

In the bimanual tasks of tapping with alternate hands and tapping a polyrhythm as well as the unimanual tasks of tracking a serial light stimulation and recalling the force pattern, these findings robustly document the idea that the movement-output chunking as the temporal component play an important role for the control of timing or force in serial movements.

While the group with autism made faster tapping movements than the normal group over the three conditions in the bimanual alternating finger-tapping, the group with mental retardation produced faster movements than the other two groups only in the 800 ms condition. Adolescents with mental retardation and autism were thus unable to spontaneously reproduce the required target intertap intervals with accuracy.

In the bimanual alternating finger-tapping, however, strong negative correlations were observed at the shorter target interval for adolescents with autism and mental retardation. In the polyrhythmic tapping task, adolescents with mental retardation and normal those further appear to adopt the integrated organization. They thus appeared to produce two or five taps with alternate hands as a movement-output chunk (Miller, 1958; Schmidt, 1988). In other words, they had pauses between sets of two or five taps with alternate hands. The adoption of an integrated organization indicated that the polyrhythm was produced as an output chunk. This indicates a link between the concepts of an integrated organization and movement-output chunking. In our preliminary experiments, on the other hand, whereas participants with mental retardation were unable to perform more complex polyrhythms than a 3:2 polyrhythm with the criteria in the practice trials, normal participants were able to produce more complex polyrhythms. Normal participants naturally produced the output chunking more tightly than mentally retarded and autistic those. This therefore allows for a speculation about the control of timing and force in serial movements: the output chunking can be regarded as a developmental milestone for the control in serial movements.

Reference

Anson, J. G. (1992). Neuromotor control and Down syndrome. In J. J. Summers (Ed.), *Approaches to the study of motor control and learning* (pp. 387-412). Amsterdam: Elsevier.

Anson, J. G., and Mawston, G. A. (2000). Patterns of muscle activation in simple reaction-time tasks. In D. J. Weeks, R. Chua, and D. Elliott (Eds.), *Perceptual-motor behavior in Down syndrome* (pp. 3-24). Champaingn, IL: Human Kinetics.

Anwar, F. (1983). The role of sensory modality for the reproduction of shape by the severely retarded. *British Journal of Developmental Psychology, 1*, 317-327.

Anwar, F., and Hermelin, B. (1979). Kinesthetic movement after-effects in children with Down syndrome. *Journal of Mental Deficiency Research, 23*, 287-297.

Baumeister, A. A., and Kellas, G. (1968). Reaction time and mental retardation. In N. E. Ellis (Ed.), *International Review of Research in Mental Retardation* (vol. 3, pp. 163-193). New York, NY: Academic Press.

Berkson,G. (1960a). An analysis of reaction time in normal and mentally retarded young men: II. Variation of complexity in reaction time tasks. *Journal of Mental Deficiency Research, 4*, 56-67.

Berkson,G. (1960b). An analysis of reaction time in normal and mentally retarded young men: III. Variation of stimulus and response complexity. *Journal of Mental Deficiency Research, 4*, 69-77.

Courchesne, E., Townsend, J., Akshoomoff, N.A., Saitoh, O., Yeung-Courchesne, R., Lincoln, A.J., James, H.E., Haas, R.H., Schreibman, L., and Lau, L. (1994a). Impairment in shifing attention in autistic and cerebellar patients. *Behavioral Neuroscience, 108*, 848-865.

Courchesne, E., Townsend, J., Akshoomoff, N.A., Yeung-Courchesne, R., Press,G.A., Murakami, J. W., Lincoln, A.J., James, H.E., Saitoh, O., Egaas, B., Haas, R.H., and Schreibman, L. (1994b). A new finding: impairment in shifting attention in autistic and cerebellar patients. In S. H. Broman, and J. Grafman (Eds.), *Atypical cognitive deficits in developmental disorders: implications for brain function* (pp. 101-137). Hillsdale, NJ: Erlbaum.

Courchesne, E., Yeung-Courchesne, R., Press, G. A., Hesselink, J. R., and Jernigan, T. L. (1988). Hypoplasia of cerebellar vermal lobules VI and VII in autism. *The New England Journal of Medicine, 318*, 1349-1354.

Crispino, L., and Bullock, T. H. (1984). Cerebellum mediates modality-specific modulation of sensory responses of the midbrain and forebrain in rat. *Proceedings of the National Academy of Sciences, 81*, 281-292.

Davis, W. E., and Kelso, J. A. S. (1982). Analysis of 'invariant characteristics' in the motor control of Down syndrome and normal subjects. *Journal of Motor Behavior, 14*, 194-212.

Davis, W. E., and Sinning, W. E. (1987). Muscle stiffness in Down syndrome and other mentally handicapped subjects: a research note. *Journal of Motor Behavior, 19*, 130-144.

Davis, W. E., Sparrow, W. A., and Ward, T. (1991). Fractioned reaction times and movement times of Down syndrome, and other adults with mental retardation. *Adapted Physical Activity Quarterly, 8,* 221-233.

Frith, U., and Frith, C. D. (1974). Specific motor disabilities in Down's syndrome. *Journal of Child Psychology and Psychiatry, 15,* 293-301.

Gentner, D. R. (1983). Keystroke timing in transcription typing. In W. E. Cooper (Ed.), *Cognitive aspects of skilled typewriting* (pp. 95-120). Berlin: Springer.

Helmuth, L. L., and Ivry, R. B. (1996). When two hands are better than one: reduced timing variability during bimanual movements. *Journal of Experimental Psychology: Human Perception and Performance, 22,* 278-293.

Hermelin, B., and O'Connor, N. (1970). *Psychological experiments with autistic children.* Oxford: Pergamon.

Hoover, J. H., Wade, M. G., and Newell, K. M. (1981). Training moderately and severely mentally retarded adults to improve reaction and movement times. *American Journal of Mental Deficiency, 85,* 389-395.

Horvat, M., Ramsey, V., Amestoy, R., and Croce, R. (2003). Muscle activation and movement responses in youth with and without mental retardation. *Research Quarterly Exercise and Sport, 74,* 319-323.

Inui, N., and Asama, K. (2003a). Timing of bimanual rhythmic finger tapping in adolescents with mental retardation or autism. *Journal of Human Movement Studies, 45,* 59-80.

Inui, N., and Asama, K. (2003b). Timing of bimanual alternating finger-tapping sequences in adolescents with mental retardation: a plot study. *Perceptual and Motor Skills, 97,* 398-400.

Inui, N., and Katsura, Y. (2002). Development of force control and timing in a finger-tapping sequence with an attenuated-force tap. *Motor Control, 6,* 333-346.

Inui, N., and Suzuki, K. (1998). Practice and serial reaction time of adolescents with autism. *Perceptual and Motor Skills, 86,* 403-410.

Inui, N., Yamanishi, M., and Tada, S. (1995). Simple reaction times and timing of serial reactions of adolescents with mental retardation, autism, and Down syndrome. *Perceptual and Motor Skills, 81,* 739-745.

Jagacinski, R. J., Marshburn, E., Klapp, S.T., and Jones, M. R. (1988). Tests of parallel versus integrated structure in polyrhythmic tapping. *Journal of Motor Behavior, 20,* 416-442.

Kanner, L. (1943). Autistic disturbances of affective contact. *Nervous Child, 2,* 217-250.

Karrer, R. (1986). Input, central, and motor segments of response time in mentally retarded and normal children. In M. G. Wade (Ed.), *Motor skill acquisition of the mentally handicapped: issues in research and training* (pp. 167-187). Amsterdam: Elsevier.

Kerr, R., and Blais, C. (1987). Down syndrome and extended practice on a complex motor task. *American Journal of Mental Deficiency, 91,* 591-597.

Kerr, R., and Blais, C. (1988). Directional probability information and Down syndrome: a training study. *American Journal on Mental Retardation, 92,* 531-538.

Klapp, S. T., Nelson, J. M., and Jagacinski, R. J. (1998). Can people tap concurrent bimanual rhythms independently ? *Journal of Motor Behavior, 30,* 301-322.

Kondo, F. (1978). The effects of cue stimuli on the reaction times of mentally retarded children: an examination of the temporal factor and the spatial factor. *The Japanese Journal of Psychology, 49*, 123-130 [in Japanese].

Krampe, R. T., Kliegl, R., Mayr, U., Engbert, R., and Vorberg, D. (2000). The fast and slow of skilled bimanual rhythm production: parallel vs. integrated timing. *Journal of Experimental Psychology: Human Perception and Performance, 26*, 206-233.

LeClair, D. A., Pollock, B. J., and Elliott, D. (1993). Movement preparation in adults with and without Down syndrome. *American Journal on Mental Retardation, 90*, 472-475.

Mawston, G. A., and Anson, J. G. (1994). Down syndrome: attention and neuromotor reaction time. *International Journal of Neuroscience, 74*, 148.

Miller, G. A. (1956). The magical number seven, plus or minus two: some limits on our capacity for processing information. *Psychological Review, 63*, 81-97.

Nieuwenhuys, R., Voogd, J., and van Huijzen, C. (1988). *The human central nervous system: a synopsis and atlas.* Berlin: Springer.

Oldfield, R. C. (1971). The assessment and analysis of handedness: the Edinburgh inventory. *Neuropsychologia, 9*, 97-113.

Peters, M., and Schwartz, S. (1989). Coordination of the two hands and effects of attentional manipulation in the production of a bimanual 2:3 polyrhythm. *Australian Journal of Psychology, 41*, 215-224.

Posner, M. I., and Petersen, S. (1990). The attention system of the human brain. *Annual Review of Neuroscience, 13*, 25-42.

Rimland, B. (1964). *Infantile autism: the syndrome and its implications for a neural theory of behavior.* Englewood Cliffs, NJ: Prentice-Hall.

Saccuzzo, D. P., and Michael, B. (1984). Speed of information-processing and structural limitations by mental retarded and dual-diagnosed retarded-schizophrenic persons. *American Journal of Mental Deficiency, 89*, 187-194.

Schmidt, R. A. (1988). *Motor control and learning: a behavioral emphasis* (Second Ed., pp. 64-65, 114-115). Champaign, IL: Human Kinetics.

Shaffer, L. H. (1978). Timing in the motor programming of typing. *Quarterly Journal of Experimental Psychology, 30*, 333-345.

Shumway-Cook, A., and Woollacott, M. H. (1985). Dynamics of postural control in the child with Down syndrome. *Physical Therapy, 65*, 1315-1322.

Simon, D. A., Elliot, D., and Anson, J. G. (2003). *Perceptual-motor behaviour in children with Down syndrome.* In G. Savelsbergh, K. Davids, J. van der Kamp, and S. J. Bennett (Eds.). *Development of movement co-ordination in children* (pp. 133-155). London: Routledge.

Summers, J. J., Ford, S., and Todd, J. A. (1993). Practice effects on the coordination of the two hands in a bimanual tapping task. *Human Movement Science, 12*, 111-133.

Summers, J. J., and Kennedy, T. M. (1992). Strategies in the production of a 5:3 polyrhythm. *Human Movement Science, 11*, 101-112.

Summers, J. J., Rosenbaum, D. A., Burns, B. D., and Ford, S. K. (1993). Production of polyrhythms. *Journal of Experimental Psychology: Human Perception and Performance, 19*, 416-428.

Un, N., and Erbahceci, F. (2000). The evaluation of reaction time on mentally retarded children. *Pediatic Rehabilitation, 4,* 1-4.

Vorberg, D., and Hambuch, R. (1978). On the temporal control of rhythmic performance. In J. Requin (Ed.), *Attention and performance VII* (pp. 535-555). Hillsdale, NJ: Erlbaum.

Vorberg, D., and Hambuch, R. (1984). Timing of two-handed rhythmic performance. *Annals of the New York Academy of Sciences, 423,* 390-406.

Williams, R. S., Hauser, S. L., Purpura, D. P., DeLong, R., and Swisher, C. N. (1980). Autism and mental retardation: neuropathological studies performed in four retarded persons with autistic behavior. *Archives of Neurology, 37,* 749-753.

Wing, A. M., and Beek, P. J. (2002). Movement timing: a tutorial. In W. Prinz and B. Hommel (Eds.), *Common mechanisms in perception and action, Attention and performance XIX* (pp. 202-226). New York, NY: Oxford University Press.

Wing, A. M., Church, R. M., and Gentner, D. R. (1989). Variability in the timing of responses during repetitive tapping with alternate hands. *Psychological Research, 51,* 28-37.

Wing, A. M., and Kristofferson, A. B. (1973). Response delays and the timing of discrete motor responses. *Perception and Psychophysics, 14,* 5-12.

In: Mental Retardation Research Advances
Editor: Elizabeth B. Heinz, pp. 35-44

ISBN: 978-1-60021-658-9
© 2007 Nova Science Publishers, Inc.

Regular Exercise as a Healthy Strategy to Reduce Oxidative Stress in Adolescents with Down Syndrome

F.J. Ordonez and *M.Rosety-Rodriguez*
School of Sport Medicine. University of Cadiz; Virgen Saliente s/n 11100
San Fernando, Cadiz, Spain

Abstract

In recent years it has been claimed trisomic cells are more sensitive to oxidative stress. This fact is of particular interest since oxidative stress has been proposed as a pathogenic mechanism of atherosclerosis, cell aging and neurodegeneration in individuals with Down syndrome.

In general population it has been recently published regular exercise may increase antioxidant system. However, far less information is available on handicapped populations such as Down syndrome.

For the reasons already mentioned we designed a research project to assess the influence of a 12-week training program on redox metabolism in adolescents with Down syndrome in order to determine its capacity to attenuate their increased oxidative damage.

Thirty-one male adolescents with Down syndrome (16.3 ± 1.1 years) performed a 12-week training program, 3 sessions/week, consisting of warm up (15 min) followed by a main part (20-35 min [increasing 5 minutes each three weeks]) at a work intensity of 60-75% of peak heart rate according to the equation HRmax=194.5-[0.56 age] (increasing 5% each three weeks) and by a cool-down period (10 min). No one of them suffered acute medical problems at that moment and had not taken part in any physical activity program in the last six months. Written informed consent was obtained from all their parents.

Blood samples were collected from an antecubital vein while participants 72-hours before the beggining of the program and after its ending. Lysed erythrocytes were

* F.J. Ordonez: Tel. +34 956 88 39 05; Fax. +34 956 88 32 30; email: franciscojavier.ordonez@uca.es

prepared by putting cells through three freeze-thaw cycles in dry ice and by the addition of five volumes of ice-cold distilled water. After centrifugation, supernatant was frozen at -20 °C until analysis.

Main outcome measurements included the assessment of lipoperoxidation -in terms of MDA content- and protein oxidation -in terms of carbonyl group content-. Antioxidant enzymes such as superoxide dismutase (SOD) glutathione peroxidase (GPX), glutathione reductase (GR), catalase (CAT) and glucose-6-phophate-dehydrogenase (G6PDH) were also assessed.

When compared to baseline values, lipoperoxidation and protein oxidation were significantly reduced. It may be explained, at least in part, since the activity of antioxidants enzymes such as glutathione persoxidase (GPX), glutathione reductase (GR) and glucose-6-phophate-dehydrogenase (G6PDH) were significantly increased after the training period.

Consquently it may be concluded regular exercise improved redox metabolism in adolescents with Down syndrome. Further studies on other handicapped populations are highly required.

Introduction

In recent years, both in vivo and in vitro studies have demonstrated the significant association between oxidative damage and different pathological disorders in general population (Burlaka et al. 2006; Nonomura et al. 2006; Yao et al. 2006). Consequently there is an increasing concern about the identification of healthy strategies that may prevent and/or attenuate its negative effects.

In this respect, it has been claimed trisomic cells are more sensitive to oxidative stress (Carratelli et al. 2001). Among the different explanations that have been proposed in the literature, SOD-catalyzed hydroxyl radical formation from the excess of H2O2 has been widely accepted.

In a more detailed way, it is generally accepted antioxidant enzyme superoxide dismutase (SOD) catalyzes the dismutation of superoxide anion ($O2^-$) to hydrogen peroxide (H2O2) and then, in a second step, glutathione peroxidase (GPX) and catalase (CAT) convert hydrogen peroxide (H2O2) to water before it may be transformed into the harmful hydroxyl radicals. Consequently, the activity of the first-step (SOD) and second-step (GPX, CAT) antioxidant enzymes, expressed as the quotient SOD/GPX+CAT, must be balanced to prevent cell damage by oxidative stress (Crosti et al. 1989).

The gene for SOD lies in humans on chromosome 21 and consequently it is conceivable either its activity is increased and above mentioned quotient got disbalanced in individuals with trisomy 21. However, instead of being beneficial, this situation is critical since the enormous pool of hydrogen peroxide may be transformed into hydroxyl radicals what may finally lead to an increased oxidative damage (Kowald et al. 2004).

In any case, this fact is of particular interest since oxidative stress has been proposed as a pathogenic mechanism of atherosclerosis, cell aging, immunological disorders and neurodegeneration in individuals with Down syndrome (Pastore et al. 2003).

Recent studies have reported the importance of the assessment of oxidative injury by mean of the determination of lipid peroxidation is increasing in the last years (Bir et al. 2006;

Steghens et al. 2005). Similarly, in vitro and in vivo studies have demonstrated protein oxidation results in the formation of carbonyl groups whose evaluation may provide a significant clue to the magnitude of oxidative stress under disease conditions (Stadtman and Levine 2000; Rosety-Rodriguez et al. 2006a).

In general population it has been recently published regular exercise may increase antioxidant enzyme system (Cutler, 2005; Elosua et al. 2003). On the contrary, exhausting exercise (Chevion et al. 2003) or overloaded training (Palazzetti et al. 2003) may increase oxidative stress and damage. However, far less information is available on handicapped populations such as Down syndrome. In this line, it would be of great interest to assess the behaviour of antioxidant enzymes such as superoxide dismutase (SOD), glutathione peroxidase (GPX), glutathione reductase (GR), catalase (CAT), glucose-6-phosphate-dehydrogenase (G6PDH) in exercised individuals with trisomy 21.

In any case the importance of blood in this research area is increasing since it may reflect changes in the antioxidant activity in other less accessible tissues (Muchova et al. 2001; Pastor et al. 1998; Rosety-Rodriguez et al. 2005; Tauler et al. 2005). Accordingly methodological procedures to assess redox metabolism in blood samples in general and erythrocytes in particular have been carefully reported and can be found elsewhere in the literature.

For the reasons already mentioned we designed a research project to assess the influence of a 12-week training program on redox metabolism in adolescents with Down syndrome in order to determine its capacity to attenuate their increased oxidative damage.

Materials and Methods

Thirty-one male adolescents with Down syndrome (16.3±1.1 years; 155.2 ± 5.7 cm; 70.8 ± 4.5 kg) performed a 12-week training program, 3 sessions/week, consisting of warm up (15 min) followed by a main part (20-35 min [increasing 5 minutes each three weeks]) at a work intensity of 60-75% of peak heart rate and by a cool-down period (10 min). According to Fernhall et al. (2001), it should be emphasized maximal heart rate for individuals with Down syndrome was predicted by the equation HRmax=194.5–[0.56 age]. It should be emphasized all these sessions were adequately supervised and controlled by long-experienced trainers.

No one of them suffered acute medical problems at that moment and had not taken part in any physical activity program in the last six months.

In order to avoid potential confounding effects, all participants received cuantitative and cualitatively a samilar diet. Cuantitatively, no significant differences were found in total Kcal intake. And cualitatively, no one of them took vitamins or antioxidants. Further no one reported toxic habits (smoking or alcohol consumption). To get these goals the role of their parents was essential, and consequently, they were adequate and carefully informed by researchers before starting our experience.

Control group included 7 age, sex and BMI (body mass index)-matched adolescents with trisomy 21 that did not performed any training program. Written informed consent was obtained from their parents. It should be emphasized our protocol was reviewed and approved by an Institutional Ethical Committee.

Blood samples were collected from an antecubital vein 72-hours before starting the 12 week training program and 72-hours after its ending. Lysed erythrocytes were prepared by putting cells through three freeze-thaw cycles in dry ice and by the addition of five volumes of ice-cold distilled water. After centrifugation, erythrocyte supernatant was frozen at -20 °C until analysis.

Main outcome measurements in our research project included the assessment of lipoperoxidation in terms of MDA (malondialdehyde; Young and Trimble, 1991) content and protein oxidation in terms of carbonyl group content (Rajesh et al. 2004). Antioxidant enzymes such as superoxide dismutase (SOD; E.C. 1.15.1.1; McCord and Fridovich, 1969) glutathione peroxidase (GPX; E.C. 1.11.1.9; Flohe and Gunzler, 1984), glutathione reductase (GR; E.C. 1.6.4.2; Goldberg and Spooner, 1992), catalase (CAT; E.C. 1.11.1.6; Beutler, 1975) and glucose-6-phophate-dehydrogenase (G6PDH E.C. 1.1.1.49; Glock and Mclean, 1953) were also assessed.

Results were expressed as mean±SD and 95% confidence intervals. A Student's *t*-test for paired data was performed to compare pre and post-test results of each parameter. In any case, significance was ascertained at $p < 0.05$.

Results

Pre and post-test values of tested variables (MDA, Carbonyl groups, SOD, CAT, GPX, GR and G6PDH) in hemolysates of adolescents with Down syndrome are listed in tables 1 and 2 respectively.

Table 1. Erythrocyte lipoperoxidation, protein oxidation and antioxidant enzyme activities in male adolescents with Down syndrome at baseline (n=31)

	Media	SD	IC 95%
MDA (μmol·l^{-1})	0.41	±0.12	[0.39-0.43] [(*)]
CARBONYL (nmol/mg protein)	1.98	±0.2	[1.94-2.02] [(*)]
SOD (U/gHb)	679.0	±82	[642.2 – 715.8]
CAT (U/gHb)	1607.0	±231	[1417.6-1797.5]
GPX (U/gHb)	24.8	±3.1	[23.1-26.5] [(*)]
GR (U/gHb)	8.8	± 0.3	[8.6 – 9.0] [(*)]
G6PDH (mU/gHb)	12.3	±1.2	[10.9-13.7] [(*)]

Nota: Results are expressed as mean SD and 95% confidence interval. MDA (Malondialdehyde). SOD (Superoxide dismutase); CAT (Catalase); GPX (Glutathione peroxidase); GR (Glutathione reductase); G6PDH (Glucose-6-phosphate-dehydrogenase). Hb (Hemoglobin).

We have also found MDA and carbonyl group contents were decreased significantly when compared to baseline. Futher, activity of antioxidant enzymes GPX, GR and G6PDH increased significantly. On the other hand, SOD and CAT did not change significantly at the end of the experiencie. No significant changes were observed in controls in any parameter assessed.

Table 2. Erythrocyte lipoperoxidation, protein oxidation and antioxidant enzyme activities in male adolescents with Down syndrome (n=31) after a 12 week aerobic training program

	Media	SD	IC 95%
MDA (μmol·l^{-1})	0.32	±0.09	[0.31-0.33] [*]
CARBONYL (nmol/mg protein)	1.16	±0.1	[1.14-1.18] [*]
SOD (U/gHb)	706.8	±91	[663.9 – 749.8]
CAT (U/gHb)	1663.2	±280	[1433.1-1893.2]
GPX (U/gHb)	29.3	±2.9	[28.1-30.5] [*]
GR (U/gHb)	10.4	± 0.5	[10.1 – 10.7] [*]
G6PDH (mU/gHb)	14.2	±1.0	[13.1-15.1] [*]

Nota: Results are expressed as mean SD and 95% confidence interval. MDA (Malondialdehyde); SOD (Superoxide dismutase); CAT (Catalase); GPX (Glutathione peroxidase); GR (Glutathione reductase); G6PDH (Glucose-6-phosphate-dehydrogenase); Hb (Hemoglobin). (*) Significant differences (p<0.05) when compared to baseline values.

Discussion

In recent years, several authors have cleraly demosntrated the role of oxidative damage in disease onset and/or progression. Fortunately, several studies have demonstrated regular exercise may improve redox metabolism by mean of decreasing biomacromolecule oxidation (lipids, proteins and DNA) and/or increasing antioxidant defense system (Elosua et al. 2003). However, to date, little attention has received this topic on handicapped populations in general and mental retardation ones in particular.

Malondialdehyde (MDA), a major end-product of oxidation of polyunsaturated fatty acids, has been frequently measured as indicator of lipid peroxidation and oxidative stress in vivo. As was hypothesized, we have observed regular exercise reduced significantly plasmatic MDA levels in male adolescents with Down syndrome. Similar results have been found in healthy children (Gonenc et al. 2000) and adults (Ozbay et al. 2002) after being exercised.

However, a 16-week aerobic training program increased plasma TBARS in adults with trisomy 21 (Monteiro et al. 1990). It may be explained, at least in part, by differences regarding the method performed to determine lipid peroxidation when compared to MDA content assessed in our study. In this respect it should be pointed out there are methodological problems with the TBARS assay, including lack of specificity and generation of artifactual TBARS under various assay conditions (Janero, 1990; Young and Trimble, 1991).

In this line, it has been recently published regular exercise may increase low-density-lipoprotein (LDL) resistance to oxidation in general population (Elosua et al. 2003). In a previous paper (Ordoñez et al. 2005a) we have reported that our 12-week training program improved significantly serum lipid profile in adolescents with trisomy 21. As was hypothesized we found that HDL-Cholesterol increased whereas LDL-Cholesterol and triglycerides decreased, what may also contribute, at least in part, to improve lipoperoxidation in exercised individuals.

In vitro and in vivo studies have demonstrated protein oxidation results in the formation of carbonyl groups whose evaluation may provide a significant clue to the magnitude of oxidative stress under disease conditions (Stadtman and Levine, 2000; Rosety-Rodriguez et al. 2006a). Accordingly, carbonylation of proteins has been considered a widespread indicator of severe oxidative damage (Dalle-Done et al. 2006).

In contrast to lipoperoxidation, to date, protein oxidation has been mostly assessed in experimental research whereas little information is available on humans in the literature. In any case, these works suggested regular and moderate exercise decreased significantly protein oxidation (Ogonovszky et al. 2005; Radak et al. 2000). On the contrary, Radak et al. (2003) reported exhaustive exercise increased carbonyl in super-marathon runners.

As was hypothesized, we have also found a 12-week exercise program reduced significantly protein oxidation, in terms of erythrocyte carbonyl group content, in male adolescents with Down syndrome (Rosety-Rodriguez et al. In Press).

In short, when compared to baseline values, lipoperoxidation and protein oxidation were significantly reduced in exercised individuals with Down syndrome.

The question arises how regular exercise may exert its action, that may finally lead to a reduction of oxidative damage in exercised-individuals. To get this goal, in the present study we assessed the influence of regular exercise on erythrocyte antioxidant enzymes such as superoxide dismutase (SOD), catalase (CAT), glutathione peroxidase (GPX), glutathione reductase (GR) and glucose-6-phosphate-dehydrogenase (G6PDH).

As was hypothesized regular exercise increased significantly erythrocyte GPX activity in adolescents with Down syndrome (Ordonez et al. 2006a).

In any case, it has been recently published that regular exercise may enhance the blood antioxidant system in general and GPX activity in particular both in human (Elosua et al. 2003) and experimental (Oztasan et al. 2004) research. On the contrary, acute exercise until exhaustion does not affect the activity of serum GPX in healthy young people (Rush and Sandiford, 2003).

To act as an antioxidant, GPX requires reduced glutathione (GSH), which is then oxidized, losing its activity. Regeneration of reduced glutathione (GSH) from oxidized glutathione (GSSG) is carried out by the enzyme glutathione reductase (GR). In order to complete this cycle, the concomitant conversion of NADPH to $NADP^+$ is essential.

This fact is of particular interest GR activity was also increased after our 12-week training program (Ordonez et al. 2006c).

Similarly, it was reported the levels of reduced glutathione (GSH) were increased after a 16-week training program in adults with Down syndrome (Monteiro et al. 1997).

As we have already stated, NADPH may play an important role in glutathione antioxidant system. The principal source of NADPH is the pentose phosphate shunt. In this respect, the activity of glucose 6-phosphate dehydrogenase (G6PDH), which is the first enzyme in the pentose phosphate pathway, may limit the rate of NADPH production and, hence, the ability of the glutathione peroxidase system to detoxify peroxides.

Fortunately, we have recently reported our 12-week training program increased sigfnificantly erythrocyte activity of G6PDH in adolescents with Down syndrome (Ordonez et al. 2005b).

On the other hand we have also found regular physical activity did not increase significantly SOD and CAT activities (Ordonez et al. 2006b; Rosety-Rodriguez et al. 2006b).

These findings suggest regular exercise may reduce oxidative damage in exercised-adolescents with trisomy 21 since it contributed to balance the quotient SOD/GPX+CAT. Accordingly, second step enzymes (mainly GPX) may convert the excess of hydrogen peroxide (H2O2), induced by increased expression of SOD, to water before it pass into hydroxyl radicals.

This fact is of particular interest since the latter may finally attack biomacromolecules (lipids and proteins) causing oxidative damage. Another observation one can make when reviewing the literature is that our series (n=31) was similar to the highest ones reported in previous studies in indiviuals with Down syndrome (Carratelli et al. 2003; Monteiro et al. 1997; Pastore et al. 2001).

Accordingly, since we have already demonstrated regular exercise improves erythrocyte antioxidant enzyme system in adolescents with Down syndrome, these programs may be highly recommended for this population. However antioxidant enzyme assessment is a complex, expensive and invasive procedure.

In order to facilitate medical-follow up of training programs by mean of an easy, economic and non-invasive procedure, it would be of interest to determine by mean of Pearson´s correlation coefficient potential associations between antioxidant enzymes and anthropometrical parameters.

Previous studies had succesfully explored the relationship of anthropometrical parameters and different parameters such as diet, exercise, disability status, and degree of social integration in individuals with Down syndrome (Fujiura et al. 1997).

In this respect we have recently found a negative but significant association between GPX activity and waist circumference (WC). Regarding body mass index (BMI) and waist to hip ratio (WHR), they were neither strongly nor significantly correlated to GPX. These results suggested anthropometrical parameters such as waist circumference are easy to perform but not strongly associated to GPX activity (Ordonez et al. 2006d). Further studies concerning other correlations with antioxidants are highly required in order to facilitate the medical follow-up of exercise programs.

Conclusion

Consquently it may be concluded regular exercise improved redox metabolism in adolescents with Down syndrome. In this line, it decreased significantly lipoperoxidation and protein oxidation what may be explained, at least in part, by a significant increase of antioxidant enzyme activities (GPX, GR and G6PDH). Further studies on this topic but focussed on other handicapped populations are highly required.

References

Bir LS, Demir S, Rota S, Koseoglu M. Increased serum malondialdehyde levels in chronic stage of ischemic stroke. *Tohoku J. Exp. Med.* 2006; 208: 33-9.

Burlaka AP, Sidorik EP, Ganusevich II, Osinsky SP. Effects of radical oxygen species and NO: formation of intracellular hypoxia and activation of matrix metalloproteinases in tumor tissues. *Exp Oncol.* 2006; 28: 49-53.

Carratelli M, Porcar, L, Ruscica M, De Simone E, Bertelli AA, Corsi MM. Reactive oxygen metabolites and prooxidant status in children with Down's syndrome. *Int. J. Clin. Pharmacol. Res.* 2001; 21: 79-84.

Chevion S, Moran DS, Heled Y, Shani Y, Regev G, Abbou B, Berenshtein E, Stadtman ER, Epstein Y. Plasma antioxidant status and cell injury after severe physical exercise. *Proc. Natl. Acad. Sci. U S A.* 2003; 100: 5119-23.

Crosti N, Bajer J, Gentile M. Catalase and glutathione peroxidase activity in cells with trisomy 21. *Clin. Genet.* 1989; 36: 107-116.

Cutler RG. Oxidative stress profiling: part I. Its potential importance in the optimization of human health. *Ann. N Y Acad. Sci.* 2005; 1055: 93-135.

Dalle-Donne I, Aldini G, Carini M, Colombo R, Rossi R, Milzani A. Protein carbonylation, cellular dysfunction, and disease progression. *J. Cell Mol. Med.* 2006; 10: 389-406.

Elosua R, Molina L, Fito M, et al. Response of oxidative stress biomarkers to a 16-week physical activity program, and to acute physical activity, in healthy young men and women. *Atherosclerosis.* 2003; 167: 327-34.

Flohe L, Gunzler WA. Assays of glutathione peroxidase. Meth Enzymol. 1984; 105: 114-21.

Fujiura GT, Fitzsimons N, Marks B, Chicoine B. Predictors of BMI among adults with Down syndrome: the social context of health promotion. *Res. Dev. Disabil.* 1997; 18: 261-274.

Glock GE, McLean P. Further studies on the properties and assay of glucose-6-phosphate dehydrogenase and 6-phosphogluconate dehydrogenase of rat liver. *Biochem. J.* 1953; 55: 400-08.

Goldberg DM, Spooner RJ. Glutathione Reductase. In: Bergmeyer HU, ed. Methods of enzymatic analysis. Weinheim: Verlag. 1992: 258-264.

Gonenc S, Acikgoz O, Semin I, Ozgonul H. The effect of moderate swimming exercise on antioxidant enzymes and lipid peroxidation levels in children. *Indian J. Physiol. Pharmacol.* 2000; 44: 340-344.

Janero DR. Malondialdehyde and thiobarbituric acid-reactivity as diagnostic indices of lipid peroxidation and peroxidative tissue injury. Free Radic Biol Med. 1990; 9: 515-540.

Meister A, Anderson ME. Glutathione. *Ann. Rev. Biochem.* 1983; 52: 711-760.

Kowald A, Klipp E. Alternative pathways might mediate toxicity of high concentrations of superoxide dismutase. *Ann. N Y Acad. Sci.* 2004; 1069: 370-374.

McCord JM, Fridovich I. Superoxide dismutase. An enzymic function for erythrocuprein (hemocuprein). *J. Biol. Chem.* 1969; 244: 6049-6055.

Monteiro CP, Varela A, Pinto M, et al. Effect of an aerobic training on magnesium, trace elements and antioxidant systems in a Down syndrome population. *Magnes Res.* 1997; 10: 65-71.

Muchova J, Sustrova M, Garaiova I, et al. Influence of age on activities of antioxidant enzymes and lipid peroxidation products in erythrocytes and neutrophils of Down syndrome patients. *Free Radic. Biol. Med.* 2001; 31: 499-508.

Nunomura A, Castellani RJ, Zhu X, Moreira PI, Perry G, Smith MA. Involvement of oxidative stress in Alzheimer disease. *J. Neuropathol. Exp. Neurol.* 2006; 65: 631-41

Ogonovszky H, Sasvari M, Dosek A, Berkes I, Kaneko T, Tahara S, Nakamoto H, Goto S, Radak Z. The effects of moderate, strenuous, and overtraining on oxidative stress markers and DNA repair in rat liver. *Can. J. Appl. Physiol.* 2005; 30: 186-95.

Ordoñez FJ, Rosety-Rodriguez M, Rosety JM, Rosety M. Anthropometric measurements as predictors of serum lipid behaviour in adolescents with Down syndrome. *Rev. Invest. Clin.* 2005a; 57: 691-694.

Ordoñez FJ, Rosety-Rodriguez M, Rosety M. A 12-week physical activity program increases glucose-6-phosphate-dehydrogenase activity in Down syndrome adolescents. *Medicina.* (B. Aires). 2005b; 65: 518-520.

Ordoñez FJ, Rosety M, Rosety-Rodriguez M. Regular physical activity increases glutathione peroxidase activity in adolescents with Down syndrome. *Clin. J. Sports Med.* 2006a; 16: 355-356.

Ordonez FJ, Rosety-Rodriguez M, Rosety M. Regular exercise did not modify significantly superoxide dismutase activity in adolescents with Down syndrome. *Br. J. Sports Med.* 2006b; 40: 717-718.

Ordoñez FJ, Rosety-Rodriguez M, Rosety M. 12 Week training program increased gluthatione reductase activity in adolescents with Down syndrome *Eur. J. Clin. Invest.* 2006c ; 36 (Suppl): 15-15.

Ordonez FJ, Rosety-Rodriguez M. Correlation between glutathione peroxidase activity and anthropometrical parameters in adolescents with Down syndrome. *Res. Dev. Disabil.* 2006d; 27:

Ordonez FJ, Rosety-Rodriguez M. Regular exercise attenuated lipid peroxidation in adolescents with down syndrome. *Clin. Biochem.* In Press

Ozbay B, Dulger H. Lipid peroxidation and antioxidant enzymes in Turkish population: relation to age, gender, exercise, and smoking. *Tohoku J. Exp. Med.* 2002; 197: 119-124.

Oztasan N, Taysi S, Gumustekin K, et al. Endurance training attenuates exercise-induced oxidative stress in erythrocytes in rat. *Eur. J. Appl. Physiol.* 2004; 91: 622-7.

Palazzetti S, Richard MJ, Favier A, Margaritis I. Overloaded training increases exercise-induced oxidative stress and damage. *Can. J. Appl. Physiol.* 2003; 28: 588-604.

Pastor MC, Sierra C, Dolade M, Navarro E, Brandi N, Cabre E. Antioxidant enzymes and fatty acid status in erythrocytes of Down's syndrome patients. *Clin. Chem.* 1998; 44: 924-9.

Pastore A, Tozzi G, Gaeta LM, Giannotti A, Bertini E, Federici G, Digilio MC, Piemonte F. 2003. Glutathione metabolism and antioxidant enzymes in children with Down syndrome. *J. Pediatr.* 2003; 142: 583-535.

Rajesh M, Sulochana KN, Coral K, Punitham R, Biswas J, Babu K, Ramakrishnan S. Determination of carbonyl group content in plasma proteins as a useful marker to assess impairment in antioxidant defense in patients with Eales' disease. *Indian. J. Ophthalmol.* 2004; 52: 139-144.

Radak Z, Sasvari M, Nyakas C, Taylor AW, Ohno H, Nakamoto H, Goto S. Regular training modulates the accumulation of reactive carbonyl derivatives in mitochondrial and cytosolic fractions of rat skeletal muscle. *Arch. Biochem. Biophys.* 2000; 383: 114-8.

Rosety-Rodriguez M, Ordóñez FJ, Rosety I, Rosety JM, Rosety M. Erythrocyte antioxidant enzymes of gilthead as early-warning bio-indicators of oxidative stress induced by malathion. *Haema.* 2005; 8: 237-240.

Rosety Rodríguez M, Ordoñez FJ, Rosety I, Frias L, Rosety MA, Rosety JM, Rosety M. 8 Week Traning program attenuates mitochondrial oxidative stress in the liver of emotional stressed rats. *Histol. Histhopathol.* 2006; 21: 1167-1170

Rosety-Rodriguez M, Ordonez FJ, Rosety M. Influence of regular exercise on erythrocyte catalase activity in adolescents with Down syndrome. *Med. Clin.* 2006; 127; 000-000.

Rosety-Rodriguez M, Ordonez FJ. Regular exercise reduces protein oxidation in adolescents with down syndrome. *Prev. Med.* In Press

Rush JW, Sandiford S. Plasma glutathione peroxidase in healthy young adults: influence of gender and physical activity. *Clin. Biochem.* 2003; 36: 345-51.

Stadtman ER, Levine RL. Protein Oxidation. *Ann. New York Acad. Sci.* 2000; 889: 191-208.

Steghens JP, Combarnous F, Arkouche W, Flourie F, Hadj-Aissa A. Influence of hemodialysis on total and free malondialdehyde measured by a new HPLC method. *Nephrol. Ther.* 2005; 1: 121-5.

Tauler P, Aguilo A, Guix P, Jimenez F, Villa G, Tur JA, Cordova A, Pons A. Pre-exercise antioxidant enzyme activities determine the antioxidant enzyme erythrocyte response to exercise. *J. Sports Sci.* 2005; 23: 5-13.

Tozzi-Ciancarelli MG, Penco M, Di Massimo C. Influence of acute exercise on human platelet responsiveness: possible involvement of exercise-induced oxidative stress. *Eur. J. Appl. Physiol.* 2002; 86: 266-272.

Yao EH, Yu Y, Fukuda N. Oxidative stress on progenitor and stem cells in cardiovascular diseases. *Curr. Pharm. Biotechnol.* 2006; 7: 101-8.

Young IS, Trimble ER. Measurement of malondialdehyde in plasma by high performance liquid chromatography with fluorimetric detection. *Ann. Clin. Biochem.* 1991; 28: 504–508.

In: Mental Retardation Research Advances
Editor: Elizabeth B. Heinz, pp. 45-58

ISBN: 978-1-60021-658-9
© 2007 Nova Science Publishers, Inc.

Chapter III

Stress and Quality of Life in Families of People with Intellectual Disabilities

Verri Annapia[*1], *Cremante Anna*[2],
Kaltchewa Dimitrina[3] *and Ronchi Guido*[4]

[1] Neurological Institute "C. Mondino" Foundation, via Mondino, 2, 27100 – Pavia;
[2] Neurological Institute "C. Mondino" Foundation, via Mondino, 2, 27100 – Pavia;
[3] Don Calabria Institute ,Milano; [4] Don Calabria Institute, Milano

Abstract

This paper reports the results of study into stress and quality of life in the parents of people with intellectual disability. Recent studies have shown that families caring for disabled members report significantly greater stress compared with families who are not providing such care. It is also known that as stress increases, the quality of life decreases.

The Questionnaire on Resources and Stress (QRS-F) (Friedrich, 1983), which is considered a general measure of adaptation and coping, was used to measure the impact of caring for a disabled person on other family members. It contains four subscales as: parent and family problems (I); pessimism (II); child characteristics (III); physical incapacitation (IV). Quality of life was measured using the Comprehensive Quality of Life Scale (Cummins, 1997).

The sample was composed by parents (55 mothers, 47 fathers) of disabled subjects with mild to severe intellectual disability (39 males, 26 females) and a control group (10 mothers and 10 fathers) caring for not-disabled family members (5 females and 5 males). It was found that stress was correlated with parental and familiar problems and a pessimistic attitude towards the situation. No differences were found between mothers and fathers although there was a tendency for mothers to give greater importance to such familiar and parental problems. Parents of male family members experience greater stress and this was more marked in the disabled sample. Moreover the relationship between

---

[*] ADDRESS FOR CORRESPONDENCE: Dr. Annapia Verri, IRCCS. Neurological Institute C. Mondino, via Mondino, 2, 27100 – Pavia (Italy); EMAIL ADDRESS: annapia.verri@mondino.it

stress, familiar problems and pessimistic attitudes increases with age of the family member.

Keywords: intellectual disability, stress, quality of life.

Introduction

The view that children with an intellectual disability (ID) induce higher levels of stress in the family than children without disabilities has underpinned much research and professional practice over the past two decades (Byrne and Cunningham, 1985; Crnic et al, 1983; Baxter 1989, Bristol and Scopler 1984; Donovan 1988). Parents of children with ID typically report more parenting stress and also mental health problems such as depression than parents of children without disabilities (Beckman 1991; Dumas et al, 1991; Dyson 1991, Emerson 2003, Friedrich and Friedrich 1981). This increased stress also tends to be chronic and persists over substantial periods of time. Parental stress may be episodic, caused by life events that may impact on any family but also from family life cycle transitions that may be particular traumatic for families of children with disabilities; these transition periods include diagnosis of the child's disabilities, starting school, change from childhood to adulthood and transition in service support from child to adult services and increasing age and infirmity of parents (Beresford 1994; Smith 1996; Kraemer and Blacher, 2001). Most parents feel that their experiences are uniquely and inherently different from those of their family and friends (Marsh, 1993), and this is reflected in a sense of isolation (Seligman and Darling, 1997). Though not all parents of children with intellectual disabilities report high levels of stress, for others the sense of difference and isolation can lead to major problems in this area (Weiss, 2002).

Parents of children with disabilities may experience fatigue, depression, lowered self-esteem, and interpersonal dissatisfaction (Marcus, 1977; Richman, 1977; Lyon and Preis, 1983; Figley, 1983; Bristol, 1984; Dyson and Fewell, 1986; Houser, 1987; Sobotor, 1989). Mothers describe themselves as unable to pursue personal goals and as having little free time (Holroyd, 1974), and they report ambivalence and grief over the amount of time devoted to the disabled child at their own expense beside that of the family (DeMyer, 1979).

Mothers of children with disabilities also experience increased moodiness, are more prone to illness (Holroyd, 1974), are acutely affected by the degree to which their child is accepted or rejected by the community (Holroyd, 1974; Bristol, 1984;), rate the behaviors of their child as stressful (Freeman et al., 1991), and report considerable family disharmony (Holroyd, 1974). These elements have direct implications for the functioning of children with ID (Hastings and Beck, 2004). For example, stressed parents respond differently to their children with behavioural problems (e.g., Conger, Patterson, and Ge, 1995; Deater-Deckard and Scarr, 1996), and when parents are suffering from depression they interact very differently with their children (Downey and Coyne, 1990).

Literature outside of the disability field shows that parents of children with ID typically have also a dysfunctional way of relating within each other and greater difficulties in communication, cohesion and adaptation (Michaels and Lewandowski, 1990). So the identification of the characteristics and the mechanisms which causes stress and discomfort of these families appear very important to find new strategies to increase the quality of life of all the family members. The evaluation of the stress and related factors was brought forward by administrating the Questionnaire on Resources and Stress of the Family (QRS-F) (Friedrich, 1983) to evaluate the aspects of family life more involved in the perception of the family stress.

This questionnaire discriminates between parents with disabled children and parents with normal children. QRS-F can also discriminate among parents with children with different pathologies, as autistic, Down syndrome, psychiatric patients (Holroyd and McArthur, 1976). Moreover there are differences between levels of stress in mothers and fathers; Holroyd (1975) has also found out that single mothers obtain higher scores than the married and that fathers have lower scores than mothers. The present research has the aim to verify also this hypothesis.

Method

Participants

A total of 102 parents of disabled subjects were solicited for participation in the present study. Participants were recruited from the sample of patients in the Neurologic Institute, IRCCS, "C. Mondino," University of Pavia, (Pavia, Italy). Of the participants, 55 were women (53.27 %) and 47 were men (46.73%) (table I-A).

Within the sample were defined three groups:

1. The first group (G1) is composed by 8 couples of parents of children with severe disability in their early age.
2. The second group (G2) is composed by 30 couples of parents of subjects in their adulthood and with mild disability.
3. The third group (G3) is composed by 17 couples of parents of subjects with severe disability and in their adulthood.

The control group (CG) in composed by 10 couples of parents with children without disabilities.

Table I/A. Description of the sample

	Fathers	Mothers	Total subjects	Sons	Daughters	Severity of the diagnosis of ID	Mean Age
G1	7	8	8	4	4	Severe	$9{,}63 \pm 1{,}19$
G2	26	30	30	17	13	Mild	$30{,}5\pm12{,}5$
G3	14	17	17	13	4	Severe	$26{,}76\pm8{,}5$
Gtot	47	55	55	34	21	Mild/severe	25.87 ± 9.81
CG	10	10	10	5	5	Normal	5.78 ± 1.48
Total	57	65	65	39	26		

The ID subjects were divided in four groups on the base of the diagnosis in the following way (table II): subjects affected by Down syndrome (n=10), subjects affected by Autistic Disorder (n=13), subjects with Infant Cerebral Palsy (ICP) (n=18) and a group of different disabilities (n=14). These groups are organized in according to results in literature. For example Eisenhower et al. (2005) found that phenotypic expressions of behaviour problems are manifested as early as age 3. These behavioural differences were paralleled by differences in maternal stress, such that mothers of children with autism are at elevated risk for high stress. We aimed to evaluate if specificity of the ID contribute to parental stress.

In the second group were taken 20 subjects (G4) to whom the ComQol has been administered (table I-B).

Table I/B. Description of the sample: subjects of G2 to whom the ComQol has been administered

	Fathers	Mothers	Total subjects	Sons	Daughters	ID	Mean Age
G4	20	20	20	13	7	mild	33.15±7,89

Table II. Ethiological diagnosis

Diagnosis	n.
Down syndrome	10
Other cromosomal disorders	4
Autistic spectrum disorder	13
ID associated with epilepsy	2
ID associated with ICP	18
ID associated with hydrocephalus	1
ID associated with Myelomeningocele	1
Tuberous Sclerosis	1
ID of unknown etiology	5
TOT	55

Instruments

Two instruments were used: the Questionnaire on Resources and Stress- Short Form (QRS-F, Friedrich et al, 1983) and the Comprehensive Quality of Life Scale (ComQOL-I5 , 5th version, Cummins, 1997).

The Friedrich short form of the Questionnaire on Resources and Stress (QRS–F) (Friedrich et al., 1983) is frequently used to study stress in families of children with disabilities (Glidden and Floyd, 1997). The original Questionnaire on Resources and Stress (QRS) (Holroyd, 1974) had 285 items true/false organised in 15 scales plus another scale which evaluates the tendency to give socially desiderable answers. This form of the questionnaire has been subject to a number of revisions that are shorter but maintain generally good reliability. While recommendations have been made for the use of different versions of the QRS with specific populations, the QRS–F is the most widely used short form (Glidden and Floyd, 1997). The QRS–F has 52 items assessing four subcomponents of parental perceptions:

I. Parent and family problems: stressful aspects of the impact of the child with disability on parents and the wider family;

II. Pessimism: parents' pessimistic beliefs about the child's future; measures the present and the future pessimism towards the possibilities of the child to become self-governing;

III. Child characteristics regards features of the child that are associated with increased demands on parents,

IV. Physical incapacity: the extent to which the child is able to perform a range of typical activities.

The Comprehensive Quality of Life Scale (ComQol; Cummins, 1997) was used to assess objective and subjective quality of life in seven domains: material well-being (possessions), health, productivity, intimacy, safety, place in the community, and emotional well-being. ComQol has been found to have good psychometric properties (Cummins et al, 1994). Subjective quality of life was assessed on two dimensions: satisfaction (responses were made on a 7-point scale ranging from delighted to terrible) and importance (responses were made on a 5-point Likert scale ranging from could not be more important to not at all important). The measurement of objective quality of life is obtained by the sum of three items for each domain. For disabled subjects a pre-test determines the extension of the Likert scale proper for the subjects.

Procedures

Packets of questionnaire were given to parents of children with ID with a brief covering letter explaining the rationale for the study. To each family two copies of the questionnaire were given (one for the mother and another for the father).

Data Analysis

The statistical analysis were executed within the total sample and the three groups identified on the base of two parameters: the age of the member with intellectual disability and the severity of the diagnosis. The following statistical analysis were used: descriptive analysis, Anova and Multivariate analysis of variance (Manova), the T-TEST for paired samples and for independent samples, linear regression.

We consider the following variables: parent sex, child sex, age of the child, type and severity of the diagnosis.

In the second part of the research the correlation between stress and quality of life was evaluated. A sample of 20 families with a mildly disabled child (13 sons, 7 daughters, mean age 33 ± 8 years) were evaluated on quality of life. These families were divided into three levels of stress :

1.   low level of stress ≤ 16;
2.   medium level of stress $16 \leq x \leq 25$;
3.   high level of stress $x \geq 25$.

No differences were found in the stress levels of mothers and fathers, so they were combined for analysis.

Statistical analysis were executed using the SPSS program.

Results

Total Sample

Parents are more stressed about familiar and parental problems (I) and stress is increased by their pessimistic perception of the situation (II), while the characteristics of the subjects (III) and the presence of physical disabilities (IV) are less important ($p<.000$).

Mother and father do not differ statistically about their stress level. In the mothers' sample stress results more increased by the presence of familiar and parental problems (I).

The *sex* of the subjects have a significant influence, so that the event to have a son increases the level of the perceived stress.

The *age* of the subjects is significantly related with the level of stress. In fact as the age of the subjects increases, the parents perceive a higher stress related to the familiar and parental problems (I) ($p< .001$) and the pessimism (II) ($p< .01$) (Figure 1).

The comparison on the base of the *diagnosis* shows that there aren't significant differences between the parents of children with Down syndrome and parents of children with autistic syndrome. On the other hand the parents of the children with infant cerebral palsy compared to the other two groups are more stressed about the physical disabilities of their children (IV) ($p< .05$). In this group both mothers and fathers refer the presence of a higher level of stress about the parental and familiar problems (I) by comparison with the parents of subjects affected by Down syndrome; moreover the parents of subjects with autistic syndrome perceive the highest level of stress about the familiar and parental problems (I). But there is not a clear statistical evidence. The fourth group of parents (children with different syndromes) show lower levels of stress, but this aspect is not statistically evident.

Results in the Groups G1, G2 and G3

Statistical analysis confirm the importance of these factors: sex of the parent, sex of the subjects with ID, age of the subjects, described in the total sample. There are some differences about the influence of the type and severity of the diagnosis.

First Group (G1)

In the group of children with severe disability the parents of children with autistic syndrome are more pessimistic compared to the parents of children with Infant cerebral palsy (p< .05). This last group compared with the parents of children with different syndromes perceive lower level of pessimism (p< .042) but higher stress in relation of the physical disabilities of the children (p< .027).

Second Group (G2)

In the group composed by parents of subjects with mild mental retardation in their adulthood, the pessimism (II) is greater in the parents of subjects affected by autism than in the parents of subjects with Infant Cerebral Palsy, while the parents of subjects with Down Syndrome report medium level of stress (p < .02). The stress which is due to the familiar and parental problems (I) is significantly higher in the parents of subjects with infant cerebral palsy especially when compared to the parents of subjects with autistic syndrome (p< .031).

Third Group (G3)

The parent of subjects with Down syndrome experiment higher level of stress compared to the parents of autistic subjects (p< .015, p< .07) and by comparison with the parents of subjects with ICP (p< .036 and p< .016); they reported more problems related to the behavioural characteristics of the children (III) and an increased pessimism (II).

Control Group (CG)

Statistical analysis confirm that parents of subjects with ID are more stressed because of familiar and parental problems; moreover they have a more pessimistic perception of the situation (p< .000). The mothers emphasise the familiar and parental problems (I) by comparison with the other aspects measured by the QRS-F (III and IV) (p< .001); in the second scale (Pessimism) they obtain lower scores than the first scale, even if not significantly different from the other factors. These results are confirmed in the group of the fathers (p< .05). The comparison based on the sex of the subjects show that the fact to have a son increases the stress in all of the two factors (p< .01).

Inter-Groups Comparison

In order to evaluate the influences of different variables, the groups were compared between them; it was pointed out the influence of:

- age of the subjects (G1 vs G2)
- severity of diagnosis (G2 vs G3);
- presence of disability (G1, G2,G3 vs CG)

The pessimism (II) increases with the age of the subjects (p< .001). Moreover a more severe diagnosis enhances the level of stress perceived (p< .000). Both mothers and fathers included in G2 and G3 obtain higher scores than the parents of the CG (p< .000), while the parents of children do not obtain different scores in the first scale when compared to the parents of the CG. The parents of the G1 obtain higher scores compared to the CG in the III and IV scales (p< .001); moreover the fathers of the G1 are more pessimism (II) than the fathers of the children without ID (p< .005).

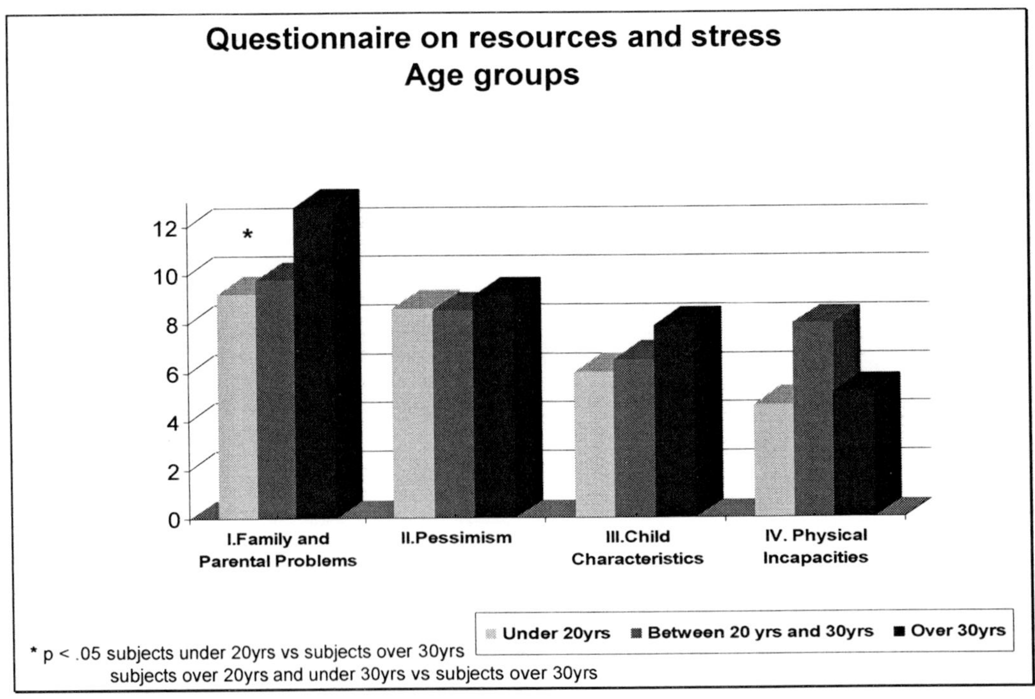

Figure 1. Age Groups. As the age of the subjects increases, the parents perceive a higher stress.

Stress and Quality of Live

About the relation between stress level and quality of life, it was found out that the quality of life changes on the basis of the sex of the subjects. In particular, in the group of males with mild disability there is a correlation between a low quality of life and a high level of stress (p < .05). Males have a lower QoL than the females in the following scales of the objective data : personal objects, health, place in community and emotional wellbeing (p< .05 and p< .000). (Figure 2)

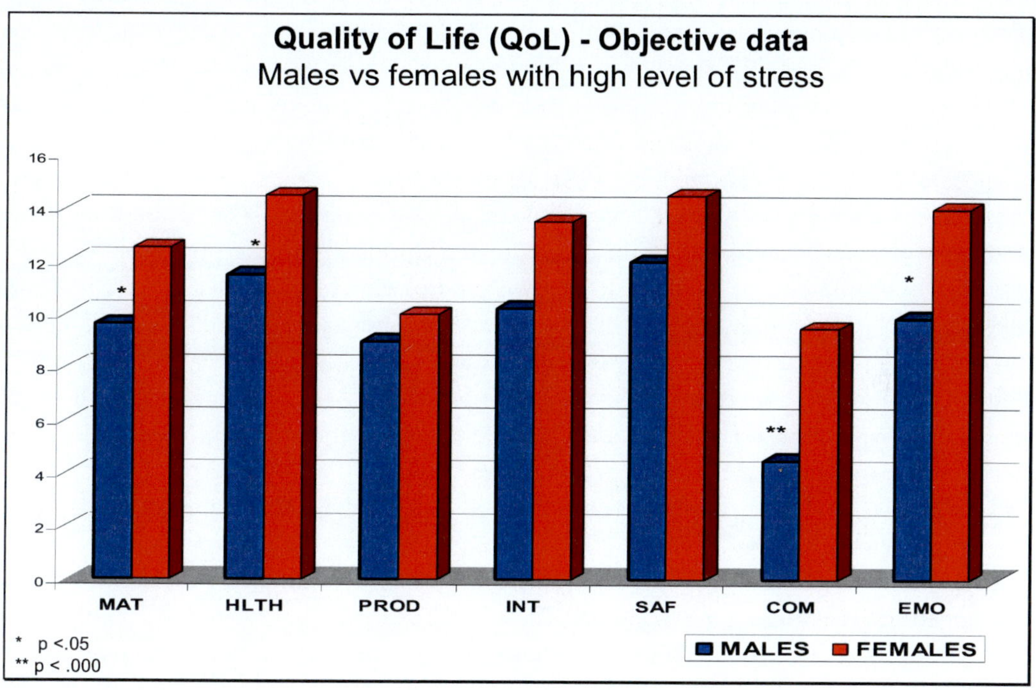

Figure 2. Quality of Life – Objective Data. Males have a lower QoL than the famales in: personal objects, health, place in community and emotional wellbeing.

Conclusion

There has been a broad consensus in the literature that stress and negative psychological effects have been considered likely outcomes for parents of children with disabilities. It becomes even more important to understand the sources of stress and the types of adaptation made in these families (Boyce et al., 1994). We investigate family responses with the respect to the presence of a member with ID. We have administrated the Questionnaire on Resources and Stress of the Family (QRS-F Friedrich, 1983) to evaluate the aspects of family life more involved in the perception of the family stress. The analysis of results in the different groups shows that stress is increased, especially by the presence of familiar and parental problems and by a pessimistic view of the situation. The difficulties related to characteristics of the subjects, the presence of physical disability and the self-help capacities are less important and do not enhance significantly the level of stress perceived by the family. A key outcome of the present review is the identification of a number of areas where more research and clinical development are required in order to strengthen the base for stress interventions with parents of people with ID. Early intervention and support may help the family to adjust and become positively involved in the care and development of the child.

Moreover mothers and fathers refer similar level of stress, even if the mothers express greater difficulties than the fathers about the familiar and parental problems.

Our results demonstrate that families with a member with disability report significantly greater stress in comparison with controls and as this stress increases the quality of life decreases. Moreover to have a son with disability appears more stressful than to have a daughter and it is probably linked to cultural factors. However Fuller (1997) shows that mothers of daughters were more likely to feel burdened by caregiving. Our study confirms that caregivers' difficulties increases as sons or daughter with ID grew chronologically older (Birenbaum, 1971; Suelze and Keenan 1981; Blacher 2001).

In our review we have analyzed the relationship between diagnosis and stress level. The parent of subjects affected by ICP are more stressed in relation to the presence of physical disabilities, while parents of children with Down syndrome and autism obtained higher scores in the scale which measures pessimistic attitudes. The interesting understanding to emerge from this study is that the group of parents of children with ICP has higher levels of stress at the growing up of children, in the scale of familiar problems. Although caregiving is a normal part of being the parent of a young child, this role takes on an entirely different significance when a child experiences functional limitations and possible long-term dependence; the task of caring for a child with complex disabilities at home might be somewhat daunting for caregivers (Raina et al. 2005).

In the families of subjects in their childhood the pessimism isn't very high and there is a more hopeful perception of the situation. These data may be interpreted by supposing that during childhood the relationship of dependence of each child from parents might mask the perception that parents have of disabilities of their own child as a stress factor. Afterwards, instead, differences compared to children which are not affected by ID are revealed and this fact comes to represent source of stress.

The evaluation of the quality of life using the Comprehensive Quality of Life Scale (ComQol; Cummins, 1997) demonstrate how a low level of quality of life correspond to a high level of stress. The variable which most determines a variation is the gender of the subjects; it was demonstrated that males with mild disability have a lower Qol than the females with mild disability. The results in literature (Fuller, 1994; Dyson, 1996) shows how families with disabled children have higher levels of stress than families with children without disability.

In conclusion, family with disable subjects often have difficult life-conditions because of the problems inside the family and the lack of an effective and strong social support. Kandel and Merrick (2003) have underlined that after the birth of a child with disability, the life of a family changes significantly and in addition to regular adaptation, the family must cope with stress, grief, disappointments and challenges, which may lead to a serious crisis or even disruption of family life.

These problems can be worsen by different life events, such as the transition to adulthood during the critical developmental period from about age 18 to 26 (Blacher, 2001); moreover they are related to the different diagnosis of disabled subjects. In this way the identification of the characteristics and the mechanism which origin stress and discomfort in these families has the aim to help them to face everyday difficulties and to find new strategies in order to increase quality of life of both disabled subjects and their families, and to enhance the number of different social services specific for the different situations and problems.

Our study is a first step in developing a more thorough understanding of sources of stress for parents of children with intellectual disability. The identification of stressors suggested avenues for future intervention.

Acknowledgements

The authors are grateful to Prof. Robert Cummins, Deakin University (Melbourne) and to Prof Lily Dyson, University of Victoria (Victoria) for their precious suggestions.

References

Baker, B.L., McIntyre, L.L., Blacher, J., Crnic, K., Edelbrock, C., and Low, C. (2003). Pre-school children with and without developmental delay: behaviour problems and parenting stress over time. *Journal of Intellectual Disability Research*, 47, 217-30.

Baxter, C., Cummins, R.-A, Yolitis, L. (2000) Parental stress attributed to family members with or without disability : a longitudinal study. *Journal of Intellectual and Developmental Disability*, 25, 105-118.

Beckman, P.-J. (1991) Comparison of mathers' and fathers' perceptions of the effect of young children with or without disabilities. *American Journal on Mental Retardation*, 95, 585-595.

Beresford, B.-A. (1994) Resources and strategies: how parent cope with the care of a disabled child. *Journal of Child Psychology and Psychiatry*, 35, 171-209.

Birenbaum, A. (1971) The mentally retarded child in the home and the family cycle. *Journal of health and social behavior*, 12, 55-65.

Blacher, J. (2001) Transition to adulthood: mental retardation, families, and culture, *American Journal of Mental Retardation*, 196, 173-88.

Boyce, G.-C., Miller, B.-C., White, K.-R. and Godfrey, M.-K.(1994) Single Parenting in Families of Children with Disabilities. *Marriage and Family Review*, 20, 389-409.

Byrne, E.-A and Cunningham, C.-C. (1985) The effects of mentally handicapped children on families: a conceptual review. *Journal of Child Psychology and Psychiatry*, 26, 847-64.

Bristol, M.-M. (1984) Family Resources and Successful Adaptation to Autistic Children. In E. Schhopler and G. B. Meisibov (Eds) The *Effects of Autism on the Family* (pp. 289–310). New York: Plenum.

Brystol, M. and Scopler, E. (1984) A developmental perspective on stress and coping in families of autistic children. In J Blancher (Ed.), *Severely handicapped young children and their families* (pp.91-112) New Jork: Academic Press.

Buelow JM, McNelis A, Shore CP, Austin JK. Stressors of parents of children with epilepsy and intellectual disability. *J. Neurosci. Nurs.* 2006 Jun;38(3):147-54, 176.

Conger, R., Patterson, G.-R. and Ge, X. (1995) It takes two to replicate: A mediational model for the impact of parents' stress on adolescent adjustment. *Child Development*, 66, 80–97.

Crnic, K.-A., Friedrich, W.-N. and Greenberg, M.-T. (1983) Adaptation of families with mentally retarded children: a model of stress, coping and family ecology. *American Journal of Mental Deficiency*, 88, 125-136.

Crnic, K.-A., Greenberg, M.T., Ragozin, A.S., Robinson, N.M. and Basham, R.B.(1983) Effects of stress and social support on mothers and premature and full-term infants. *Child Development*, 54, 209-17.

Cummins, R.-A. (1997) Comprehensive Quality of Life Scale. Adult Manual Fifth Edition Melbourne: Deakin University School of Psychology.

Cummins, R.-A., McCabe, M.-P., Gullone, E. and Romeo Y. (1994) The comprehensive quality of life scale: instrument development and psychometric evaluation on college staff and students. *Educational and Psychological Measurement*, 54, 372-382.

Deater-Deckard, K. and Scarr, S. (1996) Parenting stress among dual-earner mothers and fathers: Are there gender differences? *Journal of Family Psychology*, 10, 45–59.

DeMyer, M.-K., (1979) Parents and Children in Autism. New York:Wiley.

Donovan, A.-M. (1988) Family Stress and Ways of Coping with Adolescents Who Have Handicaps: Maternal Perceptions, *American Journal of Mental Retardation*, 92, 502–9.

Downey, G. and Coyne, J.-C. (1990) Children of depressed parents: An integrative review. *Psychological Bulletin*, 108, 50–76.

Dyson, L.and Fewell, R.-R. (1986) Sources of Stress and Adaptation of Parents of Young Handicapped Children, unpublished manuscript, University of Washington, Seattle, in M.J. Weiss, (2002) Hardiness and social support as predictors of stress in mothers of typical children, children with autism, and children with mental retardation. *Autism*, 6, 115-30.

Dumas, J.-E., Wolf, L.-C., Fissman, S.-N.and Culligan, A. (1991) Parenting stress, child behaviour problems, and dysphoria in parents of children with autism, Down syndromes, behaviour disorders, and normal development. *Exceptionality*, 2, 97-110.

Dyson, L.-L. (1991) Families of young children with handicaps: parental stress and family functioning. *American Journal on Mental Retardation*, 95, 623-29.

Dyson, L.-L. (1993) Response to presence of child with disabilities: parental stress and family functioning over time. *American Journal on Mental Retardation*, 98, 207-218.

Eisenhower, A.-S., Baker, B.-L. and Blacher, J. (2005) Preschool children with intellectual disability: syndrome specificity, behaviour problems, and maternal well-being. *Journal of Intellectual disabilities Research*, 49, 657-71.

Emerson, E. (2003) Mothers of children and adolescent with intellectual disability: social and economic situation, mental health status, and self- assessed social and psychological impact of the child difficulties." *Journal of Intellectual disabilities Research*, 47, 385-399.

Figley, C.-R. (1983) Catastrophes: An Overview of Family Reactions. In C.R. Figley and H. I. McCubbing (eds) *Stress and the Family: Coping with Catastrophe*, pp. 3–20. New York: Brunner/Mazel.

Freeman, N.L., Perry A. and Factor, D.C. (1991) Child behaviours as stressors: replicating and extending the use of the CARS as a measures of stress: a research note. *Journal of Child Psychology and Psychiatry*, 32, 1025-30.

Friedrich, W.-N and Friedrich, W.-L. (1981) Psychosocial assets of parents of handicapped and non-handicapped children. *American Journal of Mental Deficiency*, 65, 551-553.

Friedrich, W.-N., Greenberg, M.-T. and Crnic, K. (1983) A short form of the Questionnaire on Resources and stress. *American Journal of mental Deficiency*, 88, 41-8.

Glidden, L.-M., Floyd, F.-J. (1997) Disaggregating parental depression and family stress in assessing families of children with developmental disabilities: a multisample analysis. *American Journal on Mental Retardation*,102, 250-66.

Hastings, R.-P. and Beck, A. (2004) Practitioner Review: Stress intervention for parents of children with intellectual disabilities. *Journal of Child Psychology and Psychiatry*, 45, 1338-1349.

Hastings, R.-P. (2002) Parental stress and behaviour problems of children with developmental disability. *Journal of Intellectual and Developmental Disability*, 27, 149–160.

Holroyd, J. (1974) The Questionnaire on Resources and Stress: An Instrument to Measure Family Response to a Handicapped Member. *Journal of Community Psychology*, 2, 92–4.

Holroyd, J. and McArthur, D. (1976) Mental Retardation and Stress on the Parents: A Contrast between Down's Syndrome Mental Retardation and Childhood Autism, *American Journal of Mental Deficiency* , 80, 431–6.

Houser, R.-A. (1987) A Comparison of Stress and Coping by Fathers of Mentally Retarded and Non-Retarded Adolescents, unpublished doctoral dissertation, University of Pittsburgh.

Kandall, I. and Merrick, J. (2003) The birth of a child with disability. Coping by parents and siblings. *Scientific World Journal*, 20, 741-750.

Kraemer, B.-R. and Blacher, J. (2001) Transition for young adults with severe mental retardation : school preparation, parents aspectations and family involvement. *Mental Retardation*, 39, 423-435.

Lyon, S. and Preis, A. (1983) Working with Families of Severely Handicapped Persons, in M. Seligman (ed.) *The Family with a Handicapped Child*, pp. 203–32. New York: Grune and Stratton.

March, D.-T. (1993) *Families and Mental Retardation*. New York: Praeger.

Marcus, L.–M. (1997) Patterns of Coping in Families of Psychotic Children. *American Journal of Orthopsychiatry*, 47, 388–98.

Raina P, O'Donnell M, Rosenbaum P, Brehaut J, Walter SD, Russell D, Swinton M, Zhu B, Wood E. The health and well-being of caregivers of children with cerebral palsy. *Pediatrics*. 2005 Jun; 115(6): e626-36.

Richman, N. (1977) Behavior Problems in Preschool Children: Family and Social Factors. *British Journal of Psychiatry*, 131, 525–7.

Seligman, M.-E. (1991) *Learned Optimism*.New York: Knopf.

Seligman, M.-E. (2005) *La costruzione della felicità*. Che cos'è l'ottimismo, perché può migliorare la vita, Sperling andPaperback.

Seligman, M. and Darling, R.-B. (1977) *Ordinary Families, Special Children*. New York: Guilford.

Smith, G.-C. (1996) Caregiving outcomes for older mothers and adults with mental retardation: a test of the two-factors model of psychological well-being. *Psychology and Aging*, 11, 353-361.

Sobotor, W.-J. (1989) Family Coping with Stressors: A Theoretical Approach", in S .-C. Klagnbrun, G.-W. Kilman, E.-J. Clark, A.-H. Kutscher , R. Debellis, C.-A. Lambert. (eds) *Preventive Psychiatry: Early Intervention and Situational Crisis Management*, pp. 43–58. Philadelphia, PA: Charles.

Suelze, M., and Keenan, V. (1981) Changes in family support networks over the life cycle of mentally retarded persons. *American Journal of Mental Deficiency*, 86, 267-274.

Weiss, M.J. (2002) Hardiness and social support as predictors of stress in mothers of typical children, children with autism, and children with mental retardation. *Autism*, 6, 115-30.

In: Mental Retardation Research Advances
Editor: Elizabeth B. Heinz, pp. 59-74

ISBN: 978-1-60021-658-9
© 2007 Nova Science Publishers, Inc.

Chapter IV

Supporting Families of Children with Down Syndrome: What the Literature Teaches Us

---

Judy O. Berry and River J. Smith
Department of Psychology, University of Tulsa, Tulsa, OK 74104

Abstract

Down syndrome affects 1 in 800 children. These children are frequently served in early intervention programs and these first services provide a bridge for continuation of programs over the child's life course. It is well documented that these programs effectively provide needed services and help children make developmental progress. Less is known about the efficacy of support services for parents, although this is clearly a population at risk for stress. This chapter reviews research on services that parents receive, including information, emotional support, tangible help and direct psychological intervention, the effectiveness of these supports, and the importance of family resilience.

Introduction

We are exhausted by the needs of our child, yet we are called on to make huge changes and to solve all kinds of problems. This is the Catch-22 we run into when we have a child with a disability. The catch is especially onerous when our child is newborn and during times of crisis. We need so many solutions, but the solutions themselves look like problems, further demands on our scarce energy.

There is so much to learn, but we are in a survival mode: getting through the day is a great accomplishment. Those things which are most needed—new learning, creative problem solving, change—are the hardest to come by.

> Barbara Gill, mother of a son with Down syndrome
> *Changed by a Child*, 1997, p.57.

Barbara Gill is one of approximately 5000 parents each year who receive the news that their infant has Down syndrome, a genetic disorder causing developmental delays and physical anomalies, such as mental retardation, slowed speech and language, and risk for a variety of health conditions (National Institute of Child Health and Human Development, 2006). Her words remind us that this is an enormous change for families and that these families will need initial and ongoing support. Because of prenatal testing, some families will learn the diagnosis before the child is born, but almost 90% of families hear this diagnosis in the postnatal period (Skotko, 2005). Historically families of children with Down syndrome have been subject to societal stigma and isolation and children have experienced serious medical problems and deficits in educational and related services.

However, important changes have occurred. In 1929 the average lifespan for a baby born with Down syndrome was 9 years and today it is 55 years. Advances in primary care, preventive care and surgical techniques, particularly cardiac surgery, have brought about improved health and longevity. Through the 1960's segregation was the norm with families coping on their own as best they could or choosing to place their child (often in response to advice or urging from the medical community) in a segregated institutional setting. By the 1970's federal legislation opened the door for educational rights for children and adolescents with Down syndrome and other disabilities (Hardman, Drew, and Egan, 2006). More recently, emphasis has been on full inclusion in schools, in the workforce and throughout society (Bradley, 1995).

These changes are vast, and yet recent research on family support reveals that some areas of family need and the resources to meet those needs have not changed very much at all and some not nearly enough. Family support needs begin at the beginning when the child is initially diagnosed. Research that compared mothers of children with Down syndrome with mothers of children with developmental and health problems that defied diagnostic assignment (Lenhard, Breitenbach, Ebert, Schindelhauer and Henn, 2005) found greater psychological well being in the mothers of children with Down syndrome. Even though the clarity of the diagnosis can reduce stress, receiving the diagnosis is a difficult experience for parents. Skotko (2005) studied maternal response to postnatal diagnosis of Down syndrome and found past and current dissatisfaction on the part of parents concerning how the diagnosis was presented. Mothers in the United States and Spain took part in the study and the time of receiving the diagnosis ranged from 1972-2003. The experience of receiving the news left mothers frightened and anxious. Mothers were particularly concerned that physicians did not address positive aspects of having a child with Down syndrome, did not provide printed material that was current and helpful, and did not link them with other families raising children with Down syndrome. Satisfaction with how the diagnosis was presented improved over time, but improvement was small.

Hanson (2003) linked the past to the present by interviewing parents 25 years after their children participated in early intervention programs. These parents and their children were pioneers for early intervention services and the school-based services that followed. All parents interviewed reported positive gains from the early childhood experience. These gains included increased parenting competence and efficacy, learning skills to help them teach their children, parent-to-parent support and achieving a more hopeful outlook toward parenting their child. In terms of perceptions and experiences, all parents commented on positive aspects of their children and what their children bring to the family. They also talked about positive aspects of rearing a child with Down syndrome as well as difficulties and sorrows. The difficulties included medical complications, teasing and ostracism for the child and social limitations for the family. A major concern addressed by many parents was the lack of services after school ended. Supports for adults with Down syndrome, including work, social activities and community inclusion were limited and hard to come by. Parents were clear that their efforts for advocacy were essential during the entire life course of their son or daughter.

These studies provide convincing evidence that progress has been made, but problems and needs still remain. In this chapter we will first address stress and the need for support in families that include a child with Down syndrome. We will then review research on support services provided to families and the effectiveness of these services. We will conclude by addressing family resilience.

Parental Stress in Families with Children with Down Syndrome

General findings from research on families of children with developmental disabilities suggest parenting a child with a disability can lead to significant stress (Berry and Jones, 1995, Hastings and Beck, 2004; Hanson and Hanline, 1990; Lessenberry and Renfeldt, 2004). Specifically, these parents may be at higher risk for experiencing both physical and emotional difficulties, as well as increased marital conflict and social isolation when compared to parents of children without disabilities (Pelchat, Lefebure, Proulx, and Reidy, 2004). Further, parental stress has been shown to have adverse effects on child well-being in the general psychological literature and in the developmental disabilities literature (Shonkoff, Hauser-Cram, Krauss, and Upshur, 1992). Raising a child with Down syndrome provides parents with additional challenges that require various social, emotional, and economic resources above and beyond the norm. In addition, when faced with physical and developmental concerns and a shortage of resources, parents of children with Down syndrome are at risk for experiencing stress that can impact the family system (i.e., Lenhard, et. al, 2004).

Family stress theory provides a conceptual framework for understanding parental stress in families of children with Down syndrome. Family stress theory postulates that a family crisis is an interaction among a stressor, the resources a family has to cope with the stressor, and the meaning the family gives to the stressor (Peterson and Hennon, 2005; McCubbin and Patterson, 1982). This is the ABC-X stress model (Hill, 1949) in which X represents the crisis, A is the stressor, B is the resources to meet the stress and, C is the meaning attached to the stressful situation. In the context of a family with a child with developmental disabilities such as Down syndrome, stressors that elicit a "crisis" may come from various sources such as learning about a child's diagnosis or dealing with physical or developmental problems as they arise. If a family has limited support systems in place and inadequate resources to deal with these stressors, such as lack of financial and emotional support, this can be a catalyst for a break down in family functioning. Finally, the family's perception of their situation can have a detrimental impact on creating meaning and fostering the confidence and competence in caring for a child with special needs that is essential for positive adaptation (Gurlanick, 2000).

Gurlanick (2000) presented 4 major sources of stress for parents raising children with disabilities that can be conceptualized within the family stress model. These are stressors related to 1) informational needs, 2) interpersonal and family distress, 3) level of support needed for the child, and 4) parental confidence threats. Informational needs refer to the parents' need to know about their child's current health and developmental status, any anticipated complications down the road, and what services are available and how to access these services. Interpersonal and family distress may arise upon learning about the child's diagnosis and can impede positive adaptation and active coping and lead to social isolation. In terms of support, the needs of the child with disabilities can deplete family resources of time, energy, and money. Finally, confidence threats refer to the family member's perception of their ability to care for their child. Under stressful circumstances with limited resources, parents may begin to feel as though they are unable to manage the situation, which can negatively impact parental perceptions and foster pessimism.

Research specific to families raising children with Down syndrome has focused primarily on 1) whether these families are at increased risk for stress and 2) the impact of this family stress on the child's well being. Research has also shed light on specific child and family factors that may lead to family stress. It appears that while these families do experience stress, the reported level of stress is often less than family members of children with other disabilities. In addition, some families report that having a child with Down syndrome benefits the family system (Cunningham, 1996). Nonetheless, families of children with Down syndrome are likely to experience more stress than families raising children without disabilities. For example, one study found that parents of children with Down syndrome perceive more stress than parents of children without a development disability. Specifically, the stressors the families experienced were related to caregiving difficulties, child related stress such as behavior problems and parent related stress such as incompetence and role restriction (Roach, Orsmond, and Barratt, 1999). In addition, maladaptive behaviors of children are a source of stress for parents; lower levels of maladaptive behaviors and higher cognitive-linguistic functioning are linked with lower levels of maternal stress, although children with Down syndrome may be less likely to exhibit behavior problems than children with other developmental disabilities (e.g., Fidler and Hodapp, 2000).

Family Support Services and Interventions

Support services provided to families of children with Down syndrome can be placed into four broad categories. These categories are 1) information, 2) emotional support, 3) tangible support, and 4) direct psychological intervention. In addition to these support services, early intervention programs have become ideal for providing and/or linking families with support services to meet their needs. The current trend in early intervention is to target the needs of the family as a whole by providing multiple types of support rather than child focused programs alone. These efforts are promising as they address the multiple needs of the family system and acknowledge the interaction among stress, family resources, and family perception as postulated in family stress theory.

Information is often the first type of support families are offered once a diagnosis of Down syndrome is confirmed. This type of support may come from medical staff or from referrals to agencies specializing in working with children with developmental disabilities. As mentioned, a major source of stress for parents of children with developmental disabilities is unmet informational needs about the current and expected health and development of their child (Gurlanick, 2000). The information given to parents when a diagnosis is confirmed may be particularly important and can have an impact on the way in which the family perceives their child's condition and the subsequent distress they feel upon learning their child has Down syndrome. Emotional support most often comes in the form of parent-to-parent support groups or through specialized early intervention programs that target the family system. Emotional support may also be received in an informal manner from family and friends.

Tangible support may come in the form of government or grant issued stipends, medical aid, or monetary disability compensation. In addition, it may include funding for school programs and therapeutic services that target individuals with developmental disabilities. Tangible support may be particularly important for families of low socioeconomic status because it allows families to obtain direct care assistance for their child or make purchases necessary for the care of their child that would otherwise not be available. Recently, focus has been on the need to have flexible tangible support programs in place that allow parents to use money at their discretion, which can better meet the individual needs of families (Bradley, 1995). However, there are barriers to obtaining these services which include lack of information about programs and services and stringent eligibility criteria (Freedman and Capobianco, 2000).

Regarding direct psychological intervention, a vast array of services are offered. Direct psychological interventions may be specific to the child or the parent. Child specific interventions typically target problem behaviors a child is exhibiting, whereas parent specific interventions are often psychoeducational in nature and aim to alleviate the stress of raising a child with a developmental disability (Hastings and Beck 2004).

All of these types of support, alone and in combination, have value for families of children with Down syndrome. Furthermore, there is evidence to suggest that early intervention is essential because parents who report stress early on are most likely to continue to experience stress later as their child ages (Cunningham, 1996). According to Guralnick (2000), the placement of families at the center of the early intervention system is one of the major advances in the field of intervention. With this in mind, inclusion of the family system does not come without pitfalls including the difficulties inherent in the movement from a child-centered approach to a family centered approach. Families raising children with Down syndrome like all families are a heterogeneous group with varied needs, and differing needs at various points in the family lifespan.

What Families Want and Need: Research on Support Services

The following section reviews the literature on the effectiveness of the four types of support: information, emotional support, tangible support, and direct psychological intervention. In addition, effectiveness of family support within early intervention programs is addressed as these programs typically include more than on type of support.

Informational Support

The manner in which parents receive information about their child's diagnosis and the type of information given has evolved considerably over the years. In fact, research documents that health care providers are communicating with parents about their child's diagnosis earlier, are more likely to inform both parents together, and are more likely to recommend that the child stay in the home rather than be institutionalized (Pueschel, 1985). In addition, research has examined satisfaction with the initial diagnostic and educational information delivered by health care providers. An early study by Pueschel and Murphy (1976) examined the perceptions of 414 mothers' of children with Down syndrome after learning of their child's diagnosis. They discovered that a significant number of parents were dissatisfied with the information they received and the manner in which they received it. More recent research suggests similar dissatisfaction among parents. For example, Skotko and Canal (2004) examined the responses of 467 mothers of children with Down syndrome in Spain in order to determine whether postnatal informational support provided to mothers by physicians was adequate. The majority of these mothers reported that educational support and referrals provided by physicians upon receiving their child's diagnosis were insufficient. Specifically, they reported that little information was given in print form and too few referrals to support groups were made. Further, they reported that physicians spent too little time on the strengths of the child focusing primarily on the weaknesses. Based on their findings several recommendations to healthcare practitioners were made and are listed below:

1. Physicians should clearly and immediately explain results of testing.
2. Delivery of diagnosis should be done in a private setting with sensitivity and compassion.
3. Parents should be provided with factual information immediately, up to date materials should be given.
4. Counselor should be made available to families.
5. Physicians should not question the mother's decision to have child.
6. Clinics and hospitals should have referrals to parent support groups.

Skotko (2005) conducted another study examining the responses of 1,250 mothers of children with Down syndrome in the U.S. and Spain and found consistent results. Close to half the mothers who discovered their child's diagnosis in the postnatal period felt the information portrayed by the physician was highly negative. They reported they wish they would have been told earlier and given more accurate up-to-date information. In addition, mothers who received a diagnosis during the prenatal period seemed more satisfied with the information obtained by their physician and the manner in which this information was communicated. This was also true of mothers who had given birth more recently suggesting that with time there has been an improvement in the delivery of information to parents of children with Down syndrome.

Hedov, Wikblad, and Anneren (2002) examined the responses of 165 parents of children with Down syndrome in Sweden to determine if first information and support was adequate for families after receiving a diagnosis. Although nearly half the parents in the study felt they had received information about their child's condition in a timely manner, 70% of the parents in this study considered the information they were provided to be insufficient. Further, the parents felt they received more negative and less positive information about Down syndrome and that the physician's knowledge and communication of the diagnosis needed improvement.

Although the days of recommending institutionalization may be gone and some improvements have been made in delivery of diagnostic information to parents, these studies demonstrate the need for improved delivery of information to families of children with Down syndrome. Specifically, there may be a need for health practitioner training on delivery of these services and better interagency referral programs to assist with additional family needs. Given that informational services are likely to be the first services families come into contact with, it may be important to place special emphasis on this initial contact as it can be influential in shaping beliefs and attitudes families have about their child. As discussed earlier, these beliefs are important in a family's ability to adapt to the current situation.

Emotional Support

Several studies have examined the role of both formal (i.e., support groups) and informal (i.e., family and friends) support systems on parental well-being and satisfaction with their child. For example, Heritage, Rogers, and West (1994) found that parents benefited from both formal and informal support systems, with support from friends and family being no more beneficial than more formal support from physicians, support groups, and teachers. However, White and Hastings (2004) examined the responses of 33 parents of adolescents with intellectual disabilities and discovered that informal support provided by family members and friends was negatively related to parental stress, whereas no relationship was found between formal support and parent well-being suggesting that informal support may have a greater impact on parental well-being. In addition, Spiker (1982) examined mothers' perceptions of the emotional support received by parent support groups and discovered that mothers found this type of support helpful as it provided time to talk with other parents about raising a child with Down syndrome. Further, the literature supports the notion that these types of emotional support systems not only provide families with a subjective sense of well being, but also lead to enhanced family adaptation for the parent and the child in the form of better parent-child interactions, child developmental progress, and improved parental psychological and physical health (Crnic, Friedrich, and Greenberg, 1983; Hanson and Hanline, 1990; Greenberg, Seltzer, Krauss, and Kim 1997).

The role of grandparents as a source of support for parents of children with disabilities is increasingly the subject of research studies. In a study of mothers with children with intellectual disability, researchers found that less emotional support from grandparents predicted maternal depression (Heller, Hsiesh and Rowitz, 2000). The authors of a study targeting grandparent support in families with a child with Down syndrome found that grandparent support lessened stress for mothers, but not for fathers. Further, they found that conflict with grandparents increased stress for these mothers (Hastings, Thomas and Delwiche, 2002). Both studies recommended the inclusion of grandparents in discussions, interventions and future planning regarding the child with disabilities. It is of interest that the study involving parents of children with Down syndrome found different results for mothers and fathers. In the research literature, fathers have been identified as "a neglected source of information in studies of family functioning" (Cuskelly, et al, 2002, p. 159).

Tangible Support

Tangible support is often necessary for families raising a child with disabilities, however only a small proportion of state funds for individuals with developmental disabilities go towards financial support for the family (Bradley, 1995). Nonetheless, research has demonstrated that flexible financial support can alleviate stress among families raising a child with developmental disabilities (Meyers and Marcenko, 1989; Freedman et al., 2000). Several studies conducted on the effectiveness of tangible support for families have come from the state of Michigan where the Michigan Family Support Subsidy Program is in place (Meyers, et al., 1989; Herman, 1994; Herman 1991). This program provides a cash stipend of $221 for families to be used at their discretion.

One such study examined the responses of 81 families in Michigan raising a child with a severe developmental disability who received financial support through this program (Meyers et al., 1989). Mothers were interviewed over a period of time and reported less family stress and greater life satisfaction after receiving the subsidy. Although it is suggested that a "no strings attached" cash program is essential for meeting the needs of individual families, most programs do not offer this type of assistance (Bradley, 1995).

Respite care is reported to be the support service most often provided to families (Bradley, 1995). The goal of respite care is to relieve parents of their caregiving demands for a short period of time by bringing in a temporary caregiver. Research on the benefit of respite care indicates that it reduces parental stress (Chan and Sigafoos, 2001). Further, it has been argued that quality respite care provided on a regular basis may foster family adaptation and decrease out of home placement of children with disabilities (Wikler, Hanusa, and Stoycheff, 1986).

Direct Psychological Intervention

Direct psychological intervention may target the child or the parents. Interventions aimed at children are most likely to target behavioral problems. It is suggested that child focused interventions that result in reducing problematic child behaviors may enhance parental well-being (Hastings, et al., 2004). Research on child focused interventions on parental stress and well-being are promising. Several studies have demonstrated improvement in parental stress levels and well being after behavioral interventions were carried out with their children. For example, a study comparing 18 families receiving a parent training program to 18 families who did not found that parents trained in behavioral principles as a way to manage child behaviors reported, fewer child behavioral problems, lower levels of stress, and greater self-efficacy than the control group (Feldman and Werner, 2002). In addition, Wiggs and Stores (2001) examined the responses of 15 parents of children with intellectual disabilities after implementing a behavioral program aimed at alleviating child sleep problems. The results of this study showed that the program improved child and parent sleep and also reduced self-reported maternal stress levels. However, these studies are not specific to children with Down syndrome and instead target children with intellectual disabilities in general. This may be due to the low incidence of behavioral problems reported in children with Down syndrome compared to other intellectual disabilities. There has been one study examining a behavioral sleep program in children with Down syndrome which showed improvement in behavioral sleep problems, however this study did not assess the effects these improvements had on maternal well-being (Stores and Stores, 2004).

A recent article by Hastings and Beck (2004) reviews the research on the effects of direct psychology intervention on parental well-being concluding that parent focused cognitive behavioral group models are effective in reducing stress among mothers of children with intellectual disabilities. Gammon and Rose (1991) conducted a study on the effects of a cognitive behavioral group treatment program on mothers of children with developmental disabilities. In this study mothers were randomly assigned to a treatment or control group. The group focused on cognitive restructuring, enhancing problem solving and interpersonal skills, and setting individual goals. Mothers who completed the program reported a reduction in stress and improved problem solving and interpersonal skills. Kirkham and Schilling (1993) examined the efficacy of a life skills training program that included cognitive behavioral components for mothers of children with intellectual disabilities. Parents were compared to a control group who only attend a parent support group. Mothers who completed the life skills group reported lower rates of self-reported depression and stress and higher rates of social support. These gains were partially maintained after two years. Further, other studies show that similar group treatment programs that include cognitive behavioral components are effective in reducing parental stress and maternal depression (Singer, Irvin and Hawkins, 1988; Singer, Irvin, Irvine, Hawkins, and Cooley, 1989).

While child specific behavioral interventions may prove helpful in reducing parental stress, it appears that parent focused cognitive behavioral interventions aimed at providing a structured group intervention are effective at reducing parental stress. This is important because it is well documented that parental stress can negatively impact child well-being and subsequent developmental outcomes (e.g., Gurlanick, 2000). Therefore, providing direct interventions for parents aimed at alleviating parental stress and enhancing parent-child interactions will likely impact the entire family in a positive manner.

Early Intervention

Because early intervention programs are family centered, they target the developmental needs of the child and the emotional needs of family members along with their informational and resource needs (Gurlanick, 1999). Several studies have examined the impact of specific intervention programs on families of children with Down syndrome. For example, Shu, Lung, and Huang (2002) examined the effects of a home care program on the mental health of primary family caregivers. This home care program offered direct care for the child, assistance and education on solving daily care problems to parents, and referrals to community resources and supports. The results of the study indicated that with time caregivers reported an improvement in psychological well-being as a result of the services provided by the home care program.

Pelchat and colleagues (2004) assessed the longitudinal effects of an early intervention program, PRIFAM, on the adaptation of parents of children with various developmental disabilities including Down syndrome. This program was designed to provide support to members of a family with a child with developmental disabilities with the following objectives in mind:

1. To identify for each parent the maladaptive perceptions and beliefs related to the situation and reinforce those that promote adaptation and to help parents gain realistic goals for their children.
2. To help the spouses understand and support each other.
3. To promote a trusting relationship between parent and child that foster attachment.
4. To foster exchanges within the family concerning the situation and each persons role in the adaptation process.
5. To help parents keep significant relationships and utilize resources.

This program was intended to intervene at several family subsystem levels: the individual, conjugal, parental, familial, and social systems. Participants in the program were compared to a control group. Overall, the results indicated that parents who participated reported less stress, more positive perceptions about their child's disability and their situation, and were more confident in their resources.

Another study evaluated the effectiveness of a rational-emotive parent education program on parental stress of mothers of young children with Down syndrome (Greaves, 1997). This program was part of a larger early intervention program that provided services to children with disabilities and their families. The Rational-Emotive Parent Education Program (REPE) was designed to target irrational belief and the stress response that these types of beliefs often elicit. When compared to control groups the REPE program appeared to reduce parental stress. Specifically, the program seemed to decrease parents' perception of stress at post-test and the parents in the REPE program attributed less of their stress to their child's disability.

However, the entire early intervention program was effective across all groups in reducing stress related to care and management of a child with a disability.

Valuing Family Resilience

In spite of research evidence that a variety of forms of support can be beneficial to families with a child with Down syndrome, these families remain at risk for stress and problems with family functioning. And yet, the literature consistently reveals families who manage well in spite of this challenge (Berry, 2003; Hanson, 2003; Lenhard et al., 2004, Poehlmann et al., 2005). One explanation for overall positive family functioning is addressed by the concept of family resilience. Resilience, as it applies to the family system is defined as follows:

1. The property of the family system that enables it to maintain its established patterns and functioning after being challenged and confronted by risk factors: elasticity.
2. The family's ability to recover quickly from a misfortune, trauma, or transitional event causing or calling for changes in the family's pattern of functioning: buoyancy (McCubbin et al., 1997, p. 2).

Resilience provides protection for the family and facilitates family adaptation through both protective and recovery factors. Protective factors help the family to maintain integrity and functioning and to fulfill developmental tasks. Protective factors include:

- Family Traditions and Celebrations
- Family Time and Routines
- Family Hardiness
- Family Communication
- Financial Management
- Personal Compatibility and Family Accord
- Health
- Shared values Around the Use of Leisure Time
- Support Networks (McCubbin et al., 1997, p. 6)

Recovery factors help families "bounce back" and adapt in family crisis situations. Recovery factors include:

- Family Integration
- Control
- Optimism
- Mastery
- Esteem Building
- Support (McCubbin et al., 1997, p. 7)

It is of note that both protective factors and recovery factors include support for the family. This support becomes a resource, the part B of the ABC-X model of stress. In addition, both protective and recovery factors address the meaning that families attach to their situation, part C of the ABC-X model. In terms of meaning, resilient families perceive stressful events as challenging, have higher perceptions of control, and have confidence in and commitment to their families. In addition, they are aware of their strengths and are able to endorse an attitude of "stick-to-it-iveness" when obstacles appear (Maddi, 2002; Scorgie, Wilgosh, and McDonald, 1998).

The best evidence of meaning as a coping factor comes from the testimonies of parents themselves. These researchers interviewed parents and found resilience from the beginning.

> Because when a child is born with Down syndrome, you know you'd better be getting busy . . . we knew the first day that we had a challenge in front of us and that we needed to get busy and pick up the gauntlet and go (Poehlmann et al., 2005, p. 263).

These mothers were able to reflect on their experiences when writing the introduction to a book co-authored by their sons, two young men with Down syndrome.

> In looking back, we've learned that what was most important was *not* their level of intellectual achievement, but rather their personal qualities of warmth and sincerity and their contributions to their family, friends and acquaintances. In addition, we have learned the folly of attempting to predict a person's quality of life based on his or her label or condition. These boys have succeeded because they were given opportunities and allowed to take risks, and because we refused to let anyone write them off (Kingsley and Levitz, 1994, p. 5).

Conclusion

Over time family life has improved for families that include a child with Down syndrome. Diagnostic and medical treatment advances, individualized education and early intervention programs all contribute to these positive changes. So, too, do supports targeted specifically for parents. All parents need information and resources. Most parents need emotional support and tangible help beyond what can be provided informally by friends and family as well as assistance in how to include and involve others, for example grandparents, in the support network. Many parents need direct psychological intervention for themselves, for the child with Down syndrome, or for a sibling. Providers of services to children with disabilities and their families need to look to the research literature and to families to define, refine and individualize family support services and to learn what helps and what does not for each particular family. In addition, providers need to recognize and maximize family strengths. Researchers need to build on the excellent beginning provided by the studies reviewed in this chapter. More research that addresses needs and outcomes for fathers, siblings and grandparents is especially warranted. Also, a lifespan perspective is needed (i.e., Berry and Hardman, 1998) that addresses family stress, coping and resilience in families that include children, adolescents and adults with Down syndrome.

References

Berry, J. O. (2003). *Supported families.* Oklahoma City: Center for Learning and Leadership, College of Medicine, University of Oklahoma Health Sciences Center.

Berry. J.O., and Hardman, M.L. (1998). *Lifespan perspectives on the family and disability.* Austin: PRO-ED.

Berry, J. O., and Jones, W. H. (1995). The Parental Stress Scale: Initial psychometric evidence. *Journal of Social and Personal Relationships, 12,* 463-472.

Bradley, V. (1995). Support for families of children with developmental disabilities: A revolution in expectations. In Nadel and Rosenthal (Eds.) *Down syndrome living and learning in the community.* New York: Wiley.

Chan, J. and Sigafoos, J. (2001). Does respite care reduce parental stress in families with developmentally disabled children? *Child and Youth Care Forum, 30,* 253-263.

Crnic, K., Friedrich, W., and Greenberg, M. (1983). Adaptation of families with mentally retarded children: A model of stress, coping, and family ecology. *American Journal of Mental Deficiency, 88,* 125-138.

Cunningham C. (1996). Families of children with Down syndrome. *Down Syndrome Research and Practice, 4,* 87-95.

Cuskelly, M., Jobling, A., Chant, D., Bower, A., and Hayes, A. (2002). Multiple perspectives of the family life. In M. Cuskelly, A. Jobling, and S. Buckley, (Eds.). *Down syndrome across the lifespan.* London: Whurr.

Feldman, M. and Werner, S. (2002). Collateral effects of behavioral parent training on families of children with developmental disabilities and behavior disorders. *Behavioral Intervention, 17,* 75-83.

Fidler D., Hodapp, R., and Dykens, E. (2000). Stress in families of young children with Down syndrome, Williams syndrome, and Smith-Magenis syndrome. *Early Education and Development, 11,* 395-406.

Freedman, R. and Capobianco, N. (2000). The power to choose: Supports for families caring for individuals with developmental disabilities. *Health and Social Work, 25,* 59-68.

Gammon, E. and Rose, S. (1991). The Coping Skills Training Program for parents of children with developmental disabilities: An experimental evaluation. *Research on Social Work Practices, 1,* 244-256.

Gill, B. (1997). *Changed by a child.* New York: Random House.

Greaves, D. (1997). The effect of rational-emotive parent education on the stress of mothers of young children with Down syndrome. *Journal of Rational-Emotive and Cognitive-Behavior Therapy, 15,* 249-267.

Greenberg, J., Seltzer, M., Krauss, M., and Kim, H. (1997). The differential effects of social support on the psychological well-being of aging mothers of adults with mental illness or mental retardation. *Family Relations, 46,* 383-394.

Gurlanick, M. (1998). Effectiveness of early intervention for vulnerable children: A developmental perspective. *American Journal of Mental Retardation, 102,* 319-345.

Guralnick, M. (2000). Early childhood intervention: Evolution of a system. In. Wehmeyer, M. and Patton, J. (Eds.) *Mental Retardation in the 21st Century.* Austin, TX: PRO-ED.

Hardman, M., Drew, C., and Egan, M. (2006). *Human exceptionality*. Boston: Allyn and Bacon.

Hanson, M. J. (2003). Twenty-five years after early intervention: A follow-up of children with Down syndrome and their families. *Infants and Young Children, 16*, 354-365.

Hanson, M. and Hanline, J. (1990). Parenting a child with a disability: A longitudinal study of parental stress and adaptation. *Journal of Early Intervention, 14*, 234-248.

Hastings, R. and Beck, A. (2004). Practitioner Review: Stress intervention for parents of children with intellectual disabilities. *Journal of Child Psychology and Psychiatry, 45*, 1338-1394.

Hastings, R., Thomas, H., and Delwiche, N. (2002). Grandparents support from families of children with Down's syndrome. *Journal of Applied Research in Intellectual Disabilities, 15*, 97-104.

Hedov, G., Wikblad, K., and Anneren, G. (2002). First information and support provided to parents of children with Down syndrome in Sweden: Clinical goals and parental experiences. *Acta Paediatr, 91*, 1344-1349.

Heller, T., Hsieh, K., Rowitz, L. (2000). Grandparents as supports for mothers of persons with intellectual disability. *Journal of Gerontological Social Work, 33*, 23-34,

Herman, S. (1991). Use and impact of a cash subsidy program. *Mental Retardation, 29*, 253-258.

Herman, S. (1994). Cash subsidy program: Family satisfaction and need. *Mental Retardation, 32*, 416-421.

Heritage, J., Rogers, H., and West, W. (1994, Nov.). *Effects of support on the attitude of the primary care giver of a child with Down syndrome*. Paper presented at the meeting of the Southern Association for Counselor Education and Supervision. Charlotte, NC.Hill, R. (1949). *Families under stress*. New York: Harper.

Kingsley, J., and Levitz, M. (1994). *Count us in: Growing up with Down syndrome*. Orlando: Harcourt Brace.

Kirkham, M. and Schilling, R. (1990). Life skills training with mothers of handicapped children. *Journal of Social Service Research, 13*, 67-87.

Lenhard, W., Breitenbach, E., Ebert, H., Schindelhauer-Duetscher, H. and Henn, W. (2005). Psychological benefits of diagnostic certainty for mothers of children with disabilities: Lessons from Down syndrome. *American Journal of Medical Genetics, 133*, 170-175.

Levitz and Schwartz (1995). Linking parents with parents: The family connection casebook of best practices in family support. In Nadel and Rosenthal (Eds.), *Down syndrome living and learning in the community*. New York: Wiley.)

Lessenberry, B. and Renfeldt, R. (2004). Evaluating stress levels of parents of children with disabilities. *Exceptional Children, 70*, 231-244.

Maddi, S. (2002). The story of hardiness: Twenty years of theorizing, research, and practice. *Consulting Psychology Journal: Practice and Research, 54*, 173-185.

McCubbin, H. I., McCubbin, M. A., Thompson, A. I., Han, S., and Allen, C. T. (1997). Families under stress: What makes them resilient. *Journal of Family and Consumer Sciences, 2-11*.

McCubbin. H. and Patterson, J. (1982). Family adaptation to crisis. In H. McCubbin, A. Cauble, and J. Patterson (Eds.), *Family stress, coping, and social support.* Springfield: Charles C. Thomas.

Meyers, J. and Marcenko, M. (1989). Impact of a cash subsidy program for families of children with severe developmental disabilities. *Mental Retardation, 6,* 383-387.

Most, D. E., Fidler, D. J., Laforce-Booth, C., and Kelly, J. (2006). Stress trajectories in mothers of young children with Down syndrome. *Journal of Intellectual Disabilities Research, 50,* 501-514.

National Institute of Child Health and Human Development. (2006). Retrieved October 11, 2006, from http://www.nichd.nih.gov/health/topics/Down_Syndrome.cfm

Pelchat, D., Lefebvre, H., Prouix, M., and Reidy, M. (2004). Parental satisfaction with an early family intervention program. *Journal of Perinatal and Neonatal Nursing, 18,* 128-144.

Peterson, G. and Hennon, C. (2005). Conceptualizing parenting stress in the family stress theory. In P. McHenry and S. Price (Eds.), *Families and change: Coping with stressful events and change.* Thousand Oaks: Sage Publications.

Poehlmann, J., Clements, M., Addeduto, L., and Farsad, V. (2005). Family experiences associated with a child's diagnosis of Fragile X or Down syndrome: Evidence for disruption and resilience. *Mental Retardation, 43,* 255-267.

Pueschel, S. (1985). Changes in counseling practices at the birth of a child with Down syndrome. *Applied Research in Mental Retardation, 6,* 99-108.

Pueschel, S. and Murphy, A. (1976). Assessment of counseling practices at the birth of a child with Down's syndrome. *American Journal of Mental Deficiency, 81,* 523-530.

Roach, M., Orsmond, G., and Barratt, M. (1999). Mothers and fathers of children with Down syndrome: Parental stress and involvement in childcare. *American Journal on Mental Retardation, 104,* 422.436.

Scorgie, K., Wilgosh, L., and McDonald, L. (1998). Stress and coping in families of children with disabilities: An examination of recent literature. *Developmental Disabilities Bulletin, 26, 22-42.*

Singer, G., Irvin, L., and Hawkins, N. (1988). Stress management training for parents of children with severe handicaps. *Mental Retardation, 26,* 269-277.

Singer, G., Irvin, L., Irvine, B., Hawkins, N., and Cooley, E. (1989). Evaluation of community based support services for families of persons with developmental disabilities. *Journal of the Association for Persons with Severe Handicaps, 14,* 312-323.

Skotko, B. (2005). Mother of children with Down syndrome reflect on their postnatal support. *Pediatrics, 115,* 64-77.

Skotko, B. and Canal, R. (2004). Postnatal support for mothers of children with Down syndrome. *Mental Retardation, 43,* 196-212.

Shu, B. Lung, F., and Huang, C. (2002). Mental health of primary family caregivers with children with intellectual disability who receive a home care programme. *Journal of Intellectual Disability Research, 46,* 257-263.

Shonkoff, J., Hauser-Cram, P., Krauss, M., and Upshur, C. (1992). Development of infants with disabilities and their families: Implications for theory and service delivery. *Monographs of the Society for Research on Child Development, 57,* 1-153.

Spiker, D. (1982). Parent involvement in early intervention activities with their children with Down's syndrome. *Education and Training of the Mentally Retarded, 17*, 24-29.

Stores, R. and Stores, G. (2004). Evaluation of brief group administered instruction for parents to prevent or minimize sleep problems in young children with Down syndrome. *Journal of Applied Research in Intellectual Disabilities, 17*, 61-70.

Van Hooste, A. and Maes, B. (2003). Family factors in the early development of children with Down syndrome. *Journal of Early Intervention, 25*, 296-309.

White, N. and Hastings, R. (2004). Social and professional support for parents of adolescents with severe intellectual disabilities. *Journal of Applied Research in Intellectual Disabilities, 17*, 181-190.

Wiggs, L. and Stores, G. (2001). Behavioral treatment for sleep problems in children with severe intellectual disabilities and daytime challenging behavior: effects on mothers and fathers. *The British Journal of Health Psychology, 6*, 257-269.

Wikler, L., Hanusa, D., and Stoycheff, J. (1986). Home-based respite care, the child with developmental disabilities, and family stress. In C.L. Salisbury and J. Intagliata (Eds.), *Respite care: Support for persons with developmental disabilities and their families.* Baltimore: Paul Brookes.

In: Mental Retardation Research Advances
Editor: Elizabeth B. Heinz, pp. 75-87

ISBN: 978-1-60021-658-9
© 2007 Nova Science Publishers, Inc.

Chapter V

Distractor Interference Effects and Identification of Safe and Dangerous Road-Crossing Sites by Children with and without Mental Retardation

A. Alevriadou[*1] *and G. Grouios*[2]

[1]Department of Early Childhood Education, Faculty of Education in Florina,
University of Western Macedonia, Greece
[2]Department of Physical Education and Sport Sciences,
Aristotle University of Thessaloniki, Greece

Abstract

This study provides some reasoning to support the notion that individuals with mental retardation are less likely to actively inhibit response tendencies to irrelevant information in their visual field. Inherent in this idea is the notion that selective attention processes operate differently for subjects with and without mental retardation. Selection by individuals with mental retardation only involve facilitatory processes directed at the target stimulus, whereas selection by individuals without mental retardation involve both facilitatory processes directed toward the target and inhibitory processes directed against irrelevant information. The aim of the present study was to test the suppression of irrelevant information in a non-laboratory context (testing road crossing abilities of children with and without mental retardation). The sample of the study consisted of 104 young individuals. The participants were further subdivided into four groups (n=26 per group) matched on mean mental age, using the Raven's Colored Progressive Matrices: two groups with children with mental retardation (Group A and Group B) and two groups with children without mental retardation (Group C and Group D). Group A and Group C were matched on mental age at 5.6 yr.; Group B and Group D were matched on mental age at 8.0 yr. Ability to identify safe and dangerous road–crossing sites was

---

[*] Address correspondence to Dr. Anastasia Alevriadou, University of Western Macedonia, Pedagogical School of Florina, Department of Early Childhood Education, Florina, GR 53 100, Greece, or mail alevriadou@uowm.gr

assessed using computer presentations. The task featured the image of a child standing at the edge of a road facing towards the road. Two tasks were designed using a number of road-crossing sites in each one: recognition task without irrelevant information (i.e., distracting visual stimuli were removed from the scene, allowing the participant to focus on the road site) and recognition task with irrelevant information (i.e., distracting visual stimuli were included in the scene, obscuring the participant to focus on the road site). Every participant was asked to select the "safe" and "unsafe" (dangerous) road-crossing sites. Results demonstrated statistically significant differences between Groups A and C and Groups B and D in task conditions, especially in those in which irrelevant information was involved. Conclusions were drawn concerning the empirical and theoretical benefits for psychology and education, which arise from the study of safety road education in children with mental retardation.

Introduction

Attention is a multifaceted construct that is manifested in a variety of ways. Studies of visual selective attention (Broadbent, 1982; Parasuraman and Davies, 1984) have provided considerable information concerning the manner in which stimuli are selected for processing. The assumption that underlies much of the research in this area is that the environment provides individuals with a complex array of stimuli from which a subset of stimuli may be selected for processing. Selective attention implies that attention is directed toward some stimuli and away from other stimuli. The ability to narrow attention to those stimuli that are relevant to the performance of a given task and direct attention away from nonrelevant stimuli is considered to be a characteristic of optimal selective attention processing.

Since individuals with subnormal intellectual development consistently demonstrate attentional deficiencies (Bergen and Mosley, 1994; Merrill, 1990; Nugent and Mosley, 1987), selective attention processes represent a coherent focus on the search for important deficiencies in cognition associated with mental retardation. In particular, a significant number of theorists and researchers comparing the selective attention abilities of individuals with and without mental retardation have consistently shown that those with mental retardation are more distracted by the presence of irrelevant information in a stimulus array than are individuals without mental retardation (Crosby, 1972; Hagen and Huntsman, 1971). Neil and his colleagues (Neil, 1977; Neil and Westberry, 1987) and Tipper (1985) have proposed that selective attention may involve not only facilitory processes directed toward the selected target but also inhibitory processes operating on the unselected distractor stimuli.

Experimental evidence for inhibitory deficits in individuals with mental retardation has been found across many experimental tasks. In an early study, Terdal (1967) reported evidence that individuals with moderate to mild mental retardation were less able to inhibit attention to background stimuli during a simple looking task involving checkerboard stimuli. Additionally, in the presence of distractors, children with mental retardation had more difficulty in remembering information (Holowinsky and Farelly, 1988) and in inhibiting responses caused by distracting dimensions of task stimuli (Ellis, Woodley-Zanthos, Dulaney, and Palmer, 1989). A few years later, Merrill and O'Dekirk (1994), using a flanker task, found that individuals with mental retardation were affected negatively by flanking stimuli at much greater eccentricities than were individuals without mental retardation. These authors asserted that the differences observed may have resulted from the differential use of top-down processing resources across groups. Similar findings of susceptibility to distraction or interference have been reported on Stroop tasks (Ellis and Dulaney, 1991) and identity-based negative-priming tasks (e.g., Cha and Merrill, 1994). In one study, Cha (1992) measured the ability of retarded and nonretarded persons to focus attention during a visual selective attention task in which a central target stimulus letter was presented between two flanker stimuli. The results revealed that the performance of mentally retarded individuals was more influenced by the distracting effects flankers than was the performance of nonretarded individuals. In another study, Cha (1992) evaluated the degree to which retarded individuals are able to overcome the effects of the onset of distractors. The magnitude of the distractor effect differed between IQ groups. The researcher concluded that irrelevant stimuli are more powerful attractors of attention for retarded individuals than they are for nonretarded individuals. Recently, Merrill (2006) found that the failure to engage in inhibitory processes by the participants with mental retardation in tasks of selective attention was related to increased distractor interference. Taken collectively, these studies suggest that individuals with mental retardation have more difficulty than their peers without mental retardation in controlling the focus of their attention and that, at least part, this difficulty can be traced to deficits in selectively attending to relevant cues.

On the contrary, Merrill, Cha, and Moore (1994) demonstrated that individuals with and without mental retardation show similar negative-priming effects on a location-based task. Thus, individuals with mental retardation may be able to utilize top-down processing to inhibit attention to irrelevant information but did not do so in all experimental contexts (see also Crosby, 1972). Furthermore, the susceptibility of persons with mental retardation to distraction has been shown to be related to the level of task difficulty. For example, Sen and Clarke (1968) found that although adults with mental retardation were distracted by extraneous stimulation during a difficult task, they were unaffected by the same distractors when the task was easy. Similarly, Belmont and Ellis (1968) found that adults with mental retardation were not more distractible than adults without mental retardation. They suggested that some forms of distraction may have no effect or even a facilitative effect upon performance in a learning situation because they act as general arousers, resulting in greater alertness and concomitant improvements in attention.

Although there appears to be some inconsistency between studies, a particular pattern emerges that may help to explain these differences. Specifically, it may be that in tasks in which distractors are similar to the central task stimuli (i.e., the task requires more effortful processing) individuals with mental retardation show decrements in performance, whereas in tasks in which the distractors are easily distinguished from the central task stimuli, no such performance decrements are produced. Altogether, these data suggest that in some instances, individuals with mental retardation have enhanced difficulty in comparison with their peers without mental retardation in attending selectively to relevant cues (Pearson, Norton, and Farwell, 1997). The challenges facing researchers, therefore, are to identify the circumstances in which individuals with mental retardation do and do not demonstrate the ability to limit attention to task-irrelevant distractions and to develop methods and/or presentation formats that facilitate adaptive attending behavior. Additionally, the extent to which the results of laboratory-based studies of attention predict retarded individuals' behavior in educational and training settings remains to be elucidated. It is valuable, then, to determine whether it is possible to facilitate the use of mechanisms of selective attention by persons with mild mental retardation across a range of cognitive tasks.

A characteristic activity that is heavily relied on selective attention is the safe pedestrian behaviour, since one has to focus attention on the traffic environment and ignore irrelevant stimuli. Tabibi and Pfeffer (2003) indicated that attention is required for identifying road-crossing sites quickly and accurately, especially for young typically developing children. Dunbar, Lewis, and Hill (1999) found that 4- to 10-year-old typically developing children who were better at attention switching were more likely to show awareness of traffic when crossing a road, and children who maintained concentration when challenged by a distracting event, crossed the road in a "less reckless" manner. Furthermore, Hill, Lewis, and Dunbar (2000) found that 4- to 9-year-old typically developing children have difficulty paying attention to the features that make a road-crossing situation dangerous; namely, they have difficulty paying attention to relevant information and ignoring irrelevant. Unfortunately, little attention has been paid to the relationship between pedestrian skills and attention for children and adults with mental retardation. A limited number of studies have demonstrated that individuals with mild mental retardation show difficulties to find a safe place to cross the street and supported the need for pedestrian skill instruction (Matson, 1980; Page, Iwata, and Neef, 1976). There has been only one study, which shows that there is a significant relationship between attention and identification of safe and dangerous road-crossing sites in adults with mild mental retardation (Alevriadou, Angelou, and Tsakiridou, 2006).

The aim of the present study was to explore the suppression of irrelevant information of children with and without mental retardation in a non-laboratory task. For the problem at hand, a road-crossing paradigm was adopted. The task was presented by means of a table-top simulation displaying a selection of road-crossing sites varying in complexity in order to investigate the variables influencing children's ability with and without mental retardation to select safe road-crossing sites.

Method

Participants

The sample of the study consisted of 104 young individuals. To test their ability to select safe road-crossing sites, the 104 participants were further subdivided into four groups (n=26 per group) matched on mean mental age, using the Raven's Colored Progressive Matrices (Raven, 1965): two groups with mentally retarded children (Group A and Group B) and two groups with typically developing children (Group C and Group D). Group A and Group C were matched on mental age at 5.6 yr.; Group B and Group D were matched on mental age at 8.6 yr. Each pair of groups differed significantly in mean chronological age [Group A (M=7.8 yrs) and Group C (M=5.3 yrs) t=45.99, p<0.01), Group B and Group D (M=10.9 yrs) and Group C (M=8.2 yrs) t=51.19, p<0.01)]. All children with mild mental retardation were receiving special education in the nearest school in their community (inclusive education) and none were living in institutional settings. They were living in the broader area in the city of Kozani, Greece and were referred for diagnosis to the Counseling Centre for children with special needs. None of the children received any specific pedestrian skills instruction.

Group A composed of 26 children (13 boys and 13 girls) with organic mild mental retardation ranging in chronological age from 7.5 to 8.3 yrs (M=7.8 yrs, SD=0.2). Ten of the participants were premature and had anoxia at birth, two had postnatal head trauma, five had encephalitis, two were infected by the rubella in the mother, while the other seven had epilepsy. Group C consisted of 26 typically developing children (13 boys and 13 girls) with chronological ages from 5 to 5.6 yrs (M=5.3 yrs, SD=0.2). All preschoolers recruited from kindergartens. Mean mental age for the typically developing children in this group was 5.4 yrs (SD=0.3).

Group B consisted of 26 children with organic mild mental retardation (13 boys and 13 girls) ranging in chronological age from 10.5 to 11.3 years (M=10.9 yrs, SD=0.2). Ten of the participants were premature and had anoxia at birth, four had postnatal head trauma, five had encephalitis, while the other seven had epilepsy. Group D consisted of 26 typically developing children (13 boys and 13 girls) with chronological ages from 8 to 8.6 yrs (M=8.3 yrs, SD=0.2). All children were recruited from primary schools. The mean mental age for this group was 8.6 yrs (SD=0.2).

Materials

The method involved the use of a large traffic mat measuring approximately 120X100 cm. It comprised a street layout on which a range of trees, buses, and toy cars were placed to create situations similar to those individuals might encounter in the real traffic environment. The task was based on previous research on pedestrian skills (Ampofo-Boateng and Thomson, 1991; Tabibi and Pfeffer, 2002).

The recognition task featured the toy pedestrian standing at the edge of a road facing towards the road. Twenty-five road-crossing sites were represented separately, including one practice trial. Two tasks were designed using the 24 road-crossing sites: a) recognition task without irrelevant information constituted of 12 road-crossing sites in which 6 tasks represented "safe" situations (Condition 1) and 6 tasks served as "unsafe" (dangerous) situations (Condition 2) and b) recognition task with irrelevant information made up of 12 road-crossing sites in which 6 tasks represented "safe" situations (Condition 3) and 6 tasks served as "unsafe" (dangerous) situations (Condition 4). For the recognition task without irrelevant information, distracting visual information was removed from the scene (such as cats, dogs, children playing) allowing the participant to focus on the road site. Concerning the recognition task with irrelevant information, 6 unanimated distractions were included (fixed landscape) (Condition 5) as well as 6 animated distractions (Condition 6). Table 1 outlines the irrelevant information incorporated into specific road-crossing sites.

**Table 1. Road-crossing sites with irrelevant information
presented in random order to participants**

Crossing site	Irrelevant information added	Safe/Dangerous identification
Straight road	Fixed landscape (unanimated)	Safe
Zebra crossing	Fixed landscape (unanimated)	Dangerous
Blind bend	Children playing in park with a ball (animated)	Dangerous
Pelican crossing (with green man)	Cat waking in a park (animated)	Safe
Roundabout	Fixed landscape (unanimated)	Dangerous
Traffic island	Fixed landscape (unanimated)	Safe
Traffic lights on red	Fixed landscape (unanimated)	Safe
Parked cars	Road construction (animated)	Safe
Road-crossing patrol	A gardener working at a flower-bed near the road (animated)	Dangerous
Brow of a hill	Fixed landscape (unanimated)	Dangerous
Junction	Cyclist (animated)	Safe
Traffic lights on green	A street cleaner with a push broom (animated)	Dangerous

The situations were all matched as far as possible for complexity and surrounding layout. The sites included junctions, bends, parked cars or other obstructions. In constructing the sites, care was taken that each was rendered dangerous by the presence of only one of these features. Selection of the sites in both tasks was done with the aid of the Hellenic Ministry of Education (Road Safety Educational Programs). A range of possible situations was presented to independent judges who evaluated them. Only situations that showed 100 per cent agreement as to their manifest safety or danger were selected for use.

Road-crossing sites were presented in random order with a 1-min interval between trials. Trials were not time limited. Every individual was tested individually by a certified psychologist. Road-crossing sites information was recorded on a standard data collection form. Correct identification of a safe road-crossing site in each Condition was given 1 point. No point was given for identification of a safe road-crossing site.

Procedure

Informed consent was obtained before the investigation from the parents of all included children. According to our national and institutional guidelines for ethical review, institutional review board approval was not necessary. All children with mild mental retardation were examined in the Counseling Center, while typically developing children at school. The pedestrian task conditions were presented randomly to the participants. The examination was performed on individual basis. The pedestrian toy was positioned near to each of the road-crossing locations and each child was asked to judge whether should ("safe") or should not ("dangerous") cross the road. Depending on the participant's speed of performance, the task took 15 minutes to complete for groups C and D and around 25 minutes for groups A and B.

Statistical Analysis

The collected data were analyzed statistically. "Student's" t-test for independent samples was used to compare mean performance scores in task conditions between a) Group A and Group C and b) Group B and Group D. For the said purpose, statistical software package (SPSS/PC+ version 13.0, SPSS Inc., Chicago, Illinois) was used. A P-value less than 5% ($P < 0.05$) was taken as statistically significant.

Results

The comparison of the mean performance scores in task conditions between mentally retarded children (Group A) and typically developing children (Group C) are shown in table 2.

Table 2. Mean performance scores in task conditions between Group A and Group C

Task Condition	Group A	Group C	t	p
Condition 1	M=3.19	M=3.50	t=1.73	ns
Condition 2	M=3.15	M=3.42	t=1.73	ns
Condition 3	M=2.15	M=2.50	t=2.56	p<0.05
Condition 4	M=2.12	M=2.54	t=2.77	p<0.01
Condition 5	M=2.96	M=3.31	t=3.02	p<0.01
Condition 6	M=1.31	M=1.73	t=2.88	p<0.01

The comparison of the mean performance scores in task conditions between mentally retarded children (Group B) and typically developing children (Group D) are illustrated in table 3.

Table 3. Mean performance scores in task conditions between Group B and Group D

Task Condition	Group B	Group D	t	p
Condition 1	M=4.81	M=4.96	t=0.75	ns
Condition 2	M=4.54	M=4.92	t=2.07	p<0.05
Condition 3	M=2.54	M=4.04	t=9.16	p<0.01
Condition 4	M=2.50	M=4.04	t=9.38	p<0.01
Condition 5	M=3.19	M=5.04	t=10.79	p<0.01
Condition 6	M=1.85	M=3.04	t=7.097	p<0.01

Conclusion

This investigation was undertaken with the purpose of exploring the suppression of irrelevant information of children with and without mental retardation in a non-laboratory task. The present data demonstrated significant differences between the mean performance scores of the Group A and Group C in Conditions 3, 4, 5 and 6. The score of the Group A was lower than that of the Group C. This finding, in accordance with previous evidence (Cha and Merrill, 1994; Merrill and Taube, 1996) seems to suggest that individuals with mental retardation have enhanced difficulty in comparison with their typically developing mental age controls in attending selectively via the visual mode to road-crossing sites, especially when irrelevant information stimuli are involved. In other words, mentally retarded individuals are more distracted by the presence of irrelevant information stimuli than are typically developing individuals. The selection of one stimulus over another is likely to involve not only facilitatory or excitatory processes directed toward the selected target, but also inhibition or suppression processes that operate to minimize responding to non-target stimuli (Tipper, 1985). Mentally retarded participants are, thus, less efficient in suppressing non-target information than typically developing participants (Cha and Merrill, 1994). Hence, this may result in performance decrements across a variety of tasks. Research data demonstrates that 5 years old typically developing children are particularly poor at distinguishing safe and unsafe traffic locations, especially when they involve irrelevant stimuli (Ampofo-Boateng and Thomson, 1991). The absence of significant differences between the mean performance scores of the Group A and Group C in Conditions 1 and 2, may be attributed to the fact that these tasks did not involve irrelevant information. It seems that these conditions are easy for both groups A and C, although they demand judging safe and unsafe traffic sites. Additionally, both groups A and C responded more efficiently to a road-crossing target without irrelevant information as compared to one with distractors, following the same developmental pattern (Group A: Condition 1 and 2=3.19 and 3.15 vs Condition 3 and 4= 2.15 and 2.12 respectively, Group C: Condition 1 and 2=3.50 and 3.42 vs Condition 3and 4= 2.50 and 2.54 respectively).

Our findings also illustrated significant differences between the mean performance scores of the Group B and Group D in Conditions 2, 3, 4, 5 and 6. The score of the Group B was lower compared with that of the Group D. This result is in line with earlier claims that individuals with organic mental retardation (Down syndrome) have difficulties filtering irrelevant auditory (Miezejeski, 1974) or visual (Merrill and O' Dekirk, 1994) stimuli. The observed difference may be ascribed to the incapability of the individuals with mental retardation to utilize inhibitory mechanisms of selective attention (see also Houghton, Tipper, Weaver, and Shore, 1996). It seems that mentally retarded individuals exhibit poorer selection skills and smaller suppression effects than do typically developing individuals (Hagen and Huntsman, 1971), showing some kind of cognitive inertia (Ellis and Dulaney, 1991; Dulaney and Ellis, 1997). Hasher and Zacks (1988) suggested that these suppression processes may be important components of attention. If irrelevant stimuli are not effectively suppressed, they continue to demand processing resources associated with limited capacity working memory. This would reduce the functional capacity of working memory for the processing of relevant stimuli, and, as a consequence, the efficiency of processing relevant information would be reduced. Hence, inefficient stimulus suppression processes may result in performance decrements for individuals with mental retardation across a variety of tasks (Tomporowski and Tinsley, 1997).

The absence of significant differences between the mean performance scores of the Group B and Group D in Condition 1 may be assigned to the fact that this is the easiest task for both groups. Several studies have shown that typically developing children differentiate better safe than dangerous crossing sites, especially when there aren't any distractors involved (Ampofo-Boateng and Thomson, 1991; Young and Lee, 1987). The same pattern seems to exist in mentally retarded individuals.

Irrelevant information affected the ability of the individuals with, as well as without, mental retardation. This is consistent with published results on attention (Tabibi and Pfeffer, 2003), which suggest that the animated distractions (adding more visual information) may have been sufficiently demanding for all the participants (Groups A and C, B and D). An increase in irrelevant information may highlight the vulnerability of all participants to interference more. On the other hand, mentally retarded individuals experience enhanced difficulty inhibiting the influence of distractors (i.e. Condition 6 –animated irrelevant information) than typically developing individuals. This explains the fact that the performance of all groups in Condition 6 is the lowest compared with all the other Conditions. On the other hand, there are statistically significant differences between mentally retarded and typically developing individuals in both mental age groups (Group A =1.31 vs Group C=1.73, Group B=1.85 vs Group D=3.04).

As an alternative to this view, a metacognitive explanation might be supposed that the mentally retarded retardation did not judge right if the road-crossing condition was safe or dangerous. But metacognitive factors themselves cannot fully explain the whole findings. Additionally, motivational factors can also partially explain the differences found between Group B and Group D. One key factor hypothesized to affect the observed behavior in mental retardation is the history of failure in independent problem solving (Weisz, 1979). The greater history of failure that children with mental retardation experience in applying their own solutions to problems, the greater the amount of outer-directedness (reliance mainly on external cues rather than on their internal cognitive abilities to solve a task or problem) they show compared to typically developing children (Bybee and Zigler, 1998). Researchers generally report declines in outer-directedness among typically developing children at higher mental ages (Yando and Zigler, 1971; MacMillan and Wright, 1974). As typically developing children get older, they become more inner-directed, trusting their own solutions to problems. On the contrary, declines in outer-directedness are found much less consistently in older mentally retarded children (Bybee and Zigler, 1998). Again, motivational factors cannot fully explain the difference, especially between groups A and C.

In summary, our results indicate that selective attention is, at least, partially required for identifying road-crossing sites accurately. Although there are statistical significant differences in both mental age groups in favor of the typically developing participants, the differences are quantitative in nature. It seems that there are some qualitative similar patterns between participants with and without mental retardation. For example, the crossing sites that produced the most errors for all groups were the junction, the blind bend and the brow of a hill (especially when they were escorted by distractors) (this is a typical finding for typically developing children, see also Ampofo-Boateng and Thomson, 1991). Similarly, all groups, both at higher and lower mental age, had better performance in conditions involving unanimated than animated distractors. Another interesting finding is that the crossing site of the parked cars was judged automatically dangerous on the basis of the cars for both mentally retarded and typically developing individuals, especially at the lower mental age.

The present research findings highlight the need to design road-safety training programs for children with mental retardation. Presenting participants with a large traffic mat under controlled conditions facilitates the focusing of attention to the task in hand. This type of technique may have potential as a simple and attractive training device that might be used in the classroom to improve at least some aspects of mentally retarded children's road knowledge and skill. Whilst in the end there can be no substitute for training in realistic situations, it is possible that preliminary training using models might provide a basis on which in situ training might build. On the other side, the real pedestrian environment is even more demanding than the traffic mat used. It is more likely to provide interfering and distracting stimuli.

Standen, Brown, and Cromby (2001) stated that virtual environments appear to be a fruitful method of teaching skills for independent living to people with mental retardation. Standen and Brown (2005) stated that virtual reality can provide a safe setting in which to practice road safety skills that might carry too many risks in the real world especially for individuals with mental retardation. Similarly, Foot, Tolmie, Thomson, McLaren, and Whelan (1999) suggested that computer-based tasks may be useful for training in pedestrian skills. Relevant attention skills may also be trained in this way. The advantages of such tasks are that they allow control of variables, can be used to develop specific skills and are attractive to children and adults with intellectual disabilities. Alevriadou et al. (2006) conducted preliminary studies on using computer animations to teach children with intellectual disabilities how to identify safe and dangerous road-crossing sites with encouraging results. Many of these studies showed some transfer of learning from the virtual to the real world for individuals with intellectual disabilities (see also the "virtual city" by Brown, Neale, and Cobb, 1999).

Further research is needed to determine which aspects of attention are most important for safe pedestrian behavior and the type of distractions that are most deleterious for child pedestrians with and without mental retardation. Additionally, the operation of distractor interferences, which is higher in some conditions than others, indicates that one important area for future research may be to analyze the precise conditions under which group differences in selective attention processes can and cannot be obtained.

References

Alevriadou, A., Angelou, I., and Tsakiridou, E. (2006). The relationship between attention and identification of safe and dangerous road crossing sites in adults with mild ID. *Journal of Applied Research in Intellectual Disabilities*, 19(3), 239.

Ampofo-Boateng, K., and Thomson, J. (1991). Children's perception of safety and danger on the road. *British Journal of Psychology*, 82, 487-505.

Belmont, J.M., and Ellis, N.R. (1968). Effects of extraneous stimulation upon discrimination learning in normals and retardates. *American Journal of Mental Deficiency*, 72, 525-532.

Bergen, A-M. E., and Mosley, J.L. (1994). Attention and attentional shift efficiency in individuals with and without mental retardation. *American Journal on Mental Retardation*, 98, 688-743.

Broadbent, D.E. (1982). Task combination and selective intake of information. *Acta Psychologica*, 50, 253-290.

Brown, D.J. Neale, H., and Cobb, S.V. (1999). The development and evaluation of the virtual city. *International Journal of Virtual Reality*, 4, 28-41.

Bybee, J., and Zigler, E. (1998) Outer-directedness in individuals with and without mental retardation: A review. In J. Burack, R. Hodapp, and E. Zigler (Eds.), *Handbook of mental retardation and development* (pp. 434-461). Cambridge, UK: Cambridge University Press.

Cha, K-H. (1992). The effect of flanking context and its time course in focused attention processes of mentally retarded and nonretarded persons. *Dissertation Abstracts International*, 53, 2087.

Cha, K-H., and Merrill, E.C. (1994). Facilitation and inhibition effects in visual selective attention processes of persons with and without mental retardation. *American Journal on Mental Retardation*, 98, 594-600.

Crosby, K.G. (1972). Attention and distractibility in mentally retarded children. *American Journal of Mental Deficiency*, 77, 46-53.

Dulaney, C., and Ellis, N. (1997). Rigidity in the behavior of mentally retarded persons. In W. E. MacLean (Ed.), *Ellis' Handbook of mental deficiency, psychological theory and research* (pp. 175-195). Mahwah, NJ: Erlbaum.

Dunbar, G., Lewis, V., and Hill, R. (1999). Control processes and road-crossing skills. *Psychologist*, 12, 398-399.

Ellis, N.R., and Dulaney, C.L. (1991). Further evidence for cognitive inertia of persons with mental retardation. *American Journal on Mental Retardation*, 95, 613-621.

Ellis, N.R., Woodley-Zanthos, P., Dulaney, C.L., and Palmer, R.L. (1989). Automatic-effortful processing and cognitive inertia in persons with mental retardation. *American Journal on Mental Retardation*, 93, 412-423.

Foot, H., Tolmie, A., Thomson, J., McLaren, B., and Whelan K. (1999). *Recognizing the hazards. Psychologist*, 12, 400-402.

Hagen, J.W., and Huntsman, N. (1971). Selective attention and mental retardation. *Developmental Psychology*, 5, 151-160.

Hasher, L., and Zacks, R.T. (1988). Working memory, comprehension, and aging: A review and a new view. In G.H. Bower (Ed.), *The psychology of learning and motivation* (Vol. 22, pp. 193-225). San Diego: Academic Press.

Hill, R., Lewis, V., and Dunbar, G. (2000). Young children's concepts of danger. *British Journal of Developmental Psychology*, 18, 103-120.

Holowinsky, I.V., and Farrelly, J. (1988). Intentional and incidental visual memory as a function of cognitive level and color of the stimulus. *Perceptual and Motor Skills*, 66, 775-779.

Houghton, G., Tipper, S.P., Weaver, B., and Shore, D.I. (1996). Inhibition and interference in selective attention: Some tests of a neural network model. *Visual Cognition*, 3, 119-164.

MacMillan, D., and Wright, D. (1974). Outer-directedness in children of three ages as a function of experimentally induced success and failure. *Journal of Experimental Psychology*, 66, 919-925.

Matson, J.L. (1980). A controlled group study of pedestrian-skill training for the mentally retarded. *Behavior Research and Therapy*, 18, 99-106.

Merill, E.C. (1990). Resources allocation and mental retardation. In N.W. Bray (Ed.), *International Review of Research in Mental Retardation* (Vol. 16, pp. 51-88). Hillsdale, NJ: Erlbaum.

Merill, E.C. (2006). Interference and inhibition in tasks of selective attention by persons with and without mental retardation. *American Journal on Mental Retardation*, 111, 216-226.

Merrill, E.C., Cha, K-H., and Moore, A.L. (1994). The inhibition of location information by persons with and without mental retardation. *American Journal on Mental Retardation*, 99, 207-214.

Merrill, E.C., and O' Dekirk, J.M. (1994). Selective attention and mental retardation. *Cognitive Neuropsychology*, 10, 117-132.

Merrill, E.C., and Taube, M. (1996). Negative priming and mental retardation: The processing of distractor information. *American Journal on Mental Retardation*, 101, 63-71.

Miezejeski, C.M. (1974). Effect of white noise on the reaction time of mentally retarded subjects. *American Journal of Mental Deficiency*, 79, 39-43.

Neil. W.T. (1977). Inhibitory and facilitory processes in selective attention. *Journal of Experimental Psychology: Human Perception and Performance*, 3, 444-450.

Neil. W.T., and Westberry, R.L. (1987). Selective attention and the suppression of cognitive noise. *Journal of Experimental Psychology:Learning, Memory, and Cognition*, 13, 327-334.

Nugent, P.M., and Mosley, J.L. (1987). Mentally retarded and nonretarded individuals' attention allocation and capacity. *American Journal of Mental Deficiency*, 91, 598-605.

Page, T.J., Iwata, B.A., and Neef, N.A. (1976). Teaching pedestrian skills to retarded persons: Generalization from the classroom to the natural environment. *Journal of Applied Behavior Analysis,* 9, 433-444.

Parasuraman, R., and Davies, D.R. (Eds.). (1984). *Varieties of attention.* New York: Academic Press.

Pearson, D.A., Norton, A.N., and Farwell, E.C. (1997). Attention-deficit/hyperactivity in mental retardation: Nature of attention deficits. In J.A. Burack and J.T. Enns (Eds.), Attention, *development, and psychopathology* (pp. 205-231). New York, NY: Guilford Press.

Raven, J.C. (1965). *Guide to using the Colored Progressive Matrices.* London: Lewis.

Sen, A., and Clarke, A.M. (1968). Some factors affecting distractibility in the mental retardate. *American Journal of Mental Deficiency*, 73, 50-60.

Standen, P.J., and Brown, D.J. (2005). Virtual reality in the rehabilitation of people with intellectual disabilities. *Review. Cyber Psychology and Behavior*, 8(3), 272-282.

Standen, P.J., Brown, D.J., and Cromby, J.J. (2001). The effective use of virtual environments in the education and rehabilitation of students with intellectual disabilities. *British Journal of Educational Technology*, 32(3), 289-299.

Tabibi, Z., and Pfeffer, K. (2003). Choosing a safe place to cross the road: The relationship between attention and identification of safe and dangerous road-crossing sites. *Child: Care, Health and Development*, 29, 237-244.

Terdal, L.G. (1967). Stimulus satiation and mental retardation. *American Journal of Mental Deficiency*, 71, 881-885.

Tipper, S.P. (1985). The negative priming effect: Inhibitory effect of ignored primes. *Quarterly Journal of Experimental Psychology*, 37A, 571-590.

Tomporowski, P.D., and Tinsley, V. (1997). Attention in mentally retarded persons. In W.E. MacLean (Ed.), Ellis' *handbook of mental deficiency, psychological theory and research* (3rd ed., pp. 219-241). Hillsdale, NJ: Erlbaum.

Weisz, J. (1979) Perceived control and learned helplessness among mentally retarded and nonretarded children: A developmental analysis. *Developmental Psychology*, 15, 311-319.

Yando, R., and Zigler, E. (1971). Outer-directedness in the problem-solving of institutionalized and nonistitutionalized normally developing and retarded children. *Developmental Psychology*, 4, 277-288.

Young, D.S., and Lee, D.N. (1987). Training children in road crossing skills using a roadside simulation. *Accident Analysis and Prevention*, 19, 327-341.

In: Mental Retardation Research Advances
Editor: Elizabeth B. Heinz, pp. 89-103

ISBN: 978-1-60021-658-9
© 2007 Nova Science Publishers, Inc.

Chapter VI

Neurotrophic Factors in the Pathogenesis of Mental Retardation in Children

Raili Riikonen
Children`s Hospital, University of Kuopio, FINLAND

Abstract

Neurotrophic factors play an important role in early brain development. They are important for neuronal growth, differentiation, survival of neurons and synaptic formation of certain brain cells.

The aim of this study was to analyze neurotrophic factors from CSF in both in acute (severe infantile asphyxia, infantile spasms) and chronic diseases (Rett syndrome, infantile autism, white matter diseases), as well as rapidly progressive diseases (PEHO syndrome and INCL), all leading to mental retardation. It was of interest to see if they could play a role in the pathogenesis, or serve as prognostic markers.

This study shows that BDNF is increased in CSF in neonates suffering from severe asphyxia. In contrast to BDNF levels, levels of CSF NGF were largely decreased in these children. The increased BDNF might counteract neuronal damage observed in these patients following asphyxia. The level of NGF was normal in patients with normal outcome but low or negligible in those with poor outcome. CSF NGF might serve as a marker of asphyxia.

The children with cryptogenic infantile spasms had largely normal levels of NGF but the children with symptomatic spasms had low to negligible levels. The treatment with ACTH led to a greater increase of NGF in patients with good response than in those with a poor response. The therapeutic action of ACTH may be mediated by a potentiation of nerve growth promoting effect.

Patients with Rett syndrome had low concentrations of CSF NGF but normal serum concentrations compared to controls and to autistic patients. NGF is important for the function of cholinergic neurons. In Rett syndrome there seems to be a damage of cholinergic neurons of the basal forebrain.

Low levels of CSF IGF-1 was found in patients with PEHO syndrome with cerebellar atrophy and in white matter diseases. IGF-1 is important for survival of cerebellar neurons and in white matter neurons.

Low-IGF-1 levels were also found in INCL.We also showed apoptosis in brain cells with INCL. Because IGF-1 is antiapoptotic: Low IGF-1 might play a role in the loss of cortical neurons.

Conclusions: 1) Neurotrophic factors may be involved in the pathogenesis of some neurodegenerative diseases 2) Prevention and/or arrest of the process have been tested in vitro and in animal models but still await confirmation in clinical trials. 3) Trials which are ineffective in adults, could be effective earlier in life.

Introduction

There are great hopes for the therapeutic use of neurotrophic factors in adults, (in dementia, amyotrophic lateral sclerosis, Parkinson`s disease, and peripheral neuropathies [1]

In children there are still only a few studies, although the action of nerve growth factors is most intensive in the developing brain.

The aim of this study was to see if nerve growth factors could play a role in diseases of children leading to mental retardation. Both acute and chronic diseases were studied: 1) neonatal asphyxia, 2) West syndrome, 3) Rett syndrome, 4) infantile autism, 5) PEHO syndrome, 6) infantile ceroid lipofuscinosis (INCL), and 7) white matter disease.

A. What Are Neurotrophic Factors?

Neurotrophic factors are important for neuronal growth, differentiation, survival of neurons, and synaptic formation during the development of an infant brain [2]. Withdrawal of neurotrophic factors will lead to apoptosis at early ages but not later [3].

The most important neurotrophic factors are

NGF = nerve growth factor
BDNF= brain derived neurotrophic factor
GDNF= glial cell line derived neurotrophic factor
NT3/4= neurotrophin 3/4
IGF-1= insulin like growth factor-1

The pattern of expression of neurotrophic factors in the CNS and their action is quite distinct.

Neurotrophic factors have specific receptors and are located on specific chromosomes

	Specific receptor	Chromosome
NGF	TrkA	1
BDNF	TrkB	11
GDNF	Ret-c	5
NT3/4	Trk C	15/19
IGF-1	IGF-1	12

Neurotrophic factors act on specific sites in nervous system.

The most well-known neurotrophic factor NGF, *beta NGF*,is the first and best known neurotrophic factor.

NGF was first shown to act on sensory and sympathetic neurons.

Later its activity was shown in the CNS where it acts especially on the cholinergic neurons of the basal forebrain.

NGF activitates the gene expression of CHAT, the enzyme responsible for acethylcholine. It prevents degeneration of cholinergic neurons.

BDNF also acts on the cholinergic neurons but is important for survival for dopaminergic neurons in the substantia nigra, as well as GDNF.

IGF-1 and IGF-2 are members of insulin gene family.

IGF-1 acts specifically on the cerebellum, on granulose and Purkinje cells.

In the brain it is synthesized by neurons and glia cells.

Brain growth is extremely sensitive to levels of IGF-1. IGF-1 knockout gene mice show a microcephaly and demyelination in the whole brain.

Overexpression of IFG-1 leads to macrocephalia.

B. Why the Studies in Children Would Be Important?

The action of neurotrophic factors is most important in brain development.

Brain development is very active: the number of brain cells doubles from the 30th gestational week to the age of 6 months and trebles by the age of 1 year.

During early development, excess of motor and sensory neurons are produced. Only those neurons that have made a tight contact with their tissues receive sufficient amounts of neurotrophins. They continue to develop further. The other neurons are eliminated by programmed cell death (apoptosis).

The brain has a better capacity to recover from insults at early ages. This is considered to be due to increased receptor sensitivity and increased amounts of neurotrophic factors. Brain plasticity is better in young age.

Therapeutic trials with neurotrophic factors might be more important in children than in adults.

C. What Are the Earlier Studies?

The effects of neurotrophic factors have been best described in the peripheral nervous system. Much less is known about the role in the central nervous system. Pediatric studies are scanty.

1989:   Kasain and Neet [4]: detected NGF in human CSF; in one child (a child with "under-developed sympathetic nervous system" and neurological deterioration)

1996:   Lappalainen et al [5] found NGF in The CSF of children with RS by ELISA (all with mental retardation).

1997:   Suzaki et al [6] found high CSF NGF in progressive cortical atrophy and meningitis (all with mental retardation).

2000:   Calamandrei et al [7] found high serum NGF concentrations in Williams syndrome and Down syndrome (all with mental retardation).

2000:   Lipani et al [8] found low NGF in Rett syndrome in postmortem brain.

2001:   Nelson et al [9] found high BDNF and N4/5 in neonatal blood in children with autism and those with mental retardation.

2003:   Chiaretti et al [10]: Correlation between NGF expression and outcome in severe traumatic injury (and poor cognitive outcome).

The aim of our study was to see the role of neurotrophins in the pathogenesis of brain injury after acute insults and of some neurodegenerative diseases,

Further, we wanted to see if neurotrophins could be used as prognostic makers of brain injury and pave the way for rational treatment

We have studied the following diseases, both in acute and chronic diseases. The ethical Committees of the Central Hospitals of University of Kuopio and Helsinki have accepted these studies. Informed consent was given for the patients. A part of these CSF studies were taken for diagnostic evaluation. The CSF was drawn as a part of clinical investigation. CSF of the patients with INCL was taken before the genetic diagnostics was available.

D. The Finnish Study

1. Neonatal asphyxia NGF, BDNF
2. Infantile spasms NGF

PEHO syndrome IGF-1

3. INCL IGF-1
4. Rett syndrome NGF,BDNF, GDNF, IGF-1
5. Infantile autism NGF, IGF-1, IGF-2
6. White matter diseases IGF-1

1. Neonatal Asphyxia

Our patients scored less than 3 Apgar scores and/or umbilical artery ph was less than 7.1. We showed that BDNF is increased in CSF of newborns suffering from severe neonatal asphyxia [11]. In contrast to BDNF levels, levels of CSF NGF were largely decreased in these children. BDNF showed a sharp peak after asphyxia. The level of CSF NGF was low in children with neonatal asphyxia and poor prognosis, but the CSF NGF was normal in patients with neonatal asphyxia but good prognosis [12].

Hypothesis: Neonatal Asphyxia

The increased BDNF might counteract neuronal damage CSF NGF might serve as a marker of asphyxia.

Chiaretti et al 2001 [10] showed similar results after severe brain trauma: BDNF represents an early marker of brain injury.

NGF expression is indicative of a good outcome.

2. Infantile Spasms or West Syndrome

This syndrome consists of infantile spasms, hypsarrhythmia and mental retardation
Age at onset is very typical of this syndrome.
We examined levels of NGF by ELISA in the CSF from 40 children with infantile spasms and in 30 controls [13].

1. The children with cryptogenic spasms (children with no known brain pathology) had largely normal levels of NGF.
2. The infants with symptomatic aetiology had low to negligible levels.
3. The patients with symptomatic, postinfectious (postencephalitic) aetiology for their spasms had very high NGF concentrations. The difference was highly significant.

Why Are the CSF Levels in Patients with Symptomatic Spasms Are So Low?

Low levels of NGF might be due to lack of stimulatory effects.

What Stimulates NGFs?

We know from experiments that steroids stimulate NGFs. Neurons require continuous influx of steroids. CSF ACTH lower in children with symptomatic aetiology for spasms than with cryptogenic aetiology. The measurement was done before starting the therapy.

Treatment with ACTH led to a greater increase of NGF in patients with a good response than in those with a poor response. The therapeutic action of ACTH may be mediated by potentiation of nerve growth promoting activity.

During early development, neurotrophic factors play an important role in the regulation of neuronal development and the formation of synapses. The cortex of a child with infantile spasms with the defective dendritic branching resembles very much that of the immature brain. ACTH could have a "catch-up" effect on the dendrites.

Low levels in patients with symptomatic aetiology possibly reflect massive neuronal death, often seen in neuroradiological studies as atrophy.

The psychomotor regression seen in these infants and their poor response to ACTH may be due to lack of growth factors to support survival of neurones.

Highly damaged brain seems to be unable to synthetize NGF and adequately to react to injury.

Hypothesis: West Syndrome

Therapeutic actions of ACTH may be due to nerve growth promoting activity

3. Rett Syndrome

RS is believed to be a neurodevelopmental disease of girls, affecting only girls. It is characterized by normal early development but then by a failure of brain growth, loss of hand skills, stereotypias, ataxia and apraxia.

Gene mutation is linked to MECP2.

RS is believed to be a neurodevelopmental rather than a neurodegenerative disease because of lack of neurodegenerative changes in postmortem brains. "Major effect of mutations in MECP2 protein is to cause age-related distruption of synaptic proliferation and pruining in the first decade" [14].

We measured the neurotrophic factors; NGF, BDNF, GDNF, and IGF-1 from the CSF and serum [15,16].

We found low concentrations of CSF NGF but normal serum concentrations. Other neurotrophic factors did not differ from the controls.

Here we compared with autistic patients and other controls

Other growth factors were normal as well in CSF as in serum.

NGF is important for the function of cholinergic neurons of the basal forebrain.

Excitatory amino acids (glutamate) were also high in patients with RS, primary or secondary to the neuropathologic changes associated with RS, [17]. Excitatory amino acids may also play a role in the pathogenesis.

Initially, RS is often misdiagnosed as autism.

RS and autism:

Similarities

    a. Early development often regarded as normal
    b. Cognitive deficits and early delays of speech
    c. Repetative, stereotyped behaviour

However, there also many differences

    1. Microcephalia in RS [18]

Normo-or macrocephalia in autism [19,20]
2. Cholinergic neurons in RS [21] Serotoninergic neurons in autism [22]

In PET study by Chugani [22] brain serotonin synthesis capacity was distrupted in autistic children

3. Frontal cortex in RS [8, 18]
Cerebellum and hippocampus in autism [23]. Neuropathological studies have not found any alterations on the forebrain structure in autism.

4. RS: postnatal origin
Autism: early prenatal (at the time of neural tube closure) [24]

We wanted to see whether the two syndromes could be distinguished by their neurotrophin levels. We measured CSF NGF and IGF-1 levels of patients with RS and infantile autism. The CSF samples were drawn as part of clinical investigations.

The patients with RS had all (39/39 patients or 100%) classical Rett syndrome had MECP2 gene which shows that our diagnosis had been made very carefully.

Because the children with autism have multiple aetiologies, we studied the patients very carefully- (careful clinical examination, neuroimaging, chromosomal analysis, EEG, tests of blood and urine for metabolic disorders, CSF examination to exclude encephalitis and progressive encephalopathies)

Only patients with primary autism were included in our study.

CSF NGF

Patients with RS had low levels of CSF NGF. Patients with autism had normal levels of CSF NGF [15, 16].

CSF IGF-1

Patients with RS had normal levels of CSF IGF-1 compared to controls [16]. Patients with autism had low levels of CSF IGF-1 [15,16].

In RS the forebrain is more severely affected than the other cortical areas

Low CSF NGF is consistent with the evidence for loss of basal forebrain cholinergic neurons in RS:

In RS basal forebrain shows

a. reduced volume in volumetric studies the cortical forebrain volume is reduced [18]
b. reduced cholinergic neurons; in size and number [18]
c. reduced choline acetyltransferase (ChAT) [21]
d. reduced NGF concentrations post-mortem [8]
e. hypometabolism of the forebrain [24,25]

The optical density of NGF was low in postmortem brain and also the receptor (TrkA) density [8].

IGF-1 is important for early brain development, myelination, survival of cerebellar neurons (Purkinje cells, granule cells) and has antiapoptotic mechanisms. In the CNS there seems to be selective susceptibility of certain distinct cell types (granule cells, Purkinje cells, oligodendrocytes, motoneurons) to lack of IGF-1.

In autism, many studies show cerebellar development defect.

Reduced numbers of Purkinje cells in the cerebellum have been reported in almost all postmortem studies and thought to be of prenatal origin.

Hypothesis: Rett Syndrome

NGF might play a role in the survival of the cholinergic neurones of the forebrain: Imbalance between neurotrophic factors and excitatory amino acids (low CSF NGF and high CSF glutamate). MECP2 mutation might cause decreased NGF activity and impairment of synaptic development.

4. Infantile Autism

Low CSF IGF-1 concentrations in autism, may point to cerebellar abnormality [26,27].

Low CSF IGF-1 was shown in patients with cerebellar atrophy in our earlier studies.

Taken together,

Our findings are in agreement with different morphological and neurochemical findings in the two syndromes (different brain growth, affected brain areas and neurotransmitter metabolism).

Two progressive neurodegenerative diseases, PEHO syndrome and INCL, are presented in the following.

5. PEHO Syndrome

A specific type of West syndrome which is characterized by progressive encephalopathy, hypsarrhythmia and optic atrophy, oedema [28-30]. The characteristic face shows narrow forehead, epicanthal folds, short nose and small chin. There is early progressive atrophy of the cerebellum (before the age of three years). In the cerebellar cortex the molecular layer is thin, the Purkinje cells are relatively preserved but abnormally small, and the cells of the internal granular layer are almost absent. The levels of nitrate metabolites, nitrite, nitrate were markedly elevated in patients with PEHO syndrome [31]. These metabolites are important in exitoxic mechanisms and neurodegeneration.

We studied IGF-1 from CSF. IGF-1 is known to be important for cerebellar neurons.

Our results showed that the levels of IGF-1 in patients with the PEHO syndrome were significantly lower than in controls or PEHO-like syndrome; patients with similar clinical symptoms without cerebellar atrophy [29].

However, low CSF IGF-1 was not specific for PEHO syndrome. It was also seen in other progressive cerebellar atrophies [29].

6. Infantile Ceroid Lipofuscinos (INCL)

- INCL is characterized by
- normal early development,-
- deceleration of brain growth,
- early psychomotor regression
- EEG isoelectric (age 3 years)
- demyelination (age 9 months-)
- cortical neuronal loss
- chromosome 1 defect (1 p32)
- PPT defect

Infantile neuronal ceroid lipofuscinosis is a progressive encephalopathy in which the patients are severely disabled and in a "vegetative stage" by the age of 3 years. The early development is normal but then it is a deceleration of brain growth. EEG is isoelectric by the age of 3 years. The gene locus has been mapped to chromosome 1p32, and mutations in the gene encoding palmitoyl-protein-thioesterase (PPT) has been identified as the cause of INCL.

INCL is characterized by extreme cerebral atrophy, selective loss of cortical neurons, and secondary loss of axons and myelin sheaths in the white matter, and marked loss of cerebellar neurons (granule cells).

The brain of a child with INCL, small, resembles a walnut.

We found low CSF IGF-1 in patients with INCL at an early stage when myelin was starting to diminish as compared with age-matched controls [32]

When the diagnosis of INCL was made and CSF was drawn, the mean age of the children 19 months.

In NMR at this stage

1. generalized cortical atrophy
2. typical hypointensive thalamus
3. changes in white matter. The first signs of myelin loss are high-signal rims around the ventricles

Our study was the first to show that apoptotic mechanisms are involved in the death of neurons and oligodendrocytes [32].

a. At biopsy: early in the disease: apoptosis
b. At autopsy: only a few cells.

Hypothesis: INCL

The pathology may be associated with low CSF-IGF-1, because IGF-1 prevents apoptosis.

7. White Matter Diseases

We studied IGF-1 in the CSF of children with various white-matter diseases: 1) children with acute disseminated encephalomyelitis and 2) children with chronic diseases: delayed myelination, and progressive leukodystrophies. Al the children with chronic diseases had moderate to severe mental retardation. We found markedly lower concentrations of IGF-1 in the patients than in 28 controls [33] IGF-1 increases both the number of oligodendrocytes and the amount of axonal myelin produced.

HYPOTHESIS: Low CSF IGF-1 can play a role in the pathology of both acute and chronic white-matter diseases in children.

D. What Do These Findings Mean in Practice ?

Hypothesis

Neurotrophic factors decrease the brain damage caused by glutamate, nitrite metabolites and free radicals. Therapeutic approach might be possible.

E. Could NT Therapy Be Useful?

In Vitro—Yes!

Mattson et al 1989 [34] has shown that when a cell was damaged by glutamate and neurotrophic factor has been added to this pyramidal cell culture increased numbers of dendrites, and synapses were developed.

Could Neurotrophin Therapy Be Useful?

In animal experiment- Yes! Neurotrophins have therapeutic effects on:

- chemotherapy-induced peripheral neuropathy [35,36)
- myelination and brain growth [37,38,39]
- neonatal asphyxia [40]
- cerebellar ataxia [41]
- retinopathy of prematurity [42]
- cognitive impairment [43]
- Ototoxic damage [44]

In Humans—Yes! There Have Been Many Therapeutic Trials

Positive effects has been shown in

- body and brain growth [45,46,47]
- insulin resistance [48]
- amyotrophic lateral sclerosis (ALS) [49]
- head injury [50]
- peripheral neuropathy [36,37
- corneal ulcus [52]

In Children-No Data!

The problems in general have been the following:

- Blood brain barrier. Do the drugs across blood-brain barrier (BBB)?
- Side effects
- Short action of the drugs
- Can we make the neurons active?

F. Future

We could perhaps use

1. Neurotrophic factors:

IGF-1 because it a) crosses the BBB [53] b) is atoxic, and when c) combined with binding protein gives steady levels [54-56]

Patients with INCL could perhaps be good candidates for therapy .

2. Drugs stimulating the production of neurotrophic factors [57].

Interestingly; recent data suggest that several drugs already in clinical use increase the synthesis, release, or signalling of neurotrophic factors. Antidepressant drugs increase the synthesis of BDNF in the brain.

3. Viral vectors containing exogenous neurotrophic factors

G. Conclusion

1) Neurotrophic factors may be involved in the pathogenesis of some neurodegenerative diseases
2) Prevention and or arrest of the process of apoptosis have been tested in vitro and in animal models but still await confirmation in clinical trials

3) Trials which are ineffective in adults, could be effective earlier in life

We hope there will be more light in the very near future.

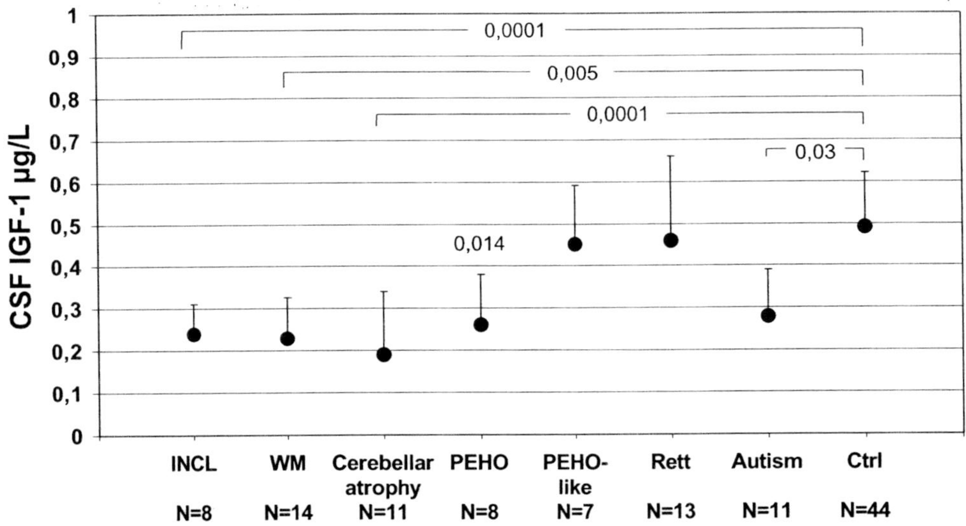

Figure 1. The concentrations of cerebrospinal fluid insulin-like growth factor-1 (IGF-1) in patients with infantile ceroid lipofuscinosis (INCL), white matter disease (WM), cerebellar atrophy, PEHO syndrome, PEHO-like syndrome, Rett syndrome, infantile autism, and controls (Ctrl).

References

[1] Hefti F. Neurotrophic factor therapy for nervous system degenerative diseases. *J. Neurobiol.* 1994; 25: 118-18.

[2] Ebendal T. Function and evolution in the NGF family and its receptors. *J. Neurosci. Res.* 1992; 32: 461-470.

[3] Sofroniew M, Cooper J. Neurotrophic mechanisms and neuronal degeneration. *Neuroscience.* 1993; 5: 285-294.

[4] Kasain M, Neet K. Nerve growth factor in human amniotic and cerebrospinal fluid. *Biofactors.* 1989; 2: 99-104.

[5] Lappalainen R, Lindholm D, Riikonen R. Low levels of nerve growth factor of children with Rett syndrome. *J. Child Neurol.* 1996; 11:1-5.

[6] Suzaki I, Hara T, Maegaki Y et al. Nerve growth factor levels in cerebrospinal fluid from patients with neurologic disorders. *J. Child Neurol.* 1997; 12: 205-207.

[7] Calamadrie G, Alleva E, Cirulli F et al. Serum NGF levels in children and adolescents with either Williams syndrome or Down syndrome. *Dev. Med. Child Neurol.* 2000; 42: 746-750.

[8] Lipani J, Bhattacharjee M, Corey D et al. Reduced nerve growth factor in Rett syndrome post-mortem brain tissue. *J. Neuropathol. Exp. Neurol.* 2000; 59: 889-895.

[9] Nelson K, Grether J, Groen L et al. Neuropeptides and neurotrophins in neonatal blood of children with autism or mental retardation. *Ann. Neurol.* 2001; 49: 597-606.

[10] Chiaretti A, Piastra M, Polidori G et al. Correlation between neurotrophic factor expression and outcome of children with severe traumatic brain injury. *Intensive Care Med.* 2003; 29: 1329-1338.

[11] Korhonen L, Riikonen R, Nawa H et al. Brain derived neurotrophic factor is increased in CSF in children suffering from asphyxia. *Neurosci. Lett.* 1998; 240: 151-154.

[12] Riikonen R, Korhonen L, Lindholm D. Cerebrospinal fluid nerve growth factor – A marker of asphyxia. *Pediatr. Neurol.* 1999; 20: 137-141.

[13] Riikonen R, Söderström S, Vanhala R et al. West syndrome: Cerebrospinal fluid nerve growth factor and effect of ACTH. *Pediatr. Neurol.* 1997; 17: 224-229.

[14] Johnston M, Jeon O, Pevsner J et al. Neurobiology of Rett syndrome, *Brain Dev.* 2001; 23 Suppl 1: S206-213.

[15] Riikonen R, Vanhala R. Levels of cerebrospinal fluid nerve growth factor differ in infantile autism and Rett syndrome. *Dev. Med. Child Neurol.* 1999; 1: 148-152

[16] Riikonen R Neurotrophic factors in the pathogenesis of Rett syndrome. *J. Child Neurol.* 2003; 18:693-697

[17] Vanhala R, Riikonen R. High levels of cerebrospinal fluid glutamate in Rett syndrome. *Pediatr. Neurol.* 1996; 15: 213-216.

[18] Armstrong D, Dunn J, Antalffy B et al. Selective dendritic alterations in the cortexof Rett syndrome. *J. Neuropathol. Exp. Neurol.* 1995; 5: 195-201

[19] Davindovitch M, Patterson B, Gartside P. Head circumference measurements in children with autism. *J. Child Neurol.* 1996: 11:389-393.

[20] Sparks B, Friedman S, Shaw D et al. Brain structural abnormalities in young children with autism spectrum disorder. *Neurology.* 2002:59: 184-192.

[21] Wenk G, Hauss-Wegzryniak B. Altered cholinergic function in the basal forebrain of girls with Rett syndrome. *Neuropediatrics.* 1999; 30:125-129.

[22] Chugani H, Muzik O, Rothermel R et al. Altered serotonin synthesis in dentathalamocortical pathway in autistic boys. *Ann. Neurol.* 1997; 42: 666-669

[23] Rapin I, Katzman R. Neurobiology of autism. *Ann. Neurol.* 1998; 43: 7-14

[24] Rodier P, Ingram J, Tisdale B et al Embryological origin for autism: developmental anomalies of the cranial motor nuclei. *J. Comp. Neurol.* 1996; 370: 27-261.

[25] Lappalainen R, Liewendahl K, Sainio K et al. Brain perfusion SPECT and EEG findings in Rett syndrome. *Acta Neurol. Scand.* 1997; 95: 44-50

[26] Vanhala R, Turpeinen U, Riikonen R. Low levels of insulin-like growth factor-I in cerebrospinal fluid in children with autism. *Dev. Med. Child Neurol.* 2001; 43: 614-616.

[27] Riikonen R, Makkonen I, Vanhala R et al- Cerebrospinal fluid insulin-like growth factors IGF-1 and IGF-2 in infantile autism. *Dev. Med. Child Neurol.* 2006; 48: 751-755.

[28] Somer M. Diagnostic criteria and genetics of the PEHO syndrome. *J. Med. Genet.* 1993; 30: 932-936.

[29] Riikonen R, Somer M, Turpeinen U. Low insulin-like growth factor (IGF-1) in cerebrospinal fluid of children with progressive encephalopathy, hypsarrhythmia, and optic atrophy (PEHO) syndrome and cerebellar degeneration. *Epilepsia.* 1999; 40: 1642-1648.

[30] Riikonen R. The PEHO syndrome. *Brain Dev.* 2001; 23:765-769.

[31] Vanhatalo S, Riikonen R. Markedly elevated nitrate/nitrite levels in the cerebrospinal fluid of children with progressive encephalopathy with edema,hypsarrhythmia and optic atrophy (PEHO syndrome). *Epilepsia.* 2000; 16:705-708.

[32] Riikonen R, Vanhanen S-L, Tyynelä J et al CSF insulin-like growth factor-1 in infantile ceroid lipofuscinosis. *Neurology.* 2000; 5: 1828-1832.

[33] Riikonen R, Turpeinen U. Cerebrospinal fluid insulin-like growth factor 1 is low in acute and chronic white-matter diseases of children. *J. Child Neurol.* 2005; 20:181-184

[34] Mattson M, Murrain M, Guthrie P, Kater S, Fibroblast growth factor and glutamate: opposing roles in the generation and degeneration of hippocampal neuroarchitecture. *J. Neurosci.* 1989; 9: 3728-3740

[35] Apfel S, Arezzo J, Lipson L, Kessler J. Nerve growth factor prevents experimental cisplatin neuropathy. *Ann. Neurol.* 1992; 31: 76-80 Chemotherapy induced neuropathy

[36] Apfel S, Arrezzo J. Lewis , Kessler J. The use of IGF-1 in the prevention of vincristine neuropathy in mice. *Ann. N Y Acad. Sci.* 1993; 692: 243-245.

[37] Carson M, Behringer R, Brister R, McMorris A. Insulin-like growth factor 1 increases brain growth and central nervous system myelination in transgenic mice. *Neuron.* 1996; 39: 114-122.

[38] Lovett-Racke A, Bittner P, Cross A et al. Regulation of experimental autoimmune encephalomyelitis with insulin-like growth factor(IGF-1) and IGF-1/IGF-binding protein-3 complex (IGF-1/IGFBP-3). *J. Clin. Invest.* 1998; 101: 1797-1804.

[39] Yao D-L, Liu X, Hudson L, Webstre H. Insulin-like growth factor -1 given subcutaneously reduces clinical deficits, decreases lesion severity and up-regulates sythesis of myelin proteins in experimental autoimmune encephalomyelitis. *Exp. Neurol.* 1996; 12:1301-1306.

[40] Holzman D, Sheldon A, Jaffe W et al. Nerve growth factor protects against hypoxic-ischemic injury. *Ann. Neurol.* 1996; 39: 114-122

[41] Fernandez A, Dela Vega G, Torres-Aleman I: Insulin-like growth factor I restores motor coordination in a rat model of cerebellar ataxia. *Proc. Natl. Acad. Sci. U S A.* 1998; 95: 1253-258.

[42] Hellström A, Perruzzi C, Meihua J et al Low IFGF-1 suppresses VEGF-survival signalling in retinal endothelial cells: Direct correlation with clinical retinopathy of prematurity. *Proc. Natl. Acad. Sci. U S A.* 2001: 98: 5804-08.

[43] Lupien S, Bluhm E, Ishii D. Systemic insulin-like growth factor-1 administration prevents cognitive impairment in diabetic rats, andbrain IGF regulates learning/memory in normal adult rats. *J. Neurosci. Res.* 2003; 74: 512-23

[44] Nakaizumi T, Kawamoto K, Minoda R, Raphael Y. Adenovirus-mediated expression of brain-dericed neurotrophic factor protects spiral ganglion neurons from ototoxic damage. *Audiol. Neurootol.* 2004; 9: 135-143

[45] Laron Z, Anin S, Klipper-Aurbach Y, Klinger B. Effects of insulin-likegrowth factor, head circumference, and body fat in patients with Laron-type dwarfism. *Lancet.* 1992; 339: 1258-61.

[46] Laron Z. The essential role of IGF-1: lessons from the long-term study and treatment of children and adults with Laron syndrome. *J. Clin. Endocrinol. Metab.* 1999; 8: 4397-4404

[47] Laron Z Insulin-like growth factor-1 (IGF-1): safety and efficacy. *Pediatr. Endocrinol. Rev.* 2004; 2 Suppl 1: 78-85.

[48] Vestergaard H, Rossen M, Urhammer S et al. Short- and long-term metabolic effects of recombinant human IGF-1 treatment in patients with severe insulin resistance and diabetes mellitus. *Eur. J. Endocrinol.* 1997; 136: 475-82

[49] Lai E, Felice K, Festoff M et al Effect of recombinant human insulin-like growth factor-1 on progression of ALS. *Neurology.* 1997; 49: 1621-30

[50] Hatton J, Rapp R, Kudsk K et al. Intravenous insulin-like growth factor-1 (IGF-1) in moderate-to-sever head injury: a phase II safety and efficacy trial. *J. Neurosurg.* 1997: 86: 779-86

[51] Apfel S, Kessler J, Adornato B et al. Recombinant human nerve growth factor in the treatment of diabetic polyneuropathy. NGF Study Group. *Neurology.* 51: 695-702.

[52] Lambiase A, Rama B, Bonini S et al. Topical treatment with nerve growth factor for corneal neurotrophic ulcers. *N. Engl. J. Med.* 1998; 338: 1222-3

[53] Pan W, Kastin A. Interactions of IGF-1 with blood-brain barrier in vivo and in situ. *Neuroendocrinology.* 2000; 72: 171-178.

[54] Lewis M, Neff N, Contreas P et al. Insulin-like growth factor-1: Potential for treatment of neuronal disorders. *Exp. Neurol.* 1993: 124: 73-88.

[55] Dore S, Kar S,Quirion R. Rediscovering an old friend; IGF-1: potential use in the treatment of neurodegenerative disease. *Trends Neurosci.* 1997; 20:326-331.

[56] Riikonen R. Insulin-like growth factor delivery across the blood-brain barrier. Potential use of IGF-1 as a drug in child neurology. *Chemotherapy.* 2006; 52: 279-281.

[57] Castren E. Neurotrophic effect of antidepressant drugs. Curr Opin Pharmacol 2004; 4: 58-64. *Neurobiology.* 2004 29:289-301.

In: Mental Retardation Research Advances
Editor: Elizabeth B. Heinz, pp. 105-146

ISBN: 978-1-60021-658-9
© 2007 Nova Science Publishers, Inc.

Chapter VII

Mental Retardation and Mental Illness: An Overview

Alka S. Ahuja[1] and Srinivas Reddy[2]
[1] Consultant Child and Adolescent Psychiatrist and Honorary Lecturer,
Gwent NHS Healthcare Trust, St. Cadoc's Hospital, Newport NP18 3XQ,
U.K. and Cardiff University, South Wales, U.K.
[2] Specialist Registrar in Child and Adolescent Psychiatry,
Gwent NHS Healthcare Trust, St. Cadoc's Hospital, Newport NP18 3XQ, U.K.

Abstract

There have been significant advances in our understanding of the pathophysiology of mental retardation in the last decade. This has been associated with a sociocultural change in conscience regarding people with mental retardation and carer support ushering a revolution in ethics of care. This chapter aims to review the current understanding of the concept of mental retardation, etiological understanding of intelligence and its impairment, assessment methods and management strategies for associated mental health disorders and disabilities. Mental retardation is identified clinically as a developmental disorder. Research in etiology of mental retardation has identified biological, environmental and psychological factors capable of producing deficits in intellectual function. The co-occurrence of psychiatric illness with mental retardation has been well established, and people with mental retardation are more likely to suffer from ill mental health (including behavioural disorders, personality disorders, autistic-spectrum disorders and attention- deficit hyperactivity disorder). These conditions are often underdiagnosed due to issues such as " diagnostic overshadowing", the tendency by which clinicians tend to overlook additional psychiatric diagnosis once a diagnosis of mental retardation is made; or "masking" in which the clinical characteristics of a mental disorder are masked by a cognitive, language or speech deficit. People with mental retardation share many mental health needs with the general population. The concept of 'normalisation', individual rights and respect for the wishes of individuals with mental retardation has complemented the deinstitutionalised community care, career support and psychopharmacological advances in psychiatry.

However, due to a variety of reasons their care has to be specifically tailored to meet these needs.

Introduction

History

Mental retardation can be found as far back in history as the therapeutic papyri of Thebes (Luxor), Egypt, around 1500 B.C. These documents clearly refer to disabilities of the mind and body due to brain damage [1]. However the status and care received by individuals with mental retardation varied greatly depending on cultures and periods of history.

In 1689, John Locke published his famous work entitled 'An Essay Concerning Human Understanding' [2]. Locke believed that an individual was born without innate ideas and described mind as a 'tabula rasa', a blank slate. This profoundly influenced the understanding of care and training provided to individuals with mental retardation. He also was the first to distinguish between mental retardation and mental illness.

A cornerstone event in the evolution of the care and treatment of the mentally retarded was the work of physician Jean-Marc-Gaspard Itard [1] who was hired in 1800 by the Director of the National Institutes for Deaf-Mutes in France to work with a boy named Victor. Victor, a young boy, had apparently lived his whole life in the woods of south central France. Based on the work of Locke and Condillac who emphasized the importance of learning through the senses, Itard developed a broad educational program for Victor to develop his senses, intellect, and emotions. After 5 years of training, Victor continued to have significant difficulties in language and social interaction though he acquired more skills and knowledge than many of Itard's contemporaries believed possible. Itard's educational approach became widely accepted and even to this day it is used in the education of the deaf.

Itard later supervised Edouard Seguin [1] who developed a comprehensive approach to the education of children with mental retardation, known as the Physiological Method [1]. Assuming a direct relationship between the senses and cognition, his approach began with sensory training including vision, hearing, taste, smell, and eye-hand coordination. In 1850, Seguin moved to the United States and became a driving force in the education of individuals with mental retardation. In 1876, he founded what would become the American Association on Metal Retardation. Many of Seguin's techniques are still in use today.

The newly developed test of intelligence developed by Binet [3] was translated in 1908 by Henry Goddard, who published an American version of the test in 1910. In 1935, Edgar Doll developed the Vineland Social Maturity Scale to assess the daily living skills/adaptive behavior of individuals suspected of having mental retardation [3]. Psychologists and educators now stepped in with medical professionals in believing that it was possible to determine who had mental retardation and provide them with appropriate training in the residential training schools. Training schools were widely established. The training schools, which were initially more educational in nature, became custodial centres breeding institutionalism. In the 1970's, a landmark class action suit in Alabama established the right to treatment of individuals living in residential facilities and purely custodial care was no longer acceptable. The United States Congress passed the Education for the Handicapped Act in 1975, now titled the Individuals with Disabilities Education Act [4], and amended in 1986. This Act guaranteed the appropriate education of all children with mental retardation and developmental disabilities, from school age through 21 years of age and provided incentives for states to develop infant and toddler service delivery systems. Today, most states in the USA guarantee intervention services to children with disabilities between birth and 21 years of age. In the United Kingdom this age is 18 years. The implications indirectly extend to include management of mental illness coexisting with mental retardation.

The terminology used for this group of individuals has varied with time. Several traditional terms denoting varying degrees of mental deficiency long predate psychiatry. In North America the broad term 'developmental delay' has become an increasingly preferred synonym by many parents and caregivers. The term developmental disability can also refer to any other physical or psychiatric delay, such as delayed puberty. Intellectual disability and learning disability are increasingly being used as a synonym for people with significantly below-average intelligence. Mental handicap is the term used by the UK Mental Health Act 1983 [5]. However the American Association on Mental Retardation [6] continues to use the term mental retardation which is adopted by the Diagnostic and Statistical Manual IV-DSM IV [7]. Due to concern about the over identification or misidentification of mental retardation, particularly in minority populations, the definition was revised in 1973 [8]. A 1977 revision [9] modified the upper Intelligence Quotient (IQ) limit to 70 - 75 to account for measurement error. IQ performances resulting in scores of 71 through 75 were only consistent with mental retardation when significant deficits in adaptive behavior were present. The recognition regarding association of mental illness with mental retardation has developed significantly ever since, Kraepelin described 'Pfropfschizophrenie' i.e. schizophrenia engrafted upon mental retardation [10]. Kraeplin also differentiated it from "oligophrenia", which is associated with low psychic or mental functioning without psychopathology [10] in people with mild retardation, suggesting a neurodevelopmental origin. In general, the types of psychopathology suffered by patients with mental retardation resemble those of normal individuals [11]. However, many studies, notably the Isle of Wight Study [12], have documented that these occur together at a greater-than-normal incidence. The current literature supports the idea that psychiatric disturbances are more common in patients with mental retardation than in persons of normal intelligence. On the other hand, the evidence regarding specific mental disorders being necessarily associated with mental retardation has been the subject of continuing controversy.

Mental Retardation and Patient Role

A diagnosis of mental retardation by itself does not amount to a disorder. A vast majority of children and adults with mental retardation live in the community with very little need of involvement from health and social services. When otherwise healthy persons with mental retardation seek help from a doctor, or are admitted to hospital, it may be assumed that they are in some perturbation of mind or as well as of body. The perception of suffering in the mind makes every patient different, even when their condition is familiar and well recognized. The mental element in any illness varies enormously with circumstance, intellectual ability and temperament. Recognition of mental retardation and its contribution to etiopathogenesis of mental illnesses may help us understand these concerns better.

Visiting a familiar doctor is usually less of an ordeal for the patient than admission to hospital as the person often retains familiarity and possibly the dignity of independence. However elements of personal distress may mask or distort the objective signs and symptoms for which the doctor is trained to look. This is more likely in this group of individuals and worsens when they are admitted as inpatients. Careful observations may need time and information from carers in interpreting symptoms. Each person thinks he is reacting normally to the predicament of illness, real or imaginary, and will expect the same degree of medical attention. This subjectivity is no different in people with mental retardation. A sensitive evaluation is needed to tease out an individual's reactions from a recognisable abnormal mental state. The intellectual abilities and developmental factors may further complicate the picture.

Nomenclature

The American Association of Mental Retardation decided by consensus in 1993 that the term 'mental retardation' was most appropriate term to describe this group of individuals [13]. It is defined as ' a disability characterized by significant limitations both in intellectual functioning and in adaptive behavior as expressed in conceptual, social, and practical adaptive skills. This disability originates before the age of 18 years'. It is used internationally and is concordant with the definition of the multidimensional International Classification of Impairments, Disabilities, and Handicaps from the World health Organisation [14]. Five assumptions essential to the application of the definition are

1. Limitations in present functioning must be considered within the context of community environments typical of the individual's age peers and culture.
2. Valid assessment considers cultural and linguistic diversity as well as differences in communication, sensory, motor, and behavioral factors.
3. Within an individual, limitations often coexist with strengths.
4. An important purpose of describing limitations is to develop a profile of needed supports.
5. With appropriate personalized supports over a sustained period, the life functioning of the person with mental retardation generally will improve.

The International statistical classification of diseases and related health problems, 10th edition - ICD 10 [15] and DSM IV [7] refer to substantial limitations in present functioning characterised by significant sub-average intellectual functioning existing concurrently with related impaired limitations in two or more of the following applicable skills areas: communication, healthcare, home living, social skills, community use, self direction, health and safety, functional, academic leisure and work and manifest before the age of 18.

This definition regards mental retardation as a state rather than as a stable trait. It does not call it a disorder and although functioning is impaired it may improve with appropriate input. Diagnostic and Statistical Manual of Mental Disorders -DSM IV [7] uses the definition put forth by the American Association on Mental Retardation. It however retains the severity level classification. The upper IQ (Intelligence quotient) limit is 70. However, it should be noted that comprehensive cognitive and adaptive skill assessment is necessary to make the diagnosis; it should not be made on the basis of an office visit or developmental screening. ICD 10 [15] characterises mental retardation as a condition resulting from a failure of the mind to develop completely. Unlike DSM-IV, ICD-10 suggests that cognitive, language; motor, social, and other adaptive behavior skills should all be used to determine the level of intellectual impairment and supports the idea of dual diagnosis, suggesting that mental retardation may be accompanied by physical or other mental disorders. Four levels of mental retardation are specified in ICD-10: mild (IQ 50 - 69), moderate (IQ 35 - 49), severe (IQ 20 - 34), and profound (IQ below 20). IQ should not be used as the only determining factor in making a diagnosis of mental retardation.

Psychopathology and Mental Retardation

Psychopathology in mental retardation may vary depending on the cognitive and intellectual ability and also on the level of communication. In addition neurological and genetic phenotypes of mental retardation may present with unique symptoms. Therefore psychopathology associated with mental retardation can be discussed in 3 ways:

1. psychopathology and developmental psychopathology of mental retardation
2. psychopathology of co morbid conditions of neurological and genetic origin
3. psychopathology of co morbid psychiatric disorders/mental illness

This chapter focuses on the characteristics and uniqueness of psychopathology of co morbid psychiatric disorders/mental illness in people with mental retardation. However, some relevant psychopathology of mental retardation and symptoms of neurological causes and genetic causes will also be discussed.

1. Psychopathology and Developmental Psychopathology of Mental Retardation

People with mental retardation have difficulty in acquisition of basic living, educational, and social skills that is apparent early in life together with evidence of a significant intellectual impairment. Some with more severe mental retardation however may have impairments of such severity that meaningful language is never acquired and there are very substantial care needs. In a significant proportion subtle signs of early developmental delay, together with evidence of learning difficulties only become apparent at school. The role of assessment is essentially to determine need and to inform the types of intervention and treatments, whether educational, medical, psychological, or social, that are likely to be effective. Systems of classification provide a useful framework for such an assessment.

Intelligence is not a unitary characteristic but is assessed on the basis of a large number of different more or less specific skills [15]. The general tendency is for skills to develop relatively to similar levels in each person but there can be large discrepancies. Some people with mental retardation can have severe impairments in one particular area, or may have a particular area of higher skill. This may present problems in determining diagnostic category to which the person with mental retardation should be classified. For a definite diagnosis, there should be a reduced level of intellectual functioning resulting in impairment in adaptive skills particularly in relation to normal social environment [15]. DSM-IV provides a framework for multiaxial diagnosis with the Axis II for personality disorders and the level of mental retardation. The focus is not primarily one of aetiology but rather of quantifying the extent of mental retardation. Adaptive functions that might be impaired depending on the level of intellectual functioning are used to help determine the level of mental retardation (mild, moderate, severe, or profound). Adaptive functioning has to be measured against what would be expected for a person of that age, and socio cultural background. The Wechsler Intelligence Scale for adults [16] and children [17] and the Vineland Adaptive Behaviour Scales [18] are validated instruments for the measurements of intellectual abilities for which there are normative data for comparison. Without the use of standardised procedures the diagnosis has to be a provisional estimate only. The diagnostic categories within mental retardation are essentially arbitrary divisions of a complex continuum [15]. The diagnostic guidelines for mild, moderate, severe and profound mental retardation generally correspond to appropriate standardised IQ rating scale scores. Challenging behaviour is a commonly used term to describe unexplained behavioural disturbance in people with mental retardation. It refers to behaviour of such an intensity, frequency and duration that the physical safety of the person or significant others are placed at risk. The term challenging behaviour was adopted from The Association for Persons with Severe Handicaps (TASH) [19]. Emerson et al [20] defines severely challenging behaviour as " Behaviour of such an intensity, frequency or duration that the physical safety of the person or others is likely to be placed in serious jeopardy, or behaviour which is likely to seriously limit or delay access to and use of ordinary community facilities". Challenging behaviour may thus restrict or limit access to, opportunities for normalised psychosocial functioning and is often a final common path of many causes.

Challenging behaviours may include aggression both verbal and physical, self-injurious behaviour, non-injurious stereo-typed behaviours. ICD 10[15] provides an option of including it with the diagnosis of mental retardation as impairment of behaviour. But this is a diagnosis clinically meaningful when all contributory psychiatric causes for such behaviour are excluded. A small number of people with mental retardation behave in ways which people without learning disabilities find difficult. For example, they may scream or hurt themselves. Some people behave like this because they are frustrated or because they cannot communicate their needs to others. The best way to deal with challenging behaviour is to find out the cause of the behaviour. This may necessitate observation by carers for a behavioural analysis. Sometimes a person with challenging behaviour may need medication if psychosocial interventions do not produce significant change.

It is difficult to assess the prevalence of challenging behaviour as this assessment is based on the social definition of challenging behaviour, individual perception of carers and the set of circumstances [21]. Between 5 and 15 per cent of people with mental retardation are reported to have some form of challenging behaviour such as aggression and self-injury which present significant challenges to carers, either because the person's own health and safety is at risk or because they place others at risk. Challenging behaviour may start in early childhood and continue into adulthood [21]. Research into challenging behaviour suggests that challenging behaviour is commoner in men, in those with specific disorders (e.g. autistic spectrum disorder) and with additional disabilities (e.g. hearing problems or communication disorders) and in the severely learning disabled.

In most cases, the challenging behaviour occurs in circumstances when a person has little control over their life or tries to exercise some powers. It may also occur because the person with mental retardation is frustrated at his or her inability to make others understand what he or she needs.

Challenging behaviour can sometimes be linked to mental health problems such as depression and evidence about the relative effectiveness of different ways to help people with challenging behaviour suggests benefits from individually planned behavioural assessments [22]. This can often be difficult, if the person has no speech or has other communication problems. Relaxation and social skills may sometimes help such people manage their anger or anxiety. Cognitive-behavioural approaches can also be useful. Use of medication, should be restricted to only those circumstances when all other measures have failed in controlling the behaviour.

2. Psychopathology of Co Morbid Conditions of Neurological and Genetic Origin

There are nearly 500 identified genetic disorders associated with mental retardation. Many of these disorders play a causal role in mental retardation. However, most of the causal relationships must be inferred [23]. The American Association on Mental Retardation subdivides the disorders that may be associated with mental retardation into three causes: prenatal causes, perinatal causes, and postnatal causes. The AAMR classification system focuses on the capabilities of retarded individuals rather than on their limitations. The categories describe the level of support required, including intermittent support, limited support, extensive support, and pervasive support. The AAMR classification mirrors the DSM-IV-TR classification. A complete list of these disorders is beyond the scope of this chapter. It should also be noted that mental retardation is both a symptom of other disorders as well as a unique syndrome or disorder. This again is inferred by our limited ability in identifying causes only in a proportion of people with mental retardation. The most common factor associated with severe mental retardation has been chromosomal abnormality, particularly Down's syndrome [24]. In approximately 20 to 30% of the individuals identified with severe mental retardation the cause has been attributed to prenatal factors, such as chromosomal abnormality. Perinatal factors such as perinatal hypoxia and obstetric complications are decreasing as are postnatal factors such as brain trauma. In 30 to 40% of cases, the cause is reported to be unknown. Other neurological conditions associated with mental retardation include epilepsy and various other neurological syndromes. Often these complicate the picture and may present as behavioural abnormalities or rarely psychiatric syndromes. Their relevance is never to be underestimated and a need for a detailed neurological assessment is important. They are also relevant in management since the medications used to treat them can interact and sometimes present with psychiatric side effects.

3. Psychopathology of Co Morbid Psychiatric Disorders/Mental Illness

Study of psychopathology among people with mental retardation presents unique challenges due to some of the following reasons:

a. Developmental and intellectual abilities may restrict expression of psychopathology
b. The unique clarity and structure of symptoms such as delusions and hallucinations may be relatively restricted
c. There are no universally agreed criteria for diagnosis though recently attempts have been made
d. Often diagnosis is based on behavioural observations and course of illness due to limitations in communication

Since its first meeting in 1964 in Montpelier, the International Association for the Scientific Study of Intellectual Disability had fostered the importance of health issues in mental retardation [25]. Mental health issues have since then evolved with the formation in recent years in the United States of the Association for Dual Diagnosis [26], and in Europe, the European Association for Mental Health in Mental Handicap [27].Further discussions about psychopathology are discussed with individual psychiatric disorders in this chapter.

Epidemiology

There are inherent problems in estimating prevalence of mental disorders in people with mental retardation. In the past various terms have been used which are ill-defined, culture-specific, and changeable social labels which are either stigmatizing or promoted as non-stigmatizing [28]. Incidence and prevalence of a heterogeneous group such as 'people with mental retardation', however defined, are determined by the varying frequencies of a wide range of disorders of different aetiology. The general health of people with mental retardation, and especially people with Down's syndrome, is poorer than that of the general population [29]. Recent statistical surveys, [30] have confirmed that epilepsy, mental illness, obesity, and general unfitness are especially common in this population.

International differences in prevalence, quality of life, morbidity, and life expectancy for people with mental retardation are grossly estimates [31]. Theoretical approaches to determining the prevalence of mental retardation uses the normal bell curve to estimate the number of individuals whose IQ falls below the established criterion score [32]. Epidemiological studies have demonstrated high rates of additional disability due to the presence of sensory and physical impairments, behavioural and psychiatric disorders, and/or a developmental profile indicative of autism [33]. Various findings relevant to prevalence of mental retardation have relevance in further studies evaluating mental illnesses in this subpopulation. Prevalence varies between similar births cohorts (concurrent age groups) in different communities. This is evident within developed countries e.g. 1.62/1000 children born in 1951-55 in Salford, United Kingdom, and 7.34/1000 children born in 1957 in Amsterdam. Greater variation is expected in developing countries, especially where there are environmental factors like iodine deficiency disease. Down syndrome is often the largest aetiological group [34]. This may be more evident in communities where traditions relating to late conception are prevalent, for example late marriage, taboos against contraception and/or abortion, and where early mortality is low. Age-specific prevalence may vary over time in the same community. Age-specific prevalence was generally low (1.8-4.0 in 1000) for children born in the early 1950s, and high (3.3-5.5 in 1000) for those born in the early 1960s, but has fallen since then. The increase was largely due to decreased early mortality and increased survival associated with better neonatal care. This phenomenon is well documented for Down syndrome from life-table studies and may be shared by other syndromes [35]. Preventive programmes for several aetiological groups including postnatal screening amniocentesis and abortion programmes have reduced Down syndrome, inherited metabolic disorders and sporadic congenital hypothyroidism creating a cumulative effect [36]. Perinatal factors probably now produce fewer neurological impairments though there is no clear evidence. Large-scale immunization has reduced secondary infectious diseases. Early identification and treatment of some syndromes has diminished residual impairments, and early stimulation and training in management has improved function. Prevalence may vary by age because of different samples of cohorts based on pre/peri and postnatal interventions which change over periods in time. Survival has increased at all ages and this may affect prevalence of different causes of mental retardation. This is more prominent among communities with better perinatal care. Prevalence and mortality data available can be used to estimate age-specific prevalence ratios. However this may be difficult when migration changes the population [37]. There are usually more males than females at all ages in the subpopulation with mental retardation. The ratio varies between 1:1 and 2:1, but with no clear pattern [38-44]. There are often no clear explanations and it could be due to vulnerability to morbidity, differential incidence and mortality. Recent studies suggest a social class gradient consistent with the known social distribution of morbidity and mortality but this may have confounding variables affecting preventable causes.

Most individuals with mild intellectual impairment will be identified as having learning disability at school, but numbers will depend upon the legal, professional, and administrative conventions of the school system. These individuals are more likely to be labeled if they also have epilepsy, communication problems, multiple physical disabilities, mental illness, or challenging behaviour, and if they are unemployed, from a low socio-economic status, a poor home environment, or have inadequate parental care. There are no representative prevalence data for these groups. Studies identifying the criteria for selection in different countries and communities which determine prevalence would help us understand prevalence rates and may guide community care planning [38-44].

Data available from developing countries suggests variable differences related to the varying spectrum of preventable organic causes, mortality, and social situations. The variability is more a marker of health, social and education than to do with economics alone. Due to methodological difficulties similar to mild mental retardation, prevalence studies of moderate mental retardation are less sensitive. For individuals with severe mental retardation (SMR), the disabilities usually necessitate special supports and services. In epidemiological studies of SMR, the condition has often been defined and identified according to the level of service need. Therefore, for SMR ascertainment prevalence is considered to be a reasonable estimate of true prevalence. Severe intellectual impairment is often recognised early. A comparative study in nine countries showed similar figures, except in Southern India [45- 46] where migration was considered a cause for high teenage figures. Precise comparative statistics between countries may not be crucial especially for mental retardation. It is vitally important to identify locally preventable etiological factors and strategically manage them. The rates of SMR however correlate better between different geographical areas than milder forms of mental retardation [38].

Prevalence of psychiatric disorders in people with mental retardation is restricted by all the drawbacks of epidemiological identification of mental retardation. In addition eliciting psychopathology needs to overcome the developmental and communication challenges of people with mental retardation. In addition studies looking at specific psychiatric disorders among people with mental retardation are relatively few [47-48].

Studies into the prevalence of psychiatric illness among adults with intellectual disability report a wide range, between 10% - 39%, depending on the sample selection and definition of psychiatric illness. Some studies include diagnoses such as behavioural disorders, pervasive developmental disorders and dementia. In addition the diagnostic criteria used and diagnostic methods vary [49]. It is not clear whether or not the rate of psychiatric illness increases with the severity of intellectual disability and also whether mental illness in general is more prevalent in people with mental retardation. Schizophrenia and psychoses in particular are present in people with severe and profound intellectual disability [50- 52]. Psychiatric morbidity is also found in 61.9% of adults with intellectual disability aged over 65 years [53]. Among adults aged 50 years and over, the prevalence of psychiatric disorders excluding dementia is 11.4% and the prevalence of dementia is 11.4% [54]. The rates of psychiatric illness as well as behavioural disorder in adults with intellectual disabilities and epilepsy are not significantly different from those in non-epileptic adults with intellectual disabilities [55-56]. The rate of functional psychiatric illness (excluding dementia and behavioural problems) in adults with severe intellectual disabilities but not Down syndrome is six times higher than in adults with intellectual disabilities and Down syndrome [57]. Controversial evidence exists as to the higher rate of depressive illness reported among people with Down syndrome compared with non Down syndrome adults with an intellectual disability [58- 59].

Studies into the prevalence of specific psychiatric illnesses amongst adults with intellectual disability indicate that some conditions are more prevalent than others in people with intellectual disability [60-63]. The point prevalence of schizophrenia is reported as between 1.3% and 3.7%. The point prevalence of affective disorders including depressive illness and mania are reported as between 1.2% and 6%.The point prevalence of anxiety related disorders in adults is reported as 6.4%. The prevalence of attention deficit hyperactivity disorder (ADHD) amongst adults with severe and profound intellectual disability (15%) is similar to children with severe intellectual disability (18%), but higher than in children with average intelligence (3%-5%) [64]. There is an association between depression and aggression with 40% of adults, adolescents and children with both intellectual disability and depression exhibiting aggression [65]. Up to 5 years after community resettlement, people with mental retardation show little change in the prevalence of psychiatric diagnoses or behavioural disturbance [66]. Outreach treatment represents an effective and efficient alternative to hospital treatment for people with mental retardation and psychiatric disorders [67- 68]. Assertive community outreach treatment or intensive care significantly decreased the bed use and hospital admission in people with borderline intelligence and psychiatric illness when compared with those who receive standard community care [69]. 17% of people with mental retardation referred to psychiatrists as emergencies presented with behavioural problems such as severe physical aggression and self-injurious behaviour [70].

Aetiopathogenesis of Mental Illness in Mental Retardation

Study of aetiological factors among people with mental retardation has provided insights into the multifactorial causative factors contributing to the aetiology of mental illness. The initial emphasis on biological causative factors including genetics has yielded good results in finding the aetiology of mental retardation. Phenotypic studies to evaluate the genotypic factors have reduced the unknown cause percentage in moderate/severe mental retardation to 20 per cent. Over 500 recognized syndromes involving genetic disorders are now recognised. However characterisation of uniqueness of phenotypic behavioural epiphenomena associated with genetic syndromes is at best suggestive and most people with mental retardation need genetic testing for diagnosis. Some genetic syndromes have characteristic behavioural symptoms which may aid in diagnosis along with characteristic dysmorphic features.

The advances in genetics, pathology, behaviour analysis, applied social research, and ethology has radically improved our knowledge of behavioural phenotypes. The most widely studied is the Down's syndrome [47]. Though the results of association between Down's syndrome and psychiatric disorders remains unclear, the debate has improved the understanding and demystifying aetiology of challenging behaviour in people with mental retardation. There is increasing evidence that such behavioural disturbances are not always related to psychiatric disorders [47]. A chain of constraining psychosocial and environmental events can be set off by a single factor which need not be necessarily negative. However the importance in understanding aetiology lies in the inherent intractability and indetectability of aetiology lending psychosocial and environmental factors as the only therapeutically modifiable factors. Such interventions have proven long term benefits and form an important component of management.

Challenging behaviours present a significant challenge in establishing aetiopathogenesis and can be described as encompassing many, if not all presentations of adjustment problems, physical illness and psychiatric disorder. A comprehensive aetiological formulation is invaluable in planning successful intervention. The behavioural disturbance augments the impairment of mental retardation resulting in increasing care needs.

The scope of this chapter is in discussing various psychiatric disorders associated with mental retardation. The various ways in which this association presents could be discussed as follows,

a.　Chance association of psychiatric disorder with mental retardation
b.　Increased incidence of psychiatric disorders among people with mental retardation
c.　Decreased incidence of psychiatric disorders among people with mental retardation

The problems in evaluating such probable associations have presented some unique challenges such as

1.　Diagnostic overshadowing- intellectual disability and communication difficulties obscure the diagnosis of a mental health disorder
2.　Importance of neurodevelopmental processes in aberrant behaviour.
3.　Specificity of aetiological association to mental retardation and psychiatric disorders
4.　Co morbid neurodevelopment disorders
5.　Lack of evidence for later/earlier onset of psychiatric illnesses
6.　Relative paucity of studies specifically studying association between mental retardation and psychiatric disorders

1. Diagnostic Overshadowing

Improved diagnostic tools have enabled clinicians to recognize affective disorder as the commonest psychiatric diagnosis in people with mental retardation [52]. The lifetime risk of schizophrenia is 3 per cent in people with mental retardation compared to 1 per cent in the ordinary population [60-62]. Historically this overlap has not been clear. The needs of the individual with both mental retardation and mental illness are still overshadowed by a primary diagnosis of mental retardation [71]. Overshadowing involves an emphasis of treatment on "mental retardation" rather than "mental illness."

2. Importance of Neurodevelopmental Processes in Aberrant Behaviour

Mental illnesses such as schizophrenia are now increasingly being viewed from a neurodevelopmental perspective. New techniques in neurological, metabolic and blood flow functional imaging along with advances in genetic testing have provided more insights into aetiological causes of mental illness. Various suggestive pathological insults and the temporal relationship between intrauterine injury and to early onset schizophrenia have been reported. A significant proportion of people with mental retardation have neurodevelopment anomalies prenatally. The nature of such changes is non specific. The extent of such a change confounding the association between mental retardation and schizophrenia remains unclear.

3. Specificity of Aetiological Association to Mental Retardation and Psychiatric Disorders

Although there is evidence to suggest neurodevelopment factors in aetiology there is a significant lack of association between the types of mental retardation and specific psychiatric disorders. There has also been an increase in survival of infants with very low birth weight and functional disorders caused by subtle neurological damage such as attention-deficit hyperactivity disorders and pervasive developmental disorder are also increasingly being diagnosed. However the specificity of association between any recognisable brain pathology and specific psychiatric illness has not been identified.

The most studied association between Down's syndrome and depression has not shown any such relationship.

4. CoMorbid Neurodevelopment Disorders

Comorbid neurodevelopment disorders often coexist with mental retardation. The commonest are pervasive developmental disorders and epilepsy. Both genetic and environmental factors play a part in the development of these conditions. One-third of toddlers with autism lose their skills at around 18 months although this may even happen in adolescence. This widely reported deterioration may yet be another example of a relatively small environmental insult destabilizing an immature or genetically predisposed brain [72].

5. Lack of Evidence for Later/Earlier Onset of Psychiatric Illnesses

The age distribution for onset of psychiatric disorders in people with mental retardation is not specific for most disorders. With the exception of adults with Down's syndrome, other adults with mental retardation are at the same risk for Alzheimer's disease as are other adults in the general population. A few rare genetic syndromes have a degenerative course associated with progressive cognitive deficits.

6. Relative Paucity of Studies Specifically Studying Association between Mental Retardation and Psychiatric Disorders

Compared to prevalence of psychiatric disorders in normal population, evidence for mental illness prevalence among people with mental retardation is lacking. Most studies looking at psychiatric morbidity have methodological problems. These relate to selection of samples and the inherent difficulties in diagnosing mental retardation in community studies. Difficulties in ascertaining diagnosis by self rating and reliance on self rating in subgroups that may be unable to communicate clearly limit the validity and generalisation of results. These factors need to be explored in each individual presenting with mental illness and mental retardation to elicit the aetiopathogenic factors. Exploring factors contributing to aetiology may require significant investment in observation and behavioural analysis but plays a significant part in managing behaviour and limit impairment. Further discussions about aetiopathogenesis are considered for individual disorders where relevant later. Psychiatric disorders are relatively more common in individuals with mental retardation than in the general population [43]. The disability resulting from psychiatric disorder and mental retardation results in handicap and impairment accounting for more than just adding up individually resulting impairments. This results predominantly from changes in behaviour through loss of social, educational and psychological opportunities. The resulting personal stress, distress for carers, and cost to the community are increasingly being quantified. However it is difficult to assess the magnitude of the problem and it remains relatively unrecognised. However large scale studies done recently have questioned the contributory risk of mental retardation to mental illness [73]. The presence of mental retardation and reasons for its increased association with psychiatric disorder needs to be explored [43]. The aetiologic role of mental retardation is at best at the level indicating mental retardation as vulnerability. Some recognised syndromes have well established association with behavioural difficulties and self harm, for example Lesch Nyhan syndrome associated with self injurious behaviour. But there is no established association with phenotypes of serious mental disorders. There are legitimate concerns regarding under recognition of dual disability. The reasons vary from diagnostic overshadowing [71] in which psychiatric disorders in persons with mental retardation are identified as simply being a feature of their intellectual handicap, to acceptance of limitations of our knowledge of psychopathology and in validating psychopathology objectively when cognitions and communication may be impaired.

Assessment and Diagnosis

Mental health professionals will be called on, at some time, to evaluate and treat individuals with mental retardation. Often this may be in crisis situations requiring emergency admissions or in inpatient facilities. It is essential, therefore, that they are familiar with the basic tools needed for assessment and treatment planning at the interface of mental retardation and psychiatric disorders. It has been estimated that 40% to 70% of individuals with mental retardation have diagnosable psychiatric disorders [74]. This subgroup of individuals, are not the only ones who come in contact with medical professionals. A person with mental retardation may present with emotional, behavioral, interpersonal, or adjustment problems that do not constitute major psychiatric disorders but that may benefit nonetheless from psychiatric input. Psychiatric care of individuals with mental retardation is most effectively rendered when a multidisciplinary team approach is used [75]. This team must take into account not only the acute problem but also the patient's relationship to long-term caregivers. A successful treatment outcome often depends in part on how well the professionals can bridge the gap between different conceptual models (medical versus rehabilitative), clinical languages, and organizational management.

There is consensus about difficulties in using current classification for people with mental retardation [75, 76]. This is due to disagreement regarding specific classification for mental retardation due to limited description of the phenomenology and variability of symptoms dependant on developmental level. The developmental cognitive aspect of psychopathology in young people adds another dimension in relevance of objectifying criteria for psychiatric disorders in young people with mental retardation [76]. With these limitations the DSM-IV [7] or the ICD-10 [15] can be used as they are evidence based systems of classification relevant to all people by the principle of generalisation. However reliability and validity of this approach when applied to children with mental retardation is still to be fully established in the subpopulation with mental retardation. These diagnostic categories require information on emotions, cognitions and perceptions which may be compromised sometimes due to difficulties in communication, especially in those with moderate and severe mental retardation. Communication difficulties including language impairment, adaptive functioning and presence of other co morbid conditions also need careful evaluation. Restrictions on dual diagnosis which are mutually exclusive (schizophrenia and Asperger's syndrome in DSM IV) are increasingly being questioned in the light of recent evidence and may need to be corrected in future classifications[7]. Classification of mental disorders using diagnostic criteria within ICD-10 or DSM-IV may be suitable for people with mild mental retardation. They lack validity and utility for people with more severe mental retardation, with autistic spectrum disorders and in those with attention deficit hyperactivity disorder associated with mild learning disabilities. Diagnostic Criteria for Psychiatric Disorders for use in adults with Learning Disabilities- DC-LD [77] provides more appropriate operationalized diagnostic criteria within a classification system specifically designed for use in adults with learning [intellectual] disabilities, and is complementary to ICD-10. It is based on the principle of broadening the diagnostic categories to avoid diagnostic confusion. It is only suitable for use by professionals trained in making psychiatric diagnosis. Some patterns of emotional and behavioural disturbance are described as being specific to persons with mental retardation, especially in DSM IV like stereotypic movement disorder. There have been descriptions of other patterns of emotional and behavioural disturbance that may occur exclusively in persons with mental retardation [76]. But such specificity is hard to validate as a specific psychiatric disorder and may face the same hurdles and criticisms of disorders specific to culture bound syndromes. They may be a marker of developmental level and intellectual ability influencing the presentation of symptoms. With these limitations some findings may be relevant as representing a decompensation or variable presentation due to cognitive and intellectual abilities. Adult patients with mild mental retardation, compared with patients with higher intellectual functioning, are more likely to have externalizing symptoms. If the people with mental retardation have psychotic symptoms, they are more likely to experience hallucinations without delusions [60]. These findings are similar to psycho-pathology in children in general and hence may represent developmental aspects of behaviour rather than being specific. It is however unclear and further research needs to clarify such issues and their relevance especially with the generally held view about disruptive conduct, withdrawal and attention and impulse control problems being more common among people with mental retardation. Population studies of children with mental retardation have shown autistic, and withdrawn behaviours to be more common in those with severe disability whereas anxiety, disruptive, and aggressive behaviours are more common in those with milder levels of mental retardation [76]. Standardized informant questionnaires that rate disturbed emotions and behaviour have been used. The Psychiatric Assessment Schedule for Adults with Developmental Disability (PAS-ADD) checklist is a screening instrument designed to assist staff in recognizing mental health problems among people with mental retardation, and consists of a checklist of life events and symptoms, scored on a four-point scale. [78]. The Diagnostic Assessment for the Severely Handicapped II is a scale that is linked to DSM-IV. The anxiety, autism and schizophrenia subscales have been validated [79]. The Cambridge Cognitive Examination is a group of tests that are included in the Cambridge Examination for Mental Disorders of the Elderly. It was originally designed to assess cognitive impairment characteristic of dementia in the elderly population [80]. Direct neuropsychological tests such as the Mini Mental State Examination are difficult to use reliably in adults with Down's syndrome [81]. Matson et al. [82] validated an instrument to measure social skills among those with severe and profound mental retardation. Their study described initial psychometric measures for the Matson Evaluation of Social Skills in individuals with Severe Retardation. The Minnesota Multiphasic Personality Inventory-168 (L) is a useful abbreviated version of the Minnesota Multiphasic Personality Inventory. It has previously been shown to have substantial validity and test-retest reliability when administered to adults and adolescent persons with mild and moderate mental retardation [83]. Factor analysis of commonly used rating scales individually identified six relatively consistent groupings of disturbance in people with mental retardation: aggression or antisocial behaviour, social withdrawal, stereotypic behaviours, hyperactive or disruptive behaviour, specific repetitive communication disturbance, and anxiety fearfulness. The Developmental Behaviour Checklist is specific for use in children and adolescents with mental retardation [84]. The existing multiaxial classification systems such as DSM IV and ICD-10 are currently used for diagnosis for people with mental retardation. Information from carers or staff from care homes along with observation and information from people with mental retardation is currently the norm in reaching diagnostic conclusions. Axis 2 on DSM IV multiaxial system is used to represent the level of MR. Information gathered from informant questionnaires may supplement and improve clinical assessment, communication and research. The clinical assessment of young people with mental retardation and psychiatric disorder requires a consideration of their developmental and cognitive abilities. Some relevant aspects influencing presentation of mental retardation and psychiatric disorder and their relative importance varies with severity of symptoms and cognitions.

Mental retardation may obscure the standard diagnostic indicators of psychiatric disorders. Especially for the psychiatrist unaccustomed to the normal manifestations of mental retardation, those manifestations may overshadow symptoms attributable to psychiatric illness [71]. Impairments in cognitive and verbal skills make it difficult for many developmentally disabled individuals to articulate abstract or global concepts such as a depressed mood. Most DSM-IV diagnoses require that the patient describe his or her internal state. Asking a person with severe mental retardation about hallucinations, delusions, or guilt may often not be productive. A clear onset of disorganized behavior may have diagnostic significance. Sovner [85] identified four aspects of mental retardation that may influence diagnosis:

a. Intellectual distortion - emotional symptoms are difficult to elicit because of deficits in abstract thinking and in receptive and expressive language skills.

b. Psychosocial masking - limited social experiences can influence the content of psychiatric symptoms (e.g. mania presenting as a belief that one can drive a car).

c. Cognitive disintegration - decreased ability to tolerate stress, leading to anxiety-induced decompensation (sometimes misinterpreted as psychosis).

d. Baseline exaggeration - increase in severity or frequency of chronic maladaptive behavior after onset of psychiatric illness.

To allow for these possible distortions, Sovner proposed that the standard diagnoses for mania and depression be modified, when applied to the developmentally disabled, to focus on biologic signs and symptoms and behavioral equivalents to subjective states.

A comprehensive cognitive assessment provides essential information required to interpret behaviour in a developmental context, make a diagnosis and plan management. The intellectual and communicative language ability of the young person will influence their perceptions and their ability to communicate their thoughts and emotions. Subjective experiences and emotions are difficult to be definitive without a subjective description by patients. This can be generalised to people with mental retardation. However symptoms of psychopathology and emotions may be indirectly expressed through developmental manifestation of behaviour similar to that seen in normal younger children [84]. The most frequent being depression manifesting as irritable behaviour. In younger persons with more severe levels of cognitive impairment, the expression of emotional and behavioural problems are more difficult to interpret and hence more often classified under unclassified or organic brain syndromes. Cognitive abilities vary individually and for example can be generalised among children with autism as to being better on performance tasks than tasks that involve visual motor skills or performing relatively poor on verbal and social comprehension tasks [86]. Recognising this helps in interpreting symptoms and diagnosis. It also contributes to planning their educational needs and other management issues. The study of motivation early in development indicated that childhood characteristics, including aspects of temperament such as emotionality and activity level, contribute to behavior [87].Consequently childhood temperamental characteristics have been identified as important predictors of psychiatric disturbance in children. This is true particularly among children with mild mental retardation compared to children with more severe retardation. No evidence exists regarding its relevance in later adulthood. Temperament may not be directly amenable to change, but may improve parental understanding and management skills, leading to better adaptation and the reduction in emotional and behavioural problems [87].

Medical assessment is a necessary component of the psychiatric assessment of people with mental retardation. It may sometimes help to establish the cause of the mental retardation and may also indicate presence of any associated medical condition that might contribute to, or complicate, the physical, emotional and behavioural problems. Young people with mental retardation have an increased risk of medical problems [48]. Other than physical complications associated with some specific syndromes, they predominantly involve the brain, such as epilepsy and cerebral palsy. Specific medical complications may be associated with known causes of mental retardation such as cardiac and bowel problems that occur in Down syndrome. Epilepsy is the most common neurological comorbidity associated with mental retardation [88]. In the US less than 1% of the general population has epilepsy. The prevalence of mental retardation is approximately 0.3-0.8%, but 20-30% of children with mental retardation have epilepsy. Approximately 35-40% of children with epilepsy also have mental retardation. Recent studies suggest that rates of psychopathology in people with mental retardation who have epilepsy are not increased except perhaps in those with poor seizure control [73]. The pathology for such association is non specific in most people with mental retardation except in some children with specific causes like tuberous sclerosis. Such lesions of tuberous sclerosis are implicated in the development of epilepsy and a range of psycho-pathological disorders including tic disorder, autism, and psychosis.

Children with mental retardation are more likely to experience adverse experiences in life compared to children in community [89]. They are more likely to undergo potential traumatic experiences like respite and institutional care, but are also a more vulnerable group susceptible to social rejection, teasing and bullying., adjusting to school and peers.

They are also more likely to be abused [89]. Cognitive abilities limit adaptability, understanding and coping abilities in socially stressful experiences and may contribute to behavioural disturbance. The potential parental experiences of emotions may involve over involvement, grief, guilt, hostility, ambivalence, and rejection. The financial burden of care, parental emotions and relationships may play an aetiological role in psychiatric presentations and need to be explored with respect to impaired attachment, relationships, and symptoms of current behavioural phenotypes [90]. Behavioural problems, perceptual and sensory deificits and communication difficulties impair attachment and parent-child interaction [90] and this may be more marked in certain subgroups of children e.g. those with autism.

Neglect, lack of stimulation, and lack of opportunity for play and social interaction can further impair the normal development. These can be relative and inappropriate depending on impairments of the child with mental retardation, for example a child with mental retardation needs to over learn some motor sequences to master activities of daily living, but parents may be doing the same level of training as for other normal children. Such impairments need to be assessed and rectified early on in the child's life to prevent difficulties later and also to help parents cope with the child better. Mothers may experience higher levels of stress with a disabled child than fathers. This may be related to more maternal involvement and responsibility for care [91] and may be culturally determined. Cultural caring responses, expectations, and attitudes may influence parenting, emotional development and behaviour of children with mental retardation [91]. Observation of child's interaction with family and carers, and a detailed history, early development and psychosocial history may help in understanding etiologic factors contributing to psychopathology and help in management of children with mental retardation and mental health problems.

Principles of Psychiatric Assessment

The components of such an assessment need to accommodate the developmental and communicative abilities of the person and should be ideally performed in a multidisciplinary setting involving carers. The principles of risk assessment also need to be followed carefully in order to avoid adverse experiences to patients. A thorough history is crucial for a psychiatric diagnosis. It can be obtained from three sources: the patient, other informants, and medical records. Some guidelines are useful for interviewing the person with mental retardation. Talking to the person helps even if it appears that he/she might not understand. A person's receptive language skills are likely to exceed his or her expressive skills. Attention to the person's developmental level may necessitate talking in a more concrete fashion, focusing on the here and now, and using words appropriate to the person's level of understanding. Leading questions are to be avoided and physical expressions and gestures to communicate with the person are helpful. Techniques such as metaphor and storytelling may also facilitate communication. Observation of the person's nonverbal interactions, especially with familiar caregivers may indicate mood and psychomotor activity along with rapport and eye contact. Informants such as the family or staff can provide information unobtainable from the patient directly. It is helpful to empathize with the informant's experience in caring for or working with the developmentally disabled person. Recent changes in the person's physical or social environment, such as a move from school to day programming or a workshop, a change of residence, loss of a favorite staff member, or anniversary dates of losses, bereavement and change of permanent carers especially in care homes may precipitate psychiatric disorders or present with behavioural problems. Circumstantial patterns such as symptoms associated with a particular setting or time of day helps to differentiate an underlying psychiatric disorder from a situational response. A longitudinal history to correlate with concurrent events such as stressors, medical problems, and medication changes may point to aetiological and maintaining factors.

Patient records are useful sources of information. Psychological evaluation with baseline data on IQ, level of adaptive functioning, language and communication skills, and ability to interact with others provides good insight. This data can be contrasted with current status to identify decompensation. Social and developmental history including prenatal history, pregnancy, birth process, and early environment, may suggest aetiological causes of mental retardation. A detailed family history including relationships and environment, history of mental retardation, mental illness, and other medical disorders is useful. Medical history needs to include cerebral palsy, sensory deficits, epilepsy, and other neurological disorders. Dysmorphic syndromes may be associated with medical problems. History of sleep, weight, and activity levels, previous consultations, laboratory findings and medication history should be included. Drug interactions can often precipitate aggression or self-injurious behavior.

Longitudinal behavioral data, when correlated with concurrent events such as environmental stresses, medical problems, and changes in medications, can contribute significantly to diagnosis and treatment. If possible, identify target behaviors that are symptoms of the underlying psychiatric disorder and may be drug responsive, such as sleep disturbances in major depression. Establish baseline rates of the target behavior(s) to monitor response to treatment.

Mental state examination is an essential step in differentiating psychiatric from medical or situational problems and to assess risk. It includes the person's general appearance, rapport with the examiner and others in the room, level and fluctuation of consciousness, psychomotor retardation or agitation, mood, range and appropriateness of affect, ability to communicate, ability to follow simple commands, memory, orientation and any observed abnormal involuntary movements such as tremors, stereotypies, automatisms, or self-injurious behavior. A thorough medical evaluation is needed to rule out an organic cause of a change in mental state or maladaptive behavior. It is especially important because people with mental retardation have an elevated rate of associated physical disabilities. The physical examination must be performed systematically and patiently. Occasionally, when the individual is uncooperative and organic pathology is strongly suspected, sedation may be necessary especially for detailed investigations. Routine laboratory work varies with age and the physical condition of the person. Electrocardiogram (ECG), measurement of electrolyte levels, complete blood count, screening blood chemistry, urinalysis, and measurement of folate and B-12 levels, syphilis serology, and thyroid function tests are commonly done depending on the differential diagnosis. Sometimes it may include an Electroencephalogram (EEG), brain imaging such as a CT or MRI, and blood level measurements, especially of anticonvulsants may be necessary. Drug interactions and medication side effects must also be considered e.g. benzodiazepines with long half-lives may accumulate, leading to drowsiness and mental clouding. Short-acting benzodiazepines may cause interdose rebound symptoms, with marked worsening of anxiety just prior to scheduled doses. Anticonvulsants may produce excessive sedation and antipsychotic drugs can have serious side effects, such as parkinsonism and akathisia that may be confused with worsening agitation. Excessive doses of antipsychotic drugs can interfere with alertness and overall performance andresponse to psychotropic medication may be idiosyncratic and often require very low doses for required response. Other medications whose effects should be monitored include antihypertensive drugs, eye drops for glaucoma (often beta-adrenergic blockers), and allergy medications (anticholinergic or antihistaminic).

As part of the multidisciplinary team approach, the evaluation may be broadened to include, as needed, consultations with the disciplines of internal medicine, gynecology, neurology and behavioral neurology, neuropsychology, pharmacology, hearing and speech therapy, physical therapy and occupational therapy.

Specific Psychiatric Disorders and Mental Retardation

Genetic Syndromes

A number of identified genetic syndromes are associated with characteristic patterns of behaviour and an increased risk of specific psychiatric disorders. Such identified behavioural phenotypes may help in diagnosis and management. Some of these are briefly described below.

Down Syndrome

Reports indicate that there is a high prevalence of psychiatric disorders and behavioural problems in people with Down syndrome [92]. Children with Down syndrome are more likely to present with externalizing disorders such as oppositional defiant disorder, conduct problems and attention-deficit problems [92]. This pattern changes in adolescence and young adulthood when persons with Down syndrome are more likely to suffer from affective disorders and dementia. A wide range of psychiatric disorders have been reported in this population, including anorexia nervosa, phobias, obsessive- compulsive disorder, mood disorders, autism, Tourette's syndrome, and schizophrenia [93-94].

Fragile X Syndrome

Fragile X syndrome is the most common genetic cause of mental retardation [95]. It is associated with characteristic behavioural problems. Uniquely a differentiation in behavioural phenotypes has been described based on sex. Boys are observed to be anxious, shy and avoiding eye contact. They may have problems with attention and hyperactivity and may sometimes present with stereotypy such as hand-flapping [95].

Girls have a similar presentation, but it is not usually as pronounced as that seen in boys. There is no evidence suggesting an association with autism. although about 5 to 10 per cent of males with fragile X have an associated autistic disorder [95]. However the behavioural signs are non specific for diagnosis on their own.

Prader-Willi Syndrome

Children with Prader-Willi syndrome have mild mental retardation and increased appetite. A significant proportion of affected children have obsessive thoughts about food and a preoccupation with seeking food [96]. They may need continuous supervision and a control over their eating habits in order to prevent life-threatening obesity [96]. They can also frequently present with other serious emotional and behavioural problems and significant proportions have obsessive compulsive symptoms. Behaviour problems such as aggression, skin picking, and oppositional defiance are also common and may be persistent [96]. The symptoms however change with age, with anxiety and low mood being more prevalent in older adolescents and adults. Risk of psychosis and pervasive developmental disorders may also be increased in some of these individuals [96].Some suggest that such an association is more likely if there is a maternal disomy of chromosome 15 which is relatively less common than the usual deletion on the long arm of the paternal chromosome 15.

Smith-Magenis Syndrome

This is due to chromosomal deletions at 17p11.2. The individuals usually have moderate levels of mental retardation and the behavioural phenotypes are characteristically hyperactive, impulsive, and aggressive. They may have an unusual minimal need for sleep [97] and are also prone to motor mannerisms such as 'self--hugging' when happy or excited. About 20 per cent present with severe self-injurious behaviours such as head banging, pushing objects into body orifices pulling nails and biting [97].

Williams Syndrome

Individuals with William's syndrome have microdeletion on chromosome 7 and usually present with moderate mental retardation. They have a specific profile of cognitive abilities with visuospatial and visuomotor deficits. Paradoxically a skill at recognizing facial features is reported in some children. Expressive language may be well developed in a small subgroup and they may present as chatterboxes, with an adult manner of speech due to the stereotypic use of phrases learnt from adult conversation [98]. In adolescence they may present with anxiety, hyperactivity, short attention span, and poor concentration.

Rett Syndrome (RS)

This condition affects only females and is characterized by hand-wringing movements, variably progressing neurological deterioration and mental retardation. The discovery of a genetic mutation (MECP2) on the X chromosome (Xq28) provided significant insight into the cause of Rett syndrome [99]. This mutation has now been found in more than 95% of those meeting criteria for typical RS and more than 50% meeting those for atypical RS. The defective gene, MECP2, or methylcytosine binding protein, is apparently lethal in males, accounting for its exclusive female presentation. Because of unusual X inactivation patterns, some females with MECP2 mutations may be normal or have mild learning disability and will not be identified unless they transmit the mutation to a daughter who develops RS. It is now known that RS can occur in males with Klinefelter syndrome (XXY) or somatic mosaicism in which some cells express the normal MECP2 and others the abnormal MECP2.The child with RS usually shows an early period of apparently normal or near normal development until 6-18 months of life. The child then loses communication skills and purposeful use of the hands and slowing of the rate of head growth becomes apparent. Soon, stereotyped hand movements and gait disturbances appear [99] with progressive deterioration.

Angelman Syndrome

Angelman syndrome is a genetic disorder correlated with mental retardation, motor impairments, lack of vocal speech, muscular hypotonia, epilepsy, and frequent smiling and laughing [100]. The most common genetic anomaly responsible for Angelman syndrome is a partial deletion of chromosome 15q11-q13 (70% of all cases). Many children with Angelman syndrome engage in repetitive and stereotyped motor behavior and in several case studies and group design studies based on parental report, researchers have found that smiling and laughing exhibited by over 80% of these individuals occurs excessively and independent of environmental context [101].

A number of other behavioural phenotypes exist and a complete description is beyond the scope of this chapter.

Organic Disorders

Dementia

Dementia is a common problem associated with mental retardation. Adults with Down syndrome have an especially increased risk of early onset of Alzheimer's disease, with nearly all developing characteristic nervous system changes by age 40[93]. After age 50, almost half of those with Down syndrome have symptoms of Alzheimer's disease. Mentally retarded adults without Down syndrome also have an increased risk of Alzheimer's disease [93]. Common symptoms of dementia among those with Down syndrome include loss of ability to adapt and increased episodes of being agitated or aggressive.

The dementia is often associated with depression, indifference, and socially inappropriate behaviors. The number of older adults with mental retardation is increasing, because life span is increasing. Life expectancy of mentally retarded people increased from 20 years in the 1930s to 60 years in 1980. Average life expectancy has increased by about 30 years for those with Down syndrome, which is the most recognizable form of mental retardation. [102]. This number is expected to double by 2030.These data help in assessing the magnitude of the problem in the absence of epidemiological studies.

Research surveys suggest that 25% of mentally retarded adults have no useful speech, and that 10% lack basic comprehension skills. Approximately half of mentally retarded adults cannot care for themselves, half have a physical disability, and half have problems getting around. These problems tend to increase in later life, because of continued mental decline and loss of mobility associated with age. One out of every 10 mentally retarded adults is totally dependent on others. These may alter the clinical presentation and also increase the disability experienced by these individuals [102]. Over 75% of adults with mental retardation live at home and are cared for by aging family members. This often leads to a crisis when parents are no longer able to provide adequate care or cannot manage a behavioral problem.

Prompt detection and treatment of mental or medical conditions improves the life expectancy and quality of life of people with mental retardation. Although the basic approach to the diagnosis and treatment of illness is no different than in anyone else, the process needs to consider the special needs of someone with mental retardation. For example, people with mental retardation typically have poor verbal skills, making it difficult for them to express how they feel or what they are thinking. Instead, mental illness often shows up as changes in behavior. Careful physical and laboratory evaluations, along with sophisticated neurological tests can often be used to determine a cause. Older adults with mental retardation who develop further intellectual deterioration or behavior problems may benefit from a referral to a specialist for an assessment.

Appropriate treatment depends on the underlying physical or mental problem. The approaches used to treat psychiatric problems are similar to those used for people without mental retardation. These include both behavioral therapy and drug treatment. Of course mental limitations may make treatment more complicated in adults with mental retardation. Evidence for use of cholinergic drugs is lacking, but may be of benefit in the early stages

Epilepsy and Mental Illness

According to current epidemiological studies, at least 1% of the general population in the United States is diagnosed with epilepsy and 10% have experienced a seizure at some point in their lifetime. Prevalence estimates for epilepsy vary in people with developmental disabilities, ranging from 12% to 30% for persons with co morbid disabilities and associated brain pathology e.g. Tuberous sclerosis [58]. Behavioral manifestations of seizures may include simple repetitive movements, such as repeated chewing, or complex motor movements and tics. However, to date, no empirical link between epileptic events and bouts of problem behavior has been documented for people with developmental disabilities. Treatment recommendations are generalised from normal population and may not always be appropriate.

Psychotic Disorders and Schizophrenia

Adults with mental retardation exhibit the same types of psychiatric disorders as adults of normal intelligence, although an accurate diagnosis is often difficult to make. Though initial reports suggested an increase in the prevalence of schizophrenia in people with mental retardation, they remain disputed. Diagnostic overshadowing, for example, in which abnormal behaviors are assumed to be the result of mental retardation rather than potential co morbid psychopathology, may obscure identification of psychiatric conditions. An examination of specific types of disorders is needed for a more complete understanding of the clinical features of psychiatric disorders in persons of varying levels of intellectual impairment [103].

The classification of psychosis based on symptomatology may present difficulties in those with mental retardation. Most information is extrapolated from studies of adults with mild mental retardation and psychosis. However difficulties in cognitive abilities and communication may mask the clinical presentation. Delusions and hallucinations are present but are usually less elaborate and poorly systematized [49]. Occasionally impulsive, aggressive, and unpredictable behaviours may dominate the clinical picture. Delusions or hallucinations may be seen as agitation, sleeplessness, or aggression. Medical problems such as chronic pain may also present as behavioral problems in people with mental retardation and will need to be differentiated from psychotic features. Catatonic features may be present in these individuals [104].

Establishing the diagnosis of sub types of schizophrenia in someone who has mental retardation can be a difficult, especially if there is severe retardation and no verbal communication. Presence of chronic persistent negative symptoms after an acute episode may aid in diagnosis rarely. The male: female ratio seems to be equal and the age of onset is similar to the general population [52]. There appears to be no specific relationship with epilepsy or chromosomal abnormalities, although paranoid syndromes are often associated with disorders of hearing and vision [52]. Acute psychosis in children with mental retardation is uncommon. In adults acute psychosis may be precipitated by stressful life events and recovery is usually complete within a few weeks [104].

Pharmacological management needs to be coordinated with a comprehensive needs assessment. Neuroleptic drugs are the most frequently prescribed agents for aggression, self-injury, and hyperactivity in people with mental retardation. Increasingly, they should be reserved for those in whom intensive behavioral intervention has failed. Atypical antipsychotic drugs in smaller doses may help to reduce side effects.

Mood Disorders

Depression

This is a frequently diagnosed mental health problem in individuals with mental retardation, with prevalence estimates equivalent to those in the general population [105]. Research in the field of mental retardation has focused primarily on the prevalence, assessment, definition, and correlates of depression, with some advances being made to treatment models for depression, both behavioral and pharmacological.

Milder forms of depression may be difficult to diagnose although dysthymia is a recognised diagnosis in this subgroup.

Studies have supported associations between depression and cognitive variables, such as hopelessness, automatic thoughts, and a low frequency of self-reinforcement [106]. The leading cognitive theories of depression such as the diathesis-stress models [107] have been generalised to all subpopulations including mental retardation. Specifically, there is disagreement whether standard criteria from DSM-IV [7] and the ICD-10 [15] should be used to diagnose depression in individuals with mental retardation or whether behavioral equivalents should be incorporated into diagnostic procedures. Behavioral equivalents for depression in individuals with mental retardation include self-injury, aggression, and screaming [108]. However the association between such behavioral equivalents and self-reported depression has not been established due to difficulties in measurement. Another reason for the controversy regarding the best strategy for diagnosing depression in persons with mental retardation is that the DSM-IV and ICD-10 criteria rely heavily on self-reports, which are suspected to be less valid in persons with mental retardation than in the general population. Individuals with severe and profound mental retardation are likely to be nonverbal and thus standard criteria may be more appropriate for individuals with mild or moderate mental retardation [108-109]. Informant report instruments commonly used in research and for screening purposes have been found to correlate poorly with self-reports of depression among individuals with mental retardation [110]. Informants usually describe valid accounts of the behavioral symptoms of depression, but report poorly on internalizing symptoms (e.g. feelings of worthlessness, suicidal ideation) because they are less readily observable. A similar trend has been observed in the general population, with parents having less awareness of their children's internalizing than externalizing symptoms [111]. Therefore validated interviews and screening procedures are required that can be administered directly to individuals with mental retardation to assess the internalizing symptoms of depression. The somatic symptoms of depression including psychomotor activity, reduced interest, increased fatigue, sleep disturbances, changes in appetite and weight may be useful indicators of depression in the absence of clear mood disturbances. An episodic illness with clear onset may help in diagnosis especially with good informants and past history.

In people with milder forms of depression focusing on psychosocial and environmental factors may benefit the individual. There are no large scale studies evaluating the treatments for depression in people with mental retardation. The guide to treatment is dependant on cognitive abilities to effect good communication for cognitive and behavioural interventions. More severe forms usually need drug treatment e.g. antidepressants. Antidepressants are used for several major psychiatric illnesses, including major depression and other depressive disorders [112]. Selective serotonin reuptake inhibitors (SSRIs) are the treatment of choice, given the more favorable side effect profile when compared with older antidepressants. However, lack of response after four to six weeks of treatment at therapeutic doses warrants reconsideration of the diagnosis and, if necessary, trials of other antidepressants such as other SSRIs, venlafaxine, trazodone, tricyclic antidepressants, or moclobemide. The majority of studies include fluoxetine [112] in treating depressed adolescents with developmental disabilities. Antidepressants should be used cautiously in this population as they may trigger a manic or hypomanic switch, especially in rapid cycling individuals or in those with mixed affective states. People with developmental disabilities are more prone to such effects of antidepressants [112].

Bipolar Disorder

Little is known about how mania manifests in people with mental retardation. Prevalence of individuals being dually diagnosed with bipolar disorder and intellectual disabilities has ranged from 0.9% to 4.8% of the intellectually disabled population [113]. These estimates vary due to the difficulties in diagnosing bipolar disorder in this population. There is no evidence suggesting an increased prevalence of bipolar disorder in mental retardation. A diagnosis of bipolar affective disorder may be difficult, especially in more severe forms of mental retardation and diagnosing bipolar disorder in this population remains challenging because of difficulties in communication, atypical presentation, and lack of clear diagnostic criteria . Methods relying on self-report of feelings may not be possible. Ruedrich (1993) suggested that the appearance or presentation of bipolar disorder in this population may be distinctly different from the presentation in the general population [113]. However such assertions have not had consistent evidence [114] and Sovner asserted that mood disorders in the intellectually disabled population are more often atypical, chronic, or rapid cycling. Self injurious behaviour and aggression are frequent symptoms. In occasional instances efficacy of mood stabilisers may be the only reliable evidence [115]. Rapid cycling pattern of bipolar disorder is often recognised in this population. A detailed monitoring of mood may provide the required evidence for diagnosis. Elated or irritable mood may be a recognisable symptom. An episodic behavioural change can be a sign of onset of mood disorder. The relationship of stressful factors precipitating onset of mood disorders remains unclear among people with mental retardation, but needs to be explored. A decreased need for sleep has been noticed to be a reliable symptom to help in differentiating behavioural problems from bipolar disorder [116]. These findings are in line with previous results suggesting that clinicians can focus on observable symptoms in cases when DSM-IV criteria are not applicable [117].

Lithium may be useful in the treatment of acute mania, cyclothymic disorder, and the prophylaxis of bipolar illness type I [112]. A number of studies reported that lithium might be beneficial in patients with developmental disabilities and concurrent aggression and mood lability [112]. However, this population is more prone to developing toxic side effects to lithium and thus requires close monitoring. Valproic acid is the treatment of choice of rapid cycling and mixed states [112]. Thus, mood stabilisers may be used in the treatment of acute mania, the prophylaxis of bipolar illness, type I, cyclothymic disorder, and challenging behaviours but the side effects need to be carefully monitored.

Anxiety Disorders

The phenomenology of clinical features and prognosis of specific anxiety disorders in children with mental retardation are very few. However clinically significant symptoms of anxiety are more common in this group compared to the general population. The prevalence rates are 10 to 12 per cent and it is equally distributed among boys and girls with mental retardation [48]. This is in contrast with the general population of children where the prevalence of anxiety disorders is about 2 to 5 per cent, affecting twice as many females. Also children with mental retardation are more likely to have simple fears characteristic of younger children such as fear of loud noises, the dark, insects, and animals [118-119]. Phobias can present in adults with mental retardation too and could be longstanding. Separation anxiety may begin in much older children with a developmental age less than 5 years. Hence it needs to be differentiated from anxieties of much later age of onset. The same may be true for early childhood phobias. Systematic desensitization approach with relaxation and modeling is helpful as part of the management plan [119].

While assessing people with mental retardation, clinicians should pay close attention to avoidant and possibly agoraphobic behaviors, particularly if they represent a change from previous behavior patterns [118]. Vague, inconsistent, or multiple somatic complaints, especially those leading to repeated visits to doctors' offices or the emergency department, should alert practitioners to consider psychiatric etiologies such as panic.

Adverse life experiences such as institutionalisation, physical and sexual maltreatment, and neglect are more common in children with mental retardation. These experiences are potentially capable of producing adjustment disorders and post-traumatic stress disorder. Vulnerability to post-traumatic stress disorder probably increases with falling IQ levels because of a reduced capacity to intellectually resolve the experience [57]. Such claims can be potentially controversial especially with unproven association between intellectual abilities and symptoms of post-traumatic stress disorder and the error may lie in ascertaining the diagnosis. A more recognised form of adjustment disorder is one of bereavement and physical illness. Often the bereavement could be a period of long absence of a carer, especially in care homes. Knowledge of past history is invaluable in raising sensitivity for such adjustment problems.

Obsessive-compulsive symptoms are common in children with mental retardation and autism. However a diagnosis of obsessive compulsive disorder needs sufficient communication skill to indicate presence of obsessional thoughts or thoughts that initiate compulsive behaviour. Insight into obsessions has been controversial, especially in children and generally not required for diagnosis. A range of behaviours can be subsumed under obsessive compulsive symptoms. These may include diverse symptoms like stereotypies and self-injurious behaviours. These are more common in children with autism and are generally considered as part of the symptoms of autism. However if such obsessions become more elaborate there are suggestions to consider treatment for obsessive compulsive disorder. A presumptive diagnosis of obsessive-compulsive disorder, based on the clear temporal emergence of compulsive repetitive behaviours, might be confirmed by a therapeutic response to pharmacological treatment [112]. There is no evidence that stereotypies act to reduce anxiety and they do not usually respond to treatments for anxiety [112].

Eating Disorders

Anorexia and bulimia nervosa are relatively rare in the context of mental retardation, particularly moderate to severe mental retardation, but mental retardation is a predisposing factor for other eating disorders such as pica and rumination. The ingestion of nonnutritive substances, pica, and the regurgitation and rechewing of food, rumination, occurs with greater frequency as the severity of cognitive disability increases. When these behaviors are a focus of clinical attention, the diagnoses should be considered.

Attention-Deficit Hyperactivity Disorder (ADHD) and Disruptive Behaviour Disorders

The diagnostic criteria for ADHD/Hyperkinetic Disorder mentioned in the DSM-IV and ICD-10 are relatively objective and are based on externally observable behaviour and hence are generally accepted as applicable to children with mental retardation. Diagnostic difficulty may be encountered in determining if the observed behaviour is 'inconsistent' with the developmental level of the child. DSM-IV does not allow a dual diagnosis of ADHD with pervasive developmental disorder [7]. This discrepancy needs more research though evidence is accumulating that they may coexist and children might benefit from treatment with stimulants [112]. Symptoms of ADHD are required to be present in at least two settings to aid in differentiating ADHD from behaviours that are reactive to a specific environment. The presence of other co morbid conditions such as anxiety and conduct disorder is not uncommon and needs to be identified and taken into account in management.

Conduct disorder and oppositional defiant disorders affect about 30 per cent of young people with mild/borderline mental retardation. They are described more commonly in boys than in girls. Studies in adults show an association between antisocial behaviour and low verbal intelligence skills. However verbal intelligence skills are strongly influenced by psychosocial and family factors [68]. Similar to ADHD both these diagnostic categories require a judgment regarding the age appropriateness of the behaviour. The issues relate to impairment in abilities to understand rights of others and be aware of the consequences of behaviour including the context of the behaviour. Children with difficulties in perception may just copy or exhibit behaviours without understanding inappropriateness or after inappropriately perceived reinforcement. A child may also be angry and uncooperative when this is the only means of communicating his or her reluctance or inability to participate in a stressful activity. These diagnoses may be inapplicable in non-verbal children or children with severe levels of mental retardation.

Tic Disorders

There is no evidence regarding increased association of tic disorder with mental retardation. However it may be difficult to differentiate tics from stereotypic movements. Communication and perceptual problems may further complicate the presentation. The general sites where tics are prominent and presence of vocalisations can help in differentiating stereotypic movements. Relatively small doses of antipsychotic such as risperidone, haloperidol or pimozide are often effective in reducing or eliminating the tics [112].

Stereotypic Movement Disorder

Persistent repetitive non-purposeful motor behaviour occurs frequently in mental retardation and is more common in those with autism. Most children do not need treatment. Interference with daily activities requiring treatment occurs in up to 3 per cent of young people with more severe levels of mental retardation [42, 43]. These behaviours may be self stimulating resulting in reinforcement, or may serve attention seeking or active avoidance communicative roles.

Pervasive Developmental Disorders

About 80 per cent of children with autism also have mental retardation [42-43]. Autism alone is associated with increased risk of emotional and behavioural problems and burden of care. The diagnosis of Asperger's disorder however is excluded by the presence of mental retardation and delayed language development [7, 15]. Children with autism also frequently present with additional co morbid symptoms such as ADHD, obsessive and compulsive behaviour, anxiety, depression, and tics. These co morbid symptoms may also respond to specific treatment [112]. Children with mental retardation may have delayed language development, stereotypic behaviours and a restricted range of interests, but these can usually be differentiated from those with autism. This distinction is dependant on reciprocal communication abilities and emotions appropriate for their developmental level [7, 15].

Self Injurious Behaviour

Self-injurious behavior (SIB) is defined as an act directed towards oneself that results in tissue damage [120]. This behavior restricts the individual's quality of life and diverts focus onto programming efforts on reducing the frequency and intensity of self-injury. This is especially the case for individuals with developmental disabilities, among who the prevalence rates of self-injurious behavior are between 5% and 16% [121].

Prevalence studies suggests that some factors such as severe or profound developmental delay, sensory or physical disability, and certain genetic disorders and syndromes are associated with increased risk of developing self-injurious behavior. Self-injurious behavior can emerge prior to 3 years of age and that some of the children continue to engage in stereotypy, self-injurious behavior or proto-self-injurious behavior after they turn 3 years of age [122].

Proto- self-injurious behavior was defined as topographically similar to common forms of self-injurious behavior, but these topographies did not produce tissue damage [122].

Berkson (2002) anecdotally noted that some topographies of self-injurious behavior (e.g., eye-poking) appeared to occur regardless of environmental variables [122], whereas others were direct responses to social changes in the environment (e.g. head-banging).

Kurtz et al. (2003) completed a relatively large-scale study to examine analogue functional analysis and treatment outcomes of SIB for young children with a wide range of functioning levels [123]. Results indicated that social consequences maintained SIB in a subgroup of people with mental retardation. A small proportion (13.8%) was non-socially mediated. The remaining (37.9%) showed an undifferentiated pattern of responding. Descriptive observations show an association with SIB and low levels of social contact.

The theoretical models proposed by Guess and Carr (1991) and Kennedy (2002) suggest that early rhythmic motor stereotypies that are characteristic of typical and delayed infant development may be precursors to some forms of emerging proto-SIB and SIB in children with developmental delay {124-125]. High frequency of repetitive motor behavior increases the probability that these behaviors will contact social contingencies and may eventually become reinforced by them.

A strategy for reducing the prevalence of SIB is to identify effective early intervention and prevention strategies for young children who are at high risk of developing SIB [122]. Motor stereotypies emerge in infancy and persist for young children with developmental delay rather than children continually developing new stereotypies throughout early childhood. In addition to topographical influences on SIB, the child's functioning level also appeared to affect the probability of SIB. For all of the children who experienced tissue damage during the study, this damage most frequently occurred in children with more severe developmental delay.

Treatment Planning

The treatment plan should include the person with mental retardation, members of multidisciplinary group, community caregivers and hospital staff. Treatment needs to be individualised. A thorough assessment of aetiological factors is an essential part of management. The treatment goals need to be formulated with enough consideration to the time and resources available. Any intervention needs to evaluate the crucial importance of variables such as consistency versus change in the person's environment, greater or lesser supervision of activities, identification of possible stressors and implementation of behavioural management strategies. Appropriate resources, therapy, activity groups to bring out the person's capacity for learning and participation should be used. The use of medications should be reserved for appropriate target disorders and syndromes. Emphasizing the possible environmental causes of problem behaviors can also help reduce the demand for indiscriminate prescription of medications and prevent side effects. Short-term administration of a benzodiazepine may sometimes be a better choice for nonspecific sedation. Medications may be needed for longer-term treatment of depression, bipolar disorder, psychotic disorders, obsessive-compulsive disorder, or attention deficit disorder. In addition, short-term pharmacologic treatment may be useful when certain symptoms have not responded to environmental interventions. In these circumstances, medications should be prescribed with essentially the same indications, contraindications, precautions, doses, and monitoring as in the general psychiatric population but with special attention to possible behavioral effects in those with mental retardation. Admission to inpatient wards for people with mental retardation needs to be carefully evaluated with regards to benefits and complications. Appropriate acute or short-term inpatient treatment, coupled with long-term treatment recommendations, has the purpose of returning the individual to his or her prior environment or other suitable community setting. Effective discharge planning strengthens the supports provided by an existing placement. Ideally, discharge planning, including plans for outpatient follow up and the provision of any additional services, should begin at the initial treatment planning meeting or even before admission. Communication is the key to effective planning. Early and continual contact with all community supports, from family to outpatient therapists, is important. The tasks of each agency and individual needs to be clear and the aims and process of any intervention needs to be realistic. This focus will help hospital staffs propose realistic aftercare treatment plans based on available resources and provider capabilities. An identified liaison service can make the transition between hospital and community smoother. An organised service planning meeting before discharge needs to consider long term issues including reviewing the course of hospitalisation and discuss how a subsequent inpatient stay can be avoided or shortened.

Health professionals should be aware of several important legal considerations. These relate to consent and human rights of people with mental retardation balancing the restrictive powers of medical professionals in treatment and care of people with mental retardation. The diagnosis of mental retardation does not by itself imply that the individual is incompetent to consent to treatment. Competence must be assessed on a case-by-case basis. In an emergency setting, life-threatening problems warrant emergency treatment, even in the absence of informed consent. In cases where competence is impaired, guardianship may need to be considered. Many states have statutes that require medical personnel to report any suspicion of abuse and have entered into binding legal agreements as a result of lawsuits initiated by plaintiffs to improve the quality of care delivered to people with mental retardation. These consent decrees may mandate procedural safeguards and specific measures of quality of treatment.

Principles of Management

Management begins with a comprehensive assessment. A multi axial diagnostic formulation based on DSM-IV or ICD-10 is designed to identify all relevant biopsychosocial factors and environmental factors relevant to aetiopathogensis and potentially useful for management. It takes account of psychiatric disorder, intellectual and cognitive abilities and deficits, temperamental factors, associated medical conditions, stress from family, peers, environment and socio-cultural context, and the current level of adaptive functioning along with impairments. A comprehensive multi-disciplinary approach to management is necessary to evaluate the complex interactions of factors contributing to the psychopathology.

Communication between professionals, parents, carers, and teachers and children with mental retardation are important means of implementing management issues and help in clearly defining roles of different members of the team [121].

Psycho Education

Parents and carers along with the person with mental retardation should form part of the team early on and should be involved as partners in the management plan to promote engagement, avoid alienation and facilitate compliance with treatment [112]. Parent education and counseling regarding the nature of the mental retardation and associated emotional and behavioural problems needs to be communicated clearly. Parents may need time to cope with their grief and may need help themselves in co-operating with management. Teachers and other carers are also required to facilitate management. More specific family therapy exploring communication and patterns of interaction, conflict resolution, and beliefs may be helpful, especially when relationships and family interactions are identifiably contributing to aetiopathology. Parent involvement in the delivery of speech therapy, and physiotherapy and behaviour modification programmes is indispensable [121].

Psychological Treatments

A wide range of psychological therapies have been explored in managing psychiatric symptoms in mental retardation. The choice however depends on intellectual abilities and symptoms that need to be managed along with patient and carer preferences. Behaviour-modification techniques based on operant conditioning principles are effective in promoting positive behaviours and reducing difficult behaviours. A detailed behavioural analysis about antecedents, details of behaviour exhibited and subsequent consequences including inadvertent reinforcers need to be clearly identified. Working with carers who can observe the behaviour would be vital in assessment and implementing a management plan in this context. An analysis of the possible function of the behaviour and changing the antecedents and consequences may prevent or reduce the behaviour. Alternatively appropriate behaviour can be reinforced by reward. However these need to be managed as part of a wider management plan involving carers and the person with mental retardation. Such strategies need to be ethically managed with consent of carers and if possible the person with mental retardation. However disruptive behaviour may also have a communicative purpose. Alternative ways of communication with pictures or other mechanisms may need to be explored. The meanings of such behaviours exhibited by people with mental retardation need to be carefully observed and analysed before specific management strategies are implemented [124].

Modified cognitive therapies are increasingly being used. These approaches take into account the level of intellectual and verbal ability of the child. Various strategies have been used including progressive muscle relaxation and breathing techniques with demonstration and imitation. They may reduce anxiety and depression [112] although the evidence for effectiveness is lacking. An understanding of intellectual abilities, developmental level and verbal comprehension abilities are important requirements though not mandatory.

Pharmacotherapy

Drugs are increasingly being used to control severe forms of behavioural disturbances. However among people with mental retardation they should be used as part of a psychosocial and educational treatment plan. Issues in pharmacotherapy include the need for informed consent from patients and carers. Evidence for the efficacy of psychotropic drugs is relatively limited in children and also among adults with mental retardation. The evidence is relatively more when use of pharmacotherapy in adults is taken into account. The principles of pharmacotherapy for intellectually normalized population need to be used taking care of adverse effect sensitivity, medical conditions and side effects of medications.

A wide range of drugs used in children with mental retardation have the capacity to produce cognitive, behavioural, and emotional side-effects, as well as mask symptoms of psychiatric disorder. Children with mental retardation are more likely to develop side effects from neuroleptics. The side effects may manifest as drowsiness, akathisia, and parkinsonian side-effects in children. Stimulants can cause irritability, anxiety, mood disturbance, and insomnia. More worrying but less prevalent are psychosis and mood disorders. Benzodiazepines may mask mood and may induce paradoxical stimulating effect in this group of children [112]. A careful consideration of the effects of current and past psychotropic medication is a necessary part of a psychiatric assessment. Sometimes it is useful to observe these individuals without medication in order to aid in assessing the behaviour and exclude aetiological contribution from drugs.

Conclusion

Mental health is a goal for all people, including those with mental retardation. There is currently a consensus that mental retardation is associated with mental illness in a greater proportion than in the general population. The previous reports of such an increased association being specific to some psychiatric disorders are currently not apparent with more methodologically sound studies. However a general increase in psychiatric morbidity needs to have a convincing explanation. The stress diathesis model provides a useful explanation and describes people with mental retardation as a vulnerable group.

All psychiatric disorders found in people with normal intelligence can theoretically present in people with mental retardation. The available evidence seems to support the hypothesis. However diagnostic constraints make more discrete classification criteria of ICD10 and DSM IV less valid, especially in people with more severe forms of mental retardation. The prevalence of vulnerability and aetiological factors that can be associated with aetiology of mental retardation has always been a speculated cause for such an increased association of mental illness with mental retardation. These range from neuropathology associated with mental retardation, social and environment adjustment problems, vulnerability to bullying and abuse and carer stress.

A greater understanding of aetiological factors present opportunities for interventions even when pharmacological interventions are limited. Psychosocial interventions including appropriate support along with input from the multidisciplinary and muliprofessional teams should never be underestimated. In addition progress in understanding psychopathology and treatment effectiveness strategies need to be individualised to help patients achieve their best potential and independence.

Prevention strategies for mental retardation are very commonly used and effective. There is however very limited evidence for prevention of mental illness among people with mental retardation. Further research is needed in many aspects of the complex interaction between mental retardation and mental illness. These relate to studying aetiology, phenomenology, cognition, and intervention strategies for mental retardation and mental illness.

References

[1]   Sheerenberger, RC. A history of mental retardation. Baltimore: Brookes Publishing Co; 1983.

[2]   Locke, J. and Woolhouse, R.S. An Essay Concerning Human Understanding-1689. London: Penguin Group; 1998.

[3]   Zenderland, L. Measuring minds: Henry Herbert Goddard and the origins of American intelligence testing. Cambridge: Cambridge University Press; 1998.

[4]   Key Provisions of the Individuals with Disabilities Education Act. In: *Special Education Manual. MICPEL;* 1995.

[5]   Dobson, F. and Michael, A. Mental Health Act. UK: Department of Health; 1983.

[6]   American Association on Mental Retardation. Mental Retardation: Definition, Classification, and Systems of Supports. 10th Edition. Washington DC: American Association on Mental Retardation; 2002.

[7]   American Psychiatric Association. Diagnostic and Statistical Manual of Classification of diseases and related health problems. 4th edition. Washington DC: American Psychiatric Association; 1994.

[8]   Grossman, HJ. Manual on terminology in mental retardation. Washington DC: American Association on Mental Deficiency; 1973.

[9]   Grossman, HJ. Manual on terminology in mental retardation. Washington DC: American Association on Mental Deficiency; 1977.

[10]   Defendorf, AR. Clinical Psychiatry, a textbook for students and physicians abstracted and adapted from the 6th German Edition of Kraepelin's *"Lehrbuch der Psychiatrie."* New York: Macmillan; 1902.

[11]   Philips, I. and Williams, N. (1975) Psychopathology and mental retardation: a study of 100 mentally retarded children I: Psychopathology. *American Journal of Psychiatry,* 132, 1265-127.

[12]   Rutter, M; Tizard, J. and Witmore, K. Education, Health, and Behaviour. London: Longman; 1970.

[13] Luckasson, R., and Spitalnick, D. M. Political and programmatic shifts of the 1992 AAMR definition of mental retardation. In: Bradley, V., Ashbaugh, J.W. and Blaney, B.C. (Eds.), *Creating individual supports for people with developmental disabilities: A mandate for change at many levels*. Baltimore: Paul H. Brookes; 1994; 81–96.

[14] World Health Organization. International Classification of Impairments, Disabilities and Handicaps. Geneva: WHO; 1980.

[15] World Health Organization. International statistical classification of diseases and related health problems. 10th revision. Geneva: WHO; 1992.

[16] Ward, S.B., Ward, T.J., Hatt, C.V., Young, D.L. and Mollner, N.R. (1995). The incidence and utility of the ACID, ACIDS, and SCAD profiles in a referred population. *Psychology in the Schools,* 32(4), 267-276.

[17] Watkins, M.W., Kush, J., and Glutting, J.J. (1997). Discriminant and predictive validity of the WISC-III ACID profile among children with learning disabilities. *Psychology in the Schools,* 34(4), 309-319.

[18] Sparrow, SS., Cicchetti, DV. and Balla, DA. Vineland Adaptive Behaviour Scales, 2nd Edition. Camberwell: ACER Press, 2005.

[19] Shaddock, A.J. and Ziber, D. (1991)Current service ideologies and responses to challenging behaviour: Social role valorization or vaporization? *Journal of Intellectual and Developmental Disability,* 17 (2), 169-175.

[20] Emerson, E., Barrett, S., Bell, C, Cummings, R., McCool, C., Toogood, A. and Mansell, J. Developing services for people with severe learning difficulties and challenging behaviour. *Report of the early work of the Special Development Team in Kent,* 1987.

[21] Qureshi, H. The Size of the Problem. In: Emerson E., McGill P. and Mansell J (Eds), *Severe Learning Disabilities and Challenging Behaviours,* Chapman and Hall; 1994.

[22] Carr, E.G., Dunlap, G., Horner, R.H., Koegel, R.L., Turnbull, A.P., Sailor, W., Anderson, J.L., Albin, R.W., Koegel, L.K., and Fox, L. (2002). Positive Behavior Support: Evolution of an Applied Science. *Journal of Positive Behavior Interventions,* 4, 16-20.

[23] McLaren, J. and Bryson, S. E. (1987) Review of recent epidemiological studies in mental retardation: prevalence, associated disorders, and etiology. *American Journal of Mental Retardation,* 92, 243-254.

[24] Rutter, M., Tizard, J., Yule, W., Graham, Y., and Whitmore, K. (1976). Isle of Wright studies 1964-1974. *Psychological Medicine,* 7, 313-332.

[25] Parmenter, T.R. (2004) Contributions of IASSID to the scientific study of intellectual disability: The past, the present, and the future. *Journal of Policy and Practice in Intellectual Disabilities,* 1, 71-78.

[26] Jacobson, J.W., Holburn, S. and Mulick, J.A. Contemporary Dual Diagnosis: MH/MR: Service Models: Volume II: Partial and Supportive Services, Kingston, New York, NADD Press; 2002.

[27] Irish College of Psychiatrists (2004). Proposed model for the delivery of a mental health service to people with intellectual disability: Occasional Paper (OP58). *Psychiatric Bulletin,* 28, 345-346.

[28] Fryers, T. Mental retardation in developing countries. In: Tantam, D and. Duncan, A. *Psychiatry for the developing world.* London: Gaskell Press; 1996; 258-90.

[29] Brown, R.I. (1998) The effects of quality of life models on the development of research and practice in the field of Down syndrome. *Downs Syndrome Research and Practice,* 5(1), 39-42.

[30] National Assembly for Wales. Welsh Health Survey 1998. Wales: *HMSO;* 1999.

[31] Roeleveld, N., Zielhuis, G.A., and Gabreels, F. (1997). The prevalence of mental retardation. *Developmental Medicine and Child Neurology,* 39, 125-32.

[32] Duncan, J., Seitz, R.J., Kolodny, J., Bor, D., Herzog, H., Ahmed, A., Newell, F.N. and Emslie, H. (2000). A neural basis for general intelligence. *Science,* 289(5478), 457-460.

[33] Cooper, S. A. (1997). Epidemiology of psychiatric disorders in elderly compared with younger adults with learning disabilities. *British Journal of Psychiatry,* 170, 375 -380.

[34] The Arc of the United States. Preventing Mental Retardation: A Guide to the Causes of Mental Retardation and Strategies for Prevention. Silver Spring, MD.2001. (http://www.thearc.org/publications/prevention.pdf).

[35] McGrother, C.W. and Marshall, B. (1990) Recent trends in incidence, morbidity and survival in Down's syndrome. *Journal of Mental Deficiency Research,* 34, 49-57.

[36] Alexander, D. (1998). Prevention of Mental Retardation: Four Decades of Research. *Mental Retardation and Developmental Disabilities Research Reviews,* 4, 50- 58.

[37] Jaffe, JH. "Mental Retardation." In: Sadock, B.J. and Sadock, V.A (Eds), Comprehensive Textbook of Psychiatry, 7th edition, Philadelphia, PA: Lippincott Williams and Wilkins; 2000.

[38] Roeleveld, N., Zielhuis, G.A. and Gabreels, F. (1997). The prevalence of mental retardation: a critical review of recent literature. *Developmental Medicine and Child Neurology,* 39,125-132.

[39] Abramowicz, H.K. and Richardson, S.A. (1975). Epidemiology of severe mental retardation in children: community studies. *American Journal of Mental Deficiency,* 80, 18-39.

[40] Dupont, A. (1989) 140 years of Danish studies on the prevalence of mental retardation. *Acta Psychiatrica Scandinavia,* 348,105-112.

[41] Fryers, T. The epidemiology of severe intellectual impairment: the dynamics of prevalence. Orlando (FL): Academic Press; 1984.

[42] Hou, J.W., Wang, T.R. and Chuang, S.M. (1998) An epidemiological and aetiological study of children with intellectual disability in Taiwan. *Journal of Intellectual Disability Research,* 42 (2), 137-143.

[43] Richardson, S.A. and Koller, H. Twenty-two years: causes and consequences of mental retardation. Cambridge (MA): Harvard University Press; 1996.

[44] Starza Smith, A. (1989). Recent trends in prevalence studies of children with severe mental retardation. *Disability Handicap and Society,* 4, 177-195.

[45] Srinath, S. and Girimaji, S.C. (1999). Epidemiology of child and adolescent mental health problems and mental retardation. *NIMHANS Journal,* 17, 355-366.

[46] Girimaji, S.R., Srinath, S. and Seshadri, S.P. (1994). A clinical study of infants presenting to a mental retardation clinic. *Indian Journal of Pediatrics,* 61(4), 373-378.

[47] Collacott, R.A., Cooper, S.A., Branford, D. and McGrother, C. (1998). Behaviour phenotype for Down's syndrome *British Journal of Psychiatry,* 172, 85 - 89.

[48] Crews, W.D., Bonaventura, S. and Rowe, F. (1994) Dual diagnosis: prevalence of psychiatric disorders in a large state residential facility for individuals with mental retardation. *American Journal of Mental Retardation,* 98 (6), 724-731.

[49] Borthwick-Duffy, S.A. (1994) Epidemiology and prevalence of psychopathology in people with mental retardation. *Journal of Consulting and Clinical Psychology,* 62(1), 17-27.

[50] Corbett, J. Psychiatric morbidity and mental retardation. In James, F.E. and Snaith, R.P. (eds) *Psychiatric Illness and Mental Handicap.* London: Royal College of Psychiatrists, Gaskell Press; 1979; 11-25.

[51] Göstason, R. (1985). Psychiatric illness among the mentally retarded: A Swedish population study. *Acta Psychiatrica Scandinavica, Suppl,* 318, 1-117.

[52] Reid, A.H. (1994). Psychiatry and learning disability. *British Journal of Psychiatry,* 164, 613-618.

[53] Cooper, S.A. (1997). Psychiatry of elderly compared to younger adults with intellectual disabilities. *Journal of Applied Research in Intellectual Disabilities,* 10(4), 303-311.

[54] Patel, P., Goldberg, D. and Moss, S. (1993) Psychiatric morbidity in older people with moderate and severe learning disability- II: The prevalence study. *British Journal of Psychiatry,* 163, 481-491.

[55] Deb, S. (1997). Mental disorder in adults with mental retardation and epilepsy. *Comprehensive Psychiatry,* 38(3), 179-184.

[56] Deb, S. and Joyce, J. (1998). Psychiatric illness and behavioural problems in adults with learning disability and epilepsy. *Behavioural Neurology,* 11(3), 125-129.

[57] Haveman, M.J., Maaskant, M.A., van Schrojenstein, H.M., Urlings, H.F.J. and Kessels, A.G.H. (1994). Mental health problems in elderly people with and without Down's syndrome. *Journal of Intellectual Disability Research,* 38(3), 341-355.

[58] Jansen, D. E., Krol, B., Groothoff, J. W., and Post, D. (2004). People with intellectual disability and their health problems: A review of comparative studies. *Journal of Intellectual Disability Research,* 48, 93-102.

[59] Collacott, R.A., Cooper, S.A. and McGrother, C. (1992). Differential rates of psychiatric disorders in adults with Down's syndrome compared with other mentally handicapped adults. *British Journal of Psychiatry,* 161, 671-674.

[60] Turner, T.H. (1989). Schizophrenia and mental handicap: an historical review, with implications for further research. Psychological Medicine, 19(2), 301-314.

[61] Lund, J. (1985). The prevalence of psychiatric morbidity in mentally retarded adults. *Acta Psychiatrica Scandinavica,* 72(6), 563-70.

[62] Hagnell, O., Öjesjö, L., Otterbeck, L. and Rorsman, B. (1993). Prevalence of mental disorders, personality traits and mental complaints in the Lundby study. *Scandinavian Journal of Social Medicine,* 21(Suppl.50), 1-76.

[63] Lund, J. (1985) Epilepsy and psychiatric disorder in the mentally retarded adults. *Acta Psychiatrica Scandinavia,* 72 (6), 557-562.

[64] Fox, R.A. and Wade, E.J. (1998). Attention deficit hyperactivity disorder among adults with severe and profound mental retardation. *Research in Developmental Disabilities,* 19(3), 275-80.

[65] Reiss, S. and Rojahn, J. (1993). Joint occurrence of depression and aggression in children and adults with mental retardation. *Journal of Intellectual Disability Research,* 37(3), 287-294.

[66] Kon, Y. and Bouras, N. (1997). Psychiatric follow-up and health services utilisation for people with learning disabilities. *British Journal of Developmental Disabilities,* 43(1), 20-26.

[67] Van Minnen, A., Hoogduin, C.A.L. and Broekman, T.G. (1997). Hospital vs. outreach treatment of patients with mental retardation and psychiatric disorders: a controlled study. *Acta Psychiatrica Scandinavica,* 95, 515-522.

[68] Holden, P. and Neff, J.A. (2000). Intensive outpatient treatment of persons with mental retardation and psychiatric disorder: a preliminary study. *Mental Retardation,* 38(1), 27-32.

[69] Tyrer, P., Hassiotis, A., Ukoumunne, O., Piachaud, J. and Harvey, K. (1999). UK 700 Group Intensive case management for patients with borderline intelligence. *Lancet,* 354, 999-1000.

[70] Kohen, D. (1993). Psychiatric emergencies in people with a mental handicap. *Psychiatric Bulletin,* 17, 587-589.

[71] Reiss, S., Levitan, G.W. and Szyszko, J. (1982). Emotional disturbance and mental retardation: Diagnostic Overshadowing. *American Journal of Mental Deficiency,* 86, 567-574.

[72] Eaves, L.C. and Ho, H.H (1996). Brief report: stability and change in cognitive and behavioral characteristics of autism through childhood. *Journal of Autism and Developmental Disorders,* 26(5), 557-569.

[73] Mathers, C., Bernard, C., Iburg, K.M., Inoue, M., Fat, D.M., Shibuya, K., Stein, C., Tomijima, N. and Xu, H. *Global Programme on Evidence for Health Policy Discussion Paper No. 54.* WHO; 2004.

[74] Szymanski, L., Madow, L. and Mallory, G. Psychiatric services to adult mentally retarded and developmentally disabled persons (Report of APA Task Force #30). Washington, DC: American Psychiatric Association; 1990.

[75] Hauser, M.J. (1997). The role of the psychiatrist in mental retardation. *Psychiatric Annals,* 27,170-174.

[76] Gillberg, C., Persson, E., Grufman, N., and Themmer, V. (1986). Psychiatric disorders in mildly and severely mentally retarded urban children and adolescents: Epidemiological aspects. *British Journal of Psychiatry,* 149, 68-74.

[77] Royal College of Psychiatrists. Diagnostic Criteria for Psychiatric Disorders for Use with Adults with Learning Disabilities (DC-LD): London: Royal College of Psychiatrists; 2001.

[78] Moss, S., Prosser, H., Costello, H., Simpson, N., Patel, P., Rowe, S., Turner, S. and Hatton, C. (1998). Reliability and validity of the PAS-ADD Checklist for detecting psychiatric disorders in adults with intellectual disability. *Journal of Intellectual Disability Research,* 42,173-183.

[79] Matson, J.L., Rush, K.S., Hamilton, M., Anderson, S.J., Bamburg, J.W., Baglio, C.S., Williams, D. and Kirkpatrick-Sanchez, S. (1999). Characteristics of depression as assessed by the Diagnostic Assessment for the Severely Handicapped-II (DASH-II). *Research in Developmental Disabilities, 20,* 305-313.

[80] Hon, J., Huppert, F.A., Holland, A.J. and Watson, P. (1999). Neuropsychological assessment of older adults with Down's syndrome: an epidemiological study using the Cambridge Cognitive Examination (CAMCOG). *British Journal of Clinical Psychology,* 38,155-165.

[81] Deb, S. and Braganza, J. (1999). Comparison of rating scales for the diagnosis of dementia in adults with Down's syndrome. *Journal of Intellectual Disability Research,* 43, 400-407.

[82] Matson, J.L., Leblanc, L.A. and Weinheimer, B. (999). Reliability of the Matson Evaluation of Social Skills in Individuals with Severe Retardation (MESSIER). *Behaviour Modification,* 23, 647-661.

[83] McDaniel, W.F. and Harris, D.W. (1999). Mental health outcomes in dually diagnosed individuals with mental retardation assessed with the MMPI-168(L): case studies. *Journal of Clinical Psychology,* 55, 487-496.

[84] Tonge, B. J., Einfeld, S. L., Krupinski, J., Mackenzie, A., McLaughlin, M., Florio, T. and Nunn, R. J. (1996). The use of factor analysis for ascertaining patterns of psychopathology in children with intellectual disability. *Journal of Intellectual Disability Research,* 40 (3), 198-207.

[85] Sovner, R. (1986). Limiting factors in using DSM-III criteria with mentally ill/mentally retarded persons. *Psychopharmacology Bulletin,* 22, 1055-1059.

[86] Iwanaga, R., Kawasaki, C. and Tsuchida, R. (2000). Brief Report: Comparison of sensory-motor and cognitive function between autism and Aspergers Syndrome in preschool children. *Journal of Autism and Developmental Disorders,* 30 (2), 169-174.

[87] Wachs, T. (1987). Specificity of environmental action as manifest in environmental correlates of infant's mastery motivation. *Developmental Psychology,* 23, 782-790.

[88] Brodtkorb, E. (1994). The diversity of epilepsy in adults with severe developmental disabilities: age at seizure onset and other prognostic factors. *Seizure,* 3(4), 277-285.

[89] Sobsey, D. Violence and abuse in the lives of people with disabilities: The end of silent acceptance? Baltimore: Paul H. Brookes Publishing Co; 1994.

[90] Turnbull, H., Buchele-Ash, A., and Mitchell, L. Abuse and neglect of children with disabilities: A policy analysis. Lawrence, Kansas: Beach Center on Families and Disability, The University of Kansas; 1994.

[91] Ong, L.C., Chandran, V. and Peng, R. (1999). Stress experienced by mothers of Malaysian children with mental retardation. *Journal of Paediatrics and Child Health,* 35 (4), 358-362.

[92] Cuskelly, M. and Dadds, M. (1992). Behavioural problems in children with Down's syndrome and their siblings. *Journal of Child Psychology and Psychiatry and Applied Disciplines,* 33, 749-761.

[93] Collacott, R.A., Cooper, S.A. and McGrother, C. (1993). Differential rates of psychiatric disorder in adults with Down syndrome compared with other mentally handicapped adults. *British Journal of Psychiatry,* 162, 848-850.

[94] Myers, B.A., Pueschel, S.M. (1991). Psychiatric disorders in persons with Down syndrome. *Journal of Nervous and Mental Disease,* 179, 609-613.

[95] O'Donnell, W.T. and Warren, S.T. (2002). A decade of molecular studies of fragile X syndrome. *Annual Review of Neuroscience,* 25,315-338.

[96] Holm, V.A., Cassidy, S.B., Butler, M.G., Hanchett, J.M., Greenswag, L.R., Whitman, B.Y. and Greenberg, F. (1993). Prader-Willi Syndrome, Consensus Diagnostic Criteria. *Pediatrics,* 91, 398-402.

[97] Girirajan, S., Vlangos, C.N., Szomju, B.B., Edelman, E, Trevors, C.D., Dupuis, L, Nezarati, M., Bunyan, D.J. and Elsea, S.H. (2006). Genotype-phenotype correlation in Smith-Magenis syndrome: evidence that multiple genes in 17p11.2 contribute to the clinical spectrum. *Genetics in Medicine,* 8(7), 417-27.

[98] Maher, B. (2001). "Music, the brain, and Williams syndrome". *The Scientist,* 15[23], 20.

[99] Kerr, A.M. and Ravine, D. (2003). Review article: breaking new ground with Rett syndrome. *Journal of Intellectual Disability Research,* 47(8), 580-7.

[100] Guirrini, R., Carrozzo, R., Rinaldi, R., and Bonanni, P. (2003). Angelman syndrome: Etiology, clinical features, diagnosis, and management of symptoms. *Paediatric Drugs,* 5, 647-661.

[101] Summers, J. A., Allison, D. B., Lynch, P. S., and Sandler, L. (1995). Behaviour problems in Angelman syndrome. *Journal of Intellectual Disability Research,* 39, 97-106.

[102] Janicki, M.P. and Dalton, A.J. Dementia, Aging, and Intellectual Disabilities: A Handbook. Philadelphia: Brunner-Mazel; 1999.

[103] Reid, A.H. (1989) Psychiatry and mental handicap: a historical perspective. *Journal of Mental Deficiency Research,* 33 (5), 363-368.

[104] Iwawaki, A. (1999) Acute psychoses in adult patients with mild mental retardation. *Seishin Shinkeigaku Zasshi,* 95 (2), 151-170.

[105] Rojahn, J. and Esbensen, A. J. Epidemiology of mood disorders in people with mental retardation. In P. Sturmey (Ed.), Mood disorders in individuals with mental retardation. Kingston, NY: NADD Press; 2005; 47-66.

[106] Esbensen, A.J. and Benson, B.A. (2005). Cognitive variables and depressed mood in adults with intellectual disabilities. *Journal of Intellectual Disability Research,* 49, 481-489.

[107] Abramson, L.Y., Metalsky, G.I., and Alloy, L. B. (1989). Hopelessness depression: A theory based subtype of depression. *Psychological Review,* 96, 358-372.

[108] Marston, G. M., Perry, D. W., and Roy, A. (1997). Manifestations of depression in people with intellectual disability. *Journal of Intellectual Disability,* 41, 476-480.

[109] McBrien, J.A. (2003) Assessment and diagnosis of depression in people with intellectual disability. *Journal of Intellectual Disability Research,* 47, 1-13.

[110] Beck, D.C., Carlson, G.A., Russell, A.T. and Brownfield, F.E. (1987). Use of depression rating instruments in developmentally and educationally delayed adolescents. *Journal of the American Academy of Child and Adolescent Psychiatry,* 26, 97-100.

[111] Cole, D.A., Tram, J.M., Martin, J.M., Hoffman, K.B., Ruiz, M.D., Jacquez, F.M. and Maschman, T.L. (2002). Individual differences in the emergence of depressive symptoms in children and adolescents: A longitudinal investigation of parent and child reports. *Journal of Abnormal Psychology*, 111, 156-165.

[112] Antochi, R., Stavrakaki, C. and Emery, P.C. (2003). Psychopharmacological treatments in persons with dual diagnosis of psychiatric disorders and developmental disabilities. *Postgraduate Medical Journal*, 79,139-146.

[113] Ruedrich, S. Bipolar mood disorders in persons with mental retardation: Assessment and diagnosis. In Fletcher, R.J and Dosen, A. (Eds*.), Mental health aspects of mental retardation: Progress in assessment and treatment.* New York: Lexington Books; 1993; 111-129.

[114] Sovner, R. (1989). The use of valproate in the treatment of mentally retarded persons with typical and atypical bipolar disorder. *Journal of Clinical Psychiatry*, 50 (Suppl.3), 40-43.

[115] Aman, M.G., Collier-Crespin, A., and Lindsay, R.L. (1989). Pharmacotherapy of disorders in mental retardation. *European Child and Adolescent Psychiatry*, 9(Suppl. 5), 98-107.

[116] Gonzalez, M. and Matson, J.L. (2006). Mania and Intellectual Disability: the course of manic symptoms in persons with intellectual disability. *American Journal on Mental Retardation*, 111 (5), 378-383.

[117] Cain, N.N., Davidson, P.W., Burhan, A.M., Andolsek, M.E., Baxter, J.T., Sullivan, L., Florescue, H., List, A. and Deutsch L. (2003). Identifying bipolar disorders in individuals with intellectual disability. *Journal of Intellectual Disability Research*, 47, 31–38.

[118] Malloy, E., Zealberg, J.J. and Paolone, T. (1998). A patient with mental retardation and possible panic disorder. *Psychiatric Services*, 49,105-106.

[119] Newman, C. and Adams, K. (2004). Dog Gone Good: managing dog phobia in a teenage boy with a learning disability. *British Journal of Learning Disabilities*, 32, 35.

[120] Tate, B.G. and Baroff, G.S. (1966). Aversive control of self-injurious behavior in a psychotic boy. *Behavior Research and Therapy*, 4, 281- 287.

[121] Schroeder, S., Rojahn, J. and Oldenquist, A. Treatment of destructive behaviors among people with mental retardation and developmental disabilities: Overview of the problem. In: *Treatment of destructive behaviors in persons with developmental disabilities* (NIH Publication No. 91–2410). Washington, DC: U. S. Department of Health and Human Services; 1991; 173-220.

[122] Berkson, G. (2002). Early development of stereotyped and self-injurious behaviors: II. Age trends. *American Journal on Mental Retardation*, 107, 468-477.

[123] Kurtz, P.F., Chin, M.D., Huete, J.M., Tarbox, R.S. F., O'Connor, J.T., Paclawskyj, T.R., and Rush, K.S. (2003). Functional analysis and treatment of self-injurious behavior in young children: A summary of 30 cases. *Journal of Applied Behavior Analysis*, 36, 205-219.

[124] Guess, D. and Carr, E.G. (1991). Emergence and maintenance of stereotypy and self-injury. *American Journal on Mental Retardation*, 96, 299-319.

[125] Kennedy, C.H. and Souza, G. (1995). Functional analysis and treatment of eye poking. *Journal of Applied Behavior Analysis, 28,* 27-37.

In: Mental Retardation Research Advances
Editor: Elizabeth B. Heinz, pp. 147-174

ISBN: 978-1-60021-658-9
© 2007 Nova Science Publishers, Inc.

Chapter VIII

Challenging Symmetry on Mental Retardation: Evidence from Williams Syndrome

Andreia Santos[1], Duncan Milne[1],
Delphine Rosset[1,2] and Christine Deruelle[1]
[1] Mediterranean Institute of Cognitive Neurosciences, CNRS, Marseille, France
[2] Autism Centre, Sainte Marguerite Hospital, Marseille, France

> "Although mentally retarded ... they have sufficient
> understanding to have acquired normal social habits"
> Williams, Barrat-Boyes and Lowe, 1961

Abstract

This paper examines the notion of symmetry on mental retardation (MR). Of the more than 1000 known genetic causes of MR, here we focus on Williams syndrome (WS) because it is characterized by an outstanding juxtaposition of deficits and preservations. Despite mild to moderate MR, WS is thought to present strengths in most social cognitive domains and in particular in face processing. Along this paper we will review studies on face and facial-emotion processing in WS. Several researchers have claimed for a link between "intact" face-processing skills and gregarious social behaviour. However, to date, this hypothesis remains unclear. Recent findings of our group showed that individuals with WS are able to decode emotions expressed in human, but not in non-human faces. This striking dissociation challenges the notion of symmetry on MR and suggests domain-specific rather than subaverage general cognitive functioning in WS. Findings are interpreted in light of a developmental rather than modular approach of cognition.

Introduction

Mental retardation (MR) is a particular state of functioning that is characterized by significant limitations both in intellectual functioning and in adaptive behaviour (AAMR, 2002). Although, it is widely accepted that MR reflects sub-average *general* intellectual functioning, strengths in *specific* cognitive domains may coexist with these limitations. Within this framework, Williams Syndrome (WS) presents a major interest. Over the last two decades the social-cognitive phenotype of WS has been described as unique and striking, with MR concurring across a peak-valley profile. Despite mild to moderate MR, marked dissociations, both within (e.g., spared visuo-perceptual but impaired visuo-constructive abilities) and between (e.g., relatively spared verbal but impaired visuo-spatial abilities) cognitive domains are commonly reported in WS. Studies investigating social behaviour in WS have also produced intriguing results. Although some features seem to be shared with other disorders with MR (e.g. anxiety and behavioural problems), the phenotype of WS is characterized by a hypersociability that is not observable in other syndromes. Together, overfriendliness, empathy and positive social outlook led many researchers to suggest that WS individuals are particularly talented on most social-cognitive domains. Interestingly, WS individuals show great interest in people's faces and relatively spared skills in discriminating facial identity. Indeed, in WS there may be greater sensitivity to facial-emotional expressions. This supposed intactness, which co-exists with MR, suggests that cognitive functioning in WS may not be as symmetrical as the notion of MR would consider and that within a MR context some cognitive domains may be spared.

This paper focuses on face-processing skills in WS since this is the domain for which many authors have claimed intactness of the functioning of a face-processing module, analogous to that found in typical development (e.g., Bellugi, Wang and Jernigan, 1994; Tager-Flusberg, Plesa-Skwerer, Faja and Joseph, 2003). First, studies in the literature on face processing will be reviewed, providing evidence both against and in favour of an "intact face module" in the WS condition. This will serve as the basis to introduce WS as a pertinent model for understanding the notion of (a)symmetry on MR. Second, the few studies available on the domain of facial-emotion processing in WS will be presented, as this ability appears to closely relate to social and face-processing abilities. Before discussing the contribution of these studies, some recent findings from our group on facial-emotion decoding in WS will be presented supporting the idea of domain-specific abilities rather than low level general cognitive functioning in WS. In conclusion, the major accounts of the studies presented will be interpreted and discussed as a challenge to the classical notion of symmetry in disorders with MR.

Mental Retardation

Introduction to Mental Retardation

MR represents the most common developmental disorder, affecting up to 2-3 percent of the population. There are different degrees of MR, ranging from mild to profound. Its onset is systematically before age of 18 years and refers to a clinical state that is developmental in origin and which affects intellectual and social functioning. According to the official definition of the American Association on Mental Retardation (AAMR, 2002), it is characterized by significant limitations both in intellectual functioning and in adaptive skills. These limitations are commonly believed to have a widespread impact in various domains, such as conceptual, social and practical. Although, it is broadly accepted that MR is characterized by general low intellectual level, in some cases these limitations coexist with strengths in specific cognitive domains. This suggests that there may be some dissociation within the atypical MR brain and that some of these functions may have been spared.

In the early 70s, Edward Zigler provided a major contribution to our understanding of MR. Rejecting the past stereotypic views, Zigler (1971) defended a "whole-person" approach of children with MR as they are more than products of low intelligence quotient. In line with this approach, cognitive disability *per se* does not account for the complex array of social and emotional developmental pathways in MR. Although more than 30 years have passed by, Zigler's proposal of integrated approaches of MR is far from reaching general consensus.

A Whole or Some Parts?

Over the past two decades, cognitive psychologists have proposed that humans possess a number of independent cognitive mechanisms rather than functioning as a "whole". These cognitive mechanisms may operate in single domains and act independently of each other (Fodor, 1983) stemming from higher level symbolic processes typically associated with general intelligence (Anderson, 1992). Within this context the question remains of whether MR is a single, general deficit touching all cognitive domains or rather the result of a specific deficit in a "cognitive-module" (e.g., Anderson and Miller, 1998). To date, this question is an issue of great controversy. Cases of brain damage (e.g., agrammatic or prosopagnosic patients) and some developmental disorders (e.g., specific language impairment) have been used to support claims about the existence of independently-functioning cognitive modules in the brain (e.g., Kress and Daum, 2003; van der Lely, 1997). Studies with infants also provided some support for the existence of these domain-specific and/or modular capacities, for example in the social-perceptual domain (e.g., Premack, 1990, Leslie and Keeble, 1987). Curiously, for our purpose, some cases of MR may also provide evidence for the interdependency of brain functions. In this context, WS presents a major interest - a rare genetic disorder that combines MR with an uneven behavioural phenotype of characteristic strengths and weaknesses. But what is WS?

Williams Syndrome

WS is a rare neurodevelopmental disorder characterized by a combination of distinctive medical, genetic, neuroanatomical and cognitive features. It was first described in the early 60s as a condition involving a constellation of cardiovascular difficulties (e.g., supravalvular aortic stenosis), peculiar facial features (e.g., wide mouths, pouting lips) and mental deficiency (Williams, Barrat-Boyes and Lowe, 1961). Curiously, this first attempt to characterize WS already makes us suspect an asymmetrical profile by describing dissociation between intellectual functioning and adaptive skills: "Although mentally retarded ... they have sufficient understanding to have acquired normal social habits" (Williams et al., 1961, pp. 1311). Insights into the nature of WS culminated in the mid-1990s with the identification of the genetic deletion responsible for it. Since then, WS is considered as a neurobiological model of special interest to study gene-brain-behaviour relationships. But why's WS so special? The following sections will highlight this question by describing several characteristic domains of the WS phenotype.

WS' (Odd) Profile

Mental Retardation

MR is clearly one of the most common features of individuals with WS. Their IQ levels, inferred from standardized measures of the Wechsler scales[1] (WAIS-III - Wechsler, 1997 and WISC-III - Wechsler, 1996), usually fall in the range of mild to moderate retardation and are about two standard deviations below the general population mean (e.g., Udwin, Yule and Martin, 1987). However, and more interestingly for our purpose, mean scores at the verbal subtests consistently overtake scores at the performance subtest and this difference often reaches 14 points, which is highly significant (Wechsler, 1996). Such disparity between the different components of IQ measure is also found in Searcy and colleagues' (2004) study which recently put forward that performance IQ increased with age in WS, but that overall IQ remain stable across ages. Thus, close observation of the IQ scores of WS individuals already corroborate the idea that intellectual disability is not a unitary condition characterized by homogeneous slowness of cognitive development, but by a variety of conditions in which some cognitive functions may be more disrupted than others.

---

[1] The Wechsler intelligence scales are general tests of intelligence standardized for use with adults (Wechsler Adult Intelligence Scale, WAIS) or with children (Wechsler Intelligence Scale for Children, WISC). They were designed to quantify Intelligence (IQ) as a global capacity of the individual to act purposefully, to think rationally, and to deal effectively with the environment. The full-scale IQ is composed by 14 subtests, comprising the Verbal (Information, Comprehension, Arithmetic, Similarities, Vocabulary, Digit Span and Letter Number Sequencing) and the Performance scales (Picture Completion, Code, Block Design, Matrix Reasoning, Picture Arrangement, Symbol Search and Object Assembly). These provide 3 scores: verbal IQ; performance IQ and a composite, single full-scale IQ score based on the combined scores. The average full-scale IQ is 100, with a standard deviation of 15 (above and below the mean). This is the average IQ range where typically developing individuals would fall.

Further evidence supporting dissociation between intellectual competences can be reached by examining more closely the cognitive profile of people with WS.

Cognitive Profile

WS presents an unique cognitive profile characterized by the striking co-existence of strengths and deficits. One of the most remarkable dissociations appears between verbal and visuo-spatial abilities. In the early 1990s, the prevailing view was that individuals with WS had normal language abilities despite severe visuo-spatial impairments and critical MR (e.g., Bellugi et al., 1994; Bellugi, Sabo and Vaid, 1988). Such a clear-cut profile has been contradicted by recent studies showing qualitatively different patterns of deficit observed within both language and visual-spatial cognition. In the domain of language, the current and nowadays dominant view considers that language development in WS mostly follows a normal, but delayed path (for a review see Karmiloff-Smith, Brown, Grice, and Paterson, 2003). Nevertheless, language of WS adults is generally grammatical and fluent, with well-developed vocabulary. Moreover, they tend to use relatively complex and syntactically correct sentences. Contrasting with this relatively spared domain, severe impairments in the visuo-spatial domain are a neuropsychological hallmark of WS. There also exists an unevenness within the visual domain of the WS profile, where weakness in visual tasks (e.g., drawings and the block design task of the Wechsler scales (Wechsler, 1996, 1997)) is contrasted with a near-normal ability to visually discriminate familiar and unfamiliar faces (e.g., Bellugi, Lichtenberger, Jones, Lai, and St. George, 2000). Several studies converge to show that when the visual stimuli involve faces, WS individuals often perform as accurately as normal controls in visual perception, recognition and discrimination tasks (Bellugi, et al., 1994; Deruelle, Rondan, Mancini, and Livet, 2003; Tager-Flusberg et al., 2003; Udwin, and Yule, 1991). Finally, it is important to note that this behavioural proficiency on face processing, as is the case for language, appears to co-exist with mild to moderate MR (Mervis, Robinson, Bertrand, Morris, Klein-Tasman, and Armstrong, 2000; Mervis, Robinson, Rowe, Becerra, and Klein-Tasman, 2004).

Behavioural Profile

Behaviour problems, such as pervasive, intense and persistent fears and anxieties, are often described in individuals with WS (e.g. Einfield, Tonge, and Florio, 1997). Such problems affect their ability to function, limiting their potential achievements. However, these are not considered as a major characteristic of the WS behavioural phenotype and can also be found in individuals with other disorders that result in MR (e.g., VanLieshout, DeMeyer, Curfs, and Fryns, 1998). Also, the intensity of reaction varies significantly across individuals. Some WS individuals may be 'on edge', uneasy, or worried, whereas others may be beset with phobias and panic states (Scheiber, 2000). Distractibility and attentional problems are also at the core of behavioural disturbance in WS. Nevertheless, the hallmark of WS behaviour is undoubtedly a marked sociability. Most of the individuals with WS exhibit an intriguing mix of social attributes. From early development they are unusually friendly, interact easily, show no fear of strangers and a strong empathy for the others (for a review see, Jones, Bellugi, Lai, Chiles, Reilly et al., 2000). They tend to be extremely outgoing to the point of being called hypersociable (e.g., Jones et al., 2000). For a long time, this notion of hypersociability and the idea of an "intact" social module in WS prevailed (Bellugi et al., 1988; Bellugi et al., 1994; Wang, Doherty, Rourke and Bellugi, 1995). This was believed to underlie strengths in specific domains such as face processing, language and theory of mind (e.g., Karmiloff-Smith, Klima, Bellugi, Grant and Baron-Cohen, 1995). Yet, the panorama is not always that positive and clear. In fact, social behaviour in WS is often maladapted and characterized by overfriendliness, oversensivity and poor peer relations (e.g., Laing, Butterworth, Ansari, Gsodl, Longhi, et al., 2002). Although sociability, empathy and overfriendliness are integral features of WS, such contradictions challenge the assumption that sociability is a unitary trait entirely spared in WS.

The Point of View of Genetics

One of the main issues of this last decade was to discover the genetic basis of these peculiar cognitive and behavioural profiles. Research on the WS genotype created a major breakthrough in understanding the origins of WS. It is now widely accepted that WS is caused by the absence of one copy of some 25 contiguous genes on chromosome 7, including the gene encoding elastin (Donnai and Karmiloff-Smith, 2000; Korenberg, Chen, Hirota, Lai, Bellugi et al., 2000). Discovery of this specific molecular profile serves as a genetic marker for WS, i.e., it is a definite way of establishing the diagnosis of WS in individuals who exhibit a wide range of physical, medical, and behavioural features included in the clinical diagnosis of WS. Genetic research also attempted at identifying specific genes that are counterparts or contribute to the manifestation of certain behavioural features of WS (e.g., Frangiskakis, Ewart, Morris, Bertrand, Robinson, Klein, et al., 1996). Recent studies based on fine grain analyses of specific areas of chromosome band 7q11.23 have suggested that the microdeletion in some of these genes may be responsible for many WS characteristics, such as MR, neonatal hypercalcemia, cardiovascular and facial anomalies (e.g., Korenberg et al., 2000). Despite major advances in this domain, detailed maps establishing the impact of this genetic disorder on brain and behaviour are still sparse. Thus, the interplay of genetic and environmental influences on the emergence of MR and specific cognitive profile in WS remains poorly understood.

The Point of View of Brain Sciences

At the structural level, several studies attempted to determine the neural markers of WS in relation to its odd profiles. Post-mortem neuroanatomical analysis showed reduced brain size (Jernigan and Bellugi, 1990), Chiari malformations (e.g., Pober and Filiano, 1995), corpus callosum shape changes (e.g., Schmitt, Eliez, Warsofsky, Bellugi and Reiss, 2001a) and altered cell size and density in primary visual cortex (Galaburda, Holinger, Bellugi and Sherman, 2002) in WS.

Studies using structural MRI also found significant brain differences between WS and typically developing individuals. These include volumetric decreases in gray and white matters of the thalamus and occipital lobes, along with an increase in the size of the amygdala and superior temporal and orbitofrontal gyri in WS (Reiss, Eckert, Rose, Karchemskiy, Kesler, Chang et al., 2004). Cerebral shape analysis also revealed reduced overall curvature of the brain in WS (Schmitt, Eliez, Bellugi, Reiss, 2001b), as well as abnormally increased gyrification in parietal and occipital lobes (Schmitt, Watts, Eliez, Bellugi, Galaburda, and Reiss, 2002) and the temporoparietal zone (Thompson, Lee, Dutton, Geaga, Hayashi, Eckert, et al., 2005). Particularly striking differences were also found in the WS corpus callosum, both in terms of shape (less curved) and volume (reduced). More precisely, while anterior callosal sections were relatively spared, reduced size was found for the splenium and the isthmus (Schmitt et al., 2001b).

Taken together these studies reveal critical differences in brain mechanisms and may help clarify the atypical neural substrate and type of brain processing in WS. Interestingly, it has been suggested that some of these anatomical findings may concur with behavioural features of WS. For instance, the overall decrease in size of the isthmus and the splenium may to some extent account for the well-known visuo-spatial deficits in this condition (Schmitt et al., 2001a, 2001b; Tomaiuolo, Di Paola, Caravale, Vicari, Petrides, Caltagirone, 2002). However, anatomo-behavioural correlates are still few and in need of further investigation.

Bringing Genes, Brain and Behaviour Together ...

The striking peak-valley profile of cognitive sparing and impairment found in WS, both across and especially within domains, provide important insights on the architecture of several cognitive systems and on the link between genes, brain and behaviour. For the purpose of this paper, the dissociations found in the cognitive domain of WS present a major interest. It is on the social-cognitive sphere that intactness was mostly defended in WS. Here we focus on one specific function believed to be "an island of sparing in WS" (Bellugi et al., 2000, pp., 19) and an integrative part of this sphere – face processing.

Face Processing

Before turning back to WS, we will first consider face-processing skills in normal development. These are thought to be important evolutionary basic skills that have helped drive the development of our social behaviour. In line with this, the human face is undoubtedly a special site to convey social and emotional information and a crucial reference for social communication. Faces are also a means for inferring intentions and desires from others. Faces are special stimuli for humans from the earliest stages of development. Newborns tend to look longer and to orient preferentially their attention to faces compared to other objects (e.g., Johnson, Dziurawiec, Ellis and Morton, 1991). This increased and early interest for faces is thought to bring about our extraordinary abilities for processing faces and facial emotions quickly and accurately (see Bruce and Young, 1986 for a review). These abilities can be assimilated to expertise phenomenon (e.g., Buckack, Gauthier and Tarr, 2006). According to several authors, expertise in face processing is closely linked to the ability to code configural properties (e.g., Rhodes, Tan, Brake and Taylor, 1989). This configural mode of processing refers to the analysis of the spatial interrelationships of facial features (i.e., eyes, nose, mouth, etc.) and is usually opposed to analytical or local mode of processing (e.g., Maurer, Le Grand, and Mondloch, 2002). Sensitivity to configural changes in face processing has been considered as evidence for face-exclusive mechanisms in normal development (e.g., Buckack et al., 2006). Curiously, this is not the case in some developmental disorders. The most striking example comes from studies in autism suggesting that the use of atypical perceptual strategies (local rather than configural processing strategies) prohibit the normal development of face-processing competences (e.g., Behrmann, Thomas, and Humphreys, 2006; Deruelle et al., 2004). Regarding WS, although the prevailing view argues for intactness of face-processing skills, some studies showed that WS rely on atypical strategies to do such processing (Deruelle, Mancini, Livet, Cassé-Perrot and de Schonen, 1999). The following sections will highlight the origin of this debate.

Face Processing in WS

The first reports of face-processing skills in WS were based on standardized face-processing tasks, such as the Benton Facial Recognition Test[2] (BFRT) and the Rivermead Face Memory task[3] (RFMT). Adults with WS were found to perform as accurately as chronological age-matched controls and even more accurately than IQ-matched individuals with Down syndrome on the BFRT (Bellugi, et al., 1994). Moreover, during experiments researchers noticed WS infants tended to look the experimenter in the eyes insistently and spent significantly more time focusing on faces than on objects (Bellugi, et al., 2000; Mervis and Bertrand, 1997). This led to the suggestion that such an early interest for faces would result in adult expertise on face-processing skills (e.g., Bellugi et al., 2000). Taken together these studies were the basis for claims of "intact" face-processing skills in WS. However, such claims were challenged by subsequent studies showing both delay and deviance in WS face processing (Karmiloff-Smith, Thomas, Annaz, Humphreys, Ewing, Brace et al., 2004). Also, near-normal face-processing abilities in WS were found to rely nevertheless on the use of atypical featural perceptual strategies (Deruelle et al., 1999; Karmiloff-Smith, 1997; Mancini, Rondan, Livet, Chabrol and Deruelle, 2006).

---

[2] The Benton Facial Recognition Test measures the ability to recognize the identity of neutral/non-emotional faces and requires the subject to select from a set of six aligned black and white photographs the face with the same identity as the reference face.

[3] The Rivermead Face Memory task is a subtest of the Rivermead Behavioural Memory Test that measures recognition and recall of faces.

Configural vs. Featural: What Strategies Do WS Individuals Use to Process Faces?

This question has been at the centre of animated debates over the past decade. Within this context, Karmiloff-Smith, one of the pioneers on the study of face processing in WS, provided a major contribution. In a preliminary study, she showed that WS individuals were able to do featural analysis but were impaired when doing configural analysis, in comparison to chronological age-matched controls (Karmiloff-Smith, 1997). Although this study included only 10 participants with WS, it had the merit of being the first to suggest that normal performance in WS might not necessarily reflect the use of normal processing strategies. Also, this study offered the opportunity to shift the attention of the scientific community from the debate of whether face-processing skills are intact or impaired, to whether its development occurs normally or atypically.

Studies from our group provide support to the initial claims of Karmiloff-Smith (1997). Face-processing skills of 12 children with Williams between the ages of 7 and 23 were compared to that of two groups of normally developing children (matched on chronological age and on mental age) across three different experiments (Deruelle et al., 1999). The first experiment focused on the ability to discriminate different aspects of faces, such as emotional expressions and gaze direction (see figure 1). The second experiment aimed at determining if participants used local or configural strategies to process faces. Finally, the third experiment assessed the ability to discriminate between local and configural transformations (see figure 2). Results revealed that while children with WS performed significantly lower than chronological age-matched controls, no such performance differences were found when compared to mental age-matched controls. Most importantly, children with WS did not show the same performance pattern as typically developing individuals did, i.e., the use of a configural face-processing mode. Contrary to control groups, WS failed to present the so-called inversion effect[4] when processing faces deprived of their usual configuration (inverted faces). In typically developing individuals this inversion effect is thought to sign configural face processing (e.g., Leder, Candrian, Huber and Bruce, 2001). Deruelle and colleagues (1999) interpreted these findings as evidence for a configural deficit in face processing in WS. More specifically, results of the third experiment described above sustained this interpretation by showing that individuals with WS discriminate local, but not configural transformations, as well as controls. Additional support to this position was also provided by a subsequent study showing that WS rely more on local rather than on configural strategies to process faces, in contrast to typically developing individuals (Karmiloff-Smith et al., 2003). Taken together these studies suggest that WS individuals do use atypical (featural) strategies to process faces while achieving near-normal levels of accuracy on face-processing tasks. This is nevertheless highly contradictory to the widespread idea that an efficient development of face processing depends on the use of configural analysis (Le Grand, Mondloch, Maurer, and Brent, 2001). Moreover, in light of the evidence from earlier studies using standardized

---

[4] The recognition of face pictures is disproportionately affected by a 180-degree rotation (inversion) in the image plane from the normal, upright viewing condition (Yin, 1969). This phenomenon is now commonly called the Face Inversion Effect. There is now agreement that the Face Inversion Effect arises from a greater difficulty to perceptually encode inverted face information (e.g. Farah, Wilson, Drain, & Tanaka, 1998).

measures (Bellugi et al., 1994), face processing is shown to be a relative strength in WS (see also Bellugi et al., 2000; Jones, Hickok, and Lai., 1998; Wang et al., 1995). However, the idea that such proficiency depends on abnormal mechanisms (featural analysis) is controversial. The question of whether configural processing is really affected in WS remains thus in need of further explanation.

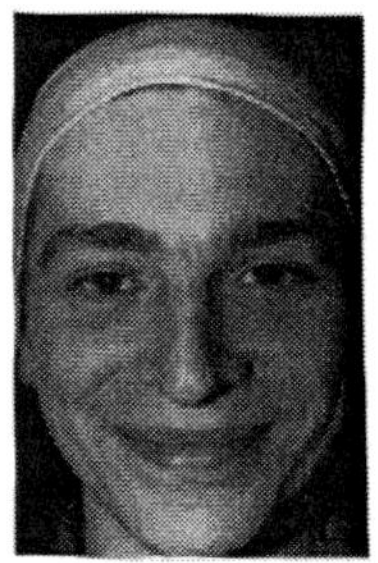

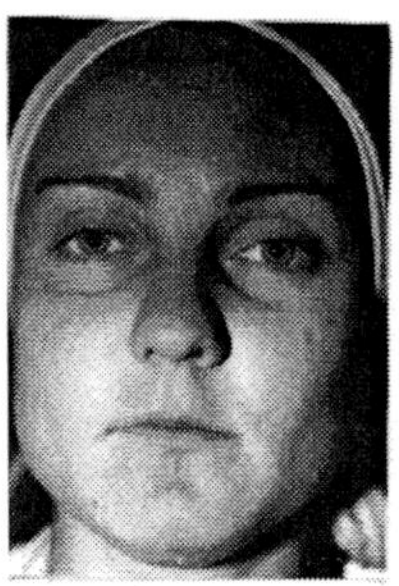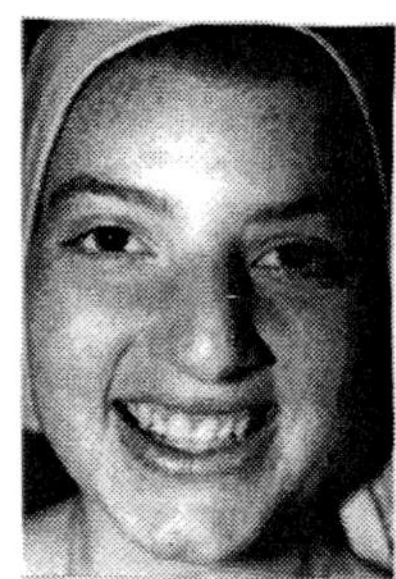

Figure 1. Example of the stimuli used by Deruelle et al. (1999) to assess the ability to discriminate different aspects of faces (e.g. emotional expressions).

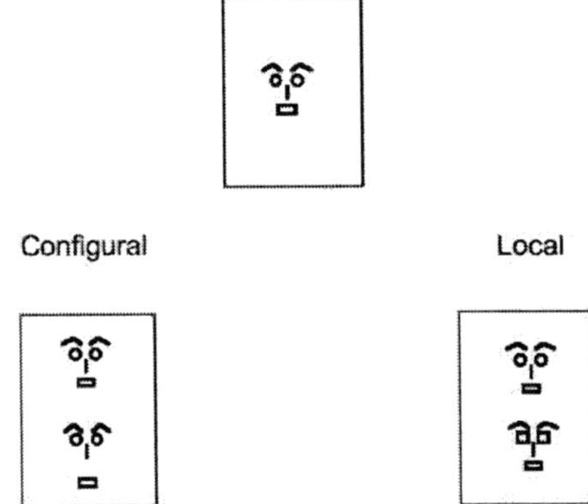

Figure 2. Example of stimuli used by Deruelle et al. (1999) to assess the ability to discriminate between local and configural transformations.

Attempting to further clarify this contradictory issue, Deruelle and colleagues (2003) designed three new experiments tapping specifically on face-processing perceptual strategies.

The first two experiments (see figure 3) contrasted the ability to match faces on the basis of high- or low-spatial frequency information (i.e., analysis based on local facial features versus on global configuration of faces, respectively). Surprisingly, results revealed that all groups of children, control (typically developing children matched on chronological age and on mental age) as well as WS (N=12) presented the same pattern of performance (i.e., they were more accurate when relying on low- rather than on high-spatial frequency). Finally, the authors tested whether children with WS differed from controls when they were to process faces on the basis of internal versus external parts of faces. Again, results suggested that children with WS, as controls, relied more on global shape (contour) than on featural components (internal). Taken together, these findings indicated that, similar to overall face-processing skills (Bellugi et al., 1988), holistic face encoding is preserved in WS (Deruelle et al., 2003). The authors interpreted the discrepancy with previous findings (Deruelle et al., 1999 and Karmiloff-Smith, 1997) as due to tasks demands. They argued that WS individuals are impaired when the task demands configural analysis (i.e;, processing of spatial relationships between elements), as it was the case in the earlier studies of Karmiloff-Smith (1997) and Deruelle et al., (1999), but exhibit intact abilities when they can perform the task on the basis of a global analysis (i.e., such as the contour), as it was the case in this latest study (Deruelle et al., 2003).

SPATIAL FREQUENCY

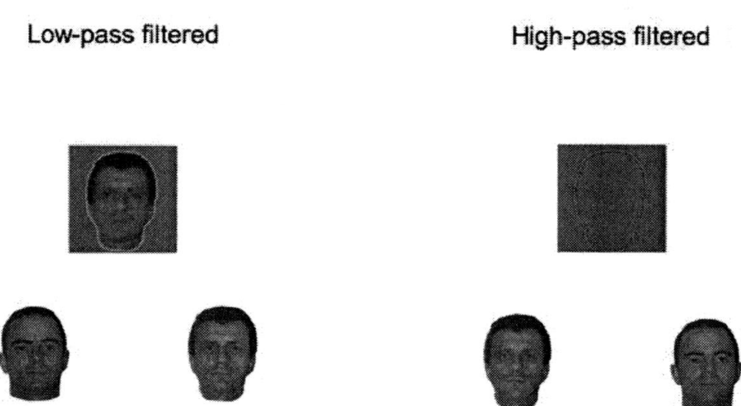

Figure 3. Example of stimuli used by Deruelle et al. (2003) to assess the ability to match faces on the basis of high or low spatial frequency information.

Further support was also provided by a study conducted by Tager-Flusberg and colleagues (2003) using the whole-part method developed in the 1990s by Tanaka and colleagues (Tanaka and Farah, 1993; Tanaka, Kay, Grinnel, Stansfield, and Szechter, 1998). This experimental paradigm focused on the distinction between holistic and feature-based face processing. Participants are presented with either a whole face or one isolated feature of faces (eyes, nose or mouth) displayed upright and inverted. They are then presented with a two-choice recognition test and are asked to select the face or the face part that best matched the target face or face parts. This method is based on the idea that if upright faces are processed holistically, the individual features of a face will be recognized more easily in the context of a whole face than in isolation. By contrast, under inverted presentations, no holistic processing advantage should be observed, neither on the whole face nor on the isolated parts conditions. Using this paradigm, Tager-Flusberg and colleagues (2003) compared the performance of 47 WS individuals to that of normally developing age-matched controls. Results clearly indicated that both groups, WS as well as controls, presented the same pattern of performance across the different conditions. Interestingly, WS individuals were found to present a whole-face advantage only under upright presentations. This was interpreted as evidence for the use of typical holistic strategies to encode and recognize faces in WS, as it happens in normal controls (Tager-Flusberg et al., 2003).

To sum, the findings of both Deruelle et al. (2003) and Tager-Flusberg et al. (2003) suggest that overall face-processing abilities are likely to be spared in WS. These findings focus on visual perceptual mechanisms for understanding face processing in WS. Investigating face processing in WS from this point of view is certainly very different from the one adopted in the earliest studies (e.g., Bellugi et al., 1988), relying more on social rather than on perceptual mechanisms to justify proficiency in this domain. But, do perceptual mechanisms account for the whole panorama of face-processing patterns observed in WS?

The first claims for intactness of face-processing skills in WS were based on the idea of an intact social module, including not only increased face processing but also increased social interest - skills that are possibly closely related. Proficiency in face processing, together with strong social motivation, has led researchers to hypothesize that relative strengths in face processing are linked to hypersociable behaviour in WS (e.g., Pober and Dykens, 1996; Jones et al., 2000). After more than one decade, has this hypothesis been validated?

Is There a Link between Face Processing and Social Skills in WS?

Contrary to what has been found in WS, some specific developmental disorders do present severe impairments in face processing. The most striking example of this comes from studies in autism. In this case, alternatively to visual perceptual impairments, pervasive problems in social interaction and reduced interest towards social stimuli were proposed as an explanation for the apparent difficulty with faces described in this condition (Grelotti, Gauthier and Schultz, 2002). Opposite performance patterns for face processing across developmental disorders as observed in autism and WS has been the issue of several comparative studies (e.g., Grelotti et al., 2002). For instance, a recent study investigating face-processing proficiency in WS compared a group of 19 individuals with WS (aged 10 to 44 years) to a group of 16 individuals with autism and to a group of 17 normal control volunteers (Rose, Lincoln, Lai, Ene, Searcy and Bellugi, 2006). These 3 groups were asked to perform a same-different face recognition task comprising three experimental conditions: upright faces with neutral expressions, upright faces with varying affective expressions (happy, sad, angry, surprised and afraid) and inverted faces with neutral expressions. The major hypothesis of this study focused on the impact of social information in face recognition abilities. It was predicted that if attention to social information does affect face recognition, the WS group would demonstrate preserved face recognition when faces vary by affective expression when compared to the autistic one, but show greater difficulty when faces were inverted. The results showed that all groups were more accurate when comparing neutral faces than when comparing faces with expressed emotions. The presence of emotional indexes in the faces seemed thus to increase the difficulty of the task. Most importantly, under this condition the WS group performed at the same level as controls. By contrast, the autistic group performed below the level of both control and WS groups, suggesting that emotional information has a negative impact on their ability to compare two faces (stimuli and target). The authors attempted to interpret these results by the well-known differences in social behaviour between individuals with WS and autism. In line with the idea that early social disinterest affects later face-processing skills in autism (e.g., Sasson, 2006) the authors suggested that the opposite would happen, i.e., that because "early in development, individuals with WS obtain normal to above-normal experience in viewing faces" this would result in "subsequent *expertise* in discrimination" (Rose et al., 2006, pp. 7). This interpretation is undoubtedly curious. Yet, rather than being *experts*, individuals with WS were found to perform at the same level as controls. This raises the doubt if the link between social interest and face-processing skills is so clear-cut. Furthermore, it seems more reliable to address this issue by testing the ability to decode social cues expressed in faces, rather than by asking participants to judge if two faces are the same or not.

In order to determine whether the positive social bias characteristic of individuals with WS interferes with facial-emotion decoding, Gagliardi and colleagues (Gagliardi, Frigerio, Burt, Cazzaniga, Perret and Borgatti, 2003) used a newly developed test of facial-expression recognition (Animated Full Facial Expression Comprehension Test – AFFECT). Performance of a WS group (N=26) was compared to 2 groups of typically developing individuals (one matched on chronological age and another on mental age). One original contribution of this study was the finding that despite performing at normal levels on the BFRT, individuals with WS were nevertheless poorer in their overall performance for recognizing facial expression than controls of the same age and indistinguishable from controls matched on intellectual level. Because changes in configuration of the face are an important part of expressions, these differences were interpreted as resulting from a lack of configural ability in WS. Finally, results showed no positive labelling bias in the WS group's interpretation of facial expressions. Thus, this study failed to provide validation to the idea of a link between increased positive social bias in WS and the interpretation of proficiency in facial expressions.

More recently, Plesa-Skwerer and colleagues (Plesa-Skwerer, Faja, Schofield, Verballis and Tager-Flusberg, 2005) conducted a study aimed at further investigating perception of emotional expressions in WS. Contrary to previous studies, the authors hypothesized that the WS group would show impairments in emotion labelling relative to typically developing individuals. Moreover, it was predicted that, compared to individuals with learning/intellectual disabilities (matched on chronological and mental age), individuals with WS would not present more facilities to label emotions, despite their gregarious social behaviour. Results corroborated these two predictions suggesting that emotion recognition is neither an increased nor spared ability in WS. This is in contradiction with the initial studies claiming that most social-cognitive abilities are generally impaired in this population

(Karmiloff-Smith et al., 1995). However, this hypothesis linking relative strengths in face processing and increased social interest cannot be refuted on the basis of the only two studies that tested facial-emotion processing in WS. It remains thus, to date, a hypothesis needing confirmation.

We conducted a study aimed at determining the impact of social relevance in face-processing abilities, as an attempt to participate at this heated and continuing debate. In order to extend face-processing assessment beyond identity processing we used a facial-emotion recognition task. This task included three different types of faces believed to vary in terms of social value: photographs of real faces, human cartoon faces and non-human cartoon faces. It was hypothesized that increased motivation towards social stimuli underlies face-processing skills in WS. Thus, a face's *social status* should have a greater impact on the performances of WS participants than on typically developing individuals. Before describing and discussing the findings of this study we will present the underling methodological aspects.

Who Was Included?

This study included 17 children and adolescents with WS (13 female and 4 male) aged 7 to 19 years ($M = 13.3$; $SD = 3.4$). The diagnosis of WS was confirmed for all participants by both clinical evaluation (neurologist and neuropsychologist) and a FISH test (fluorescent *in situ* hybridization) for microdeletion on one copy of the gene for elastin on chromosome 7. Furthermore, all participants fulfilled the clinical diagnostic criteria set out by Preus (1984). IQ standardized measures (WAIS-III (Wechsler, 1997) or WISC-III (Wechsler, 1996), according to the subject's age) were used to assess intellectual functioning and to confirm MR diagnosis. Full-scale IQ scores ranged from 40 to 81 ($M = 56.7$; $SD = 11.5$), verbal IQ scores ranged from 46 to 91 ($M = 65.3$; $SD = 13.8$) and performance IQ scores ranged from 46 to 80 ($M = 55.2$; $SD = 9.3$). IQ profile was thus characterized by a clear dissociation between verbal and performance abilities. This in agreement with several previous studies on WS (e.g. Jarrold, Baddeley, and Hewes, 1998). Mental age, inferred from Wechsler' IQ measures, was inferior to chronological age and ranged from 4 to 11 years ($M = 7.4$; $SD = 2.2$). Participants were recruited via Regional Williams Syndrome Associations and all attended schools or specialized centres at the time of testing. In order to verify that face processing in WS was independent from intellectual functioning, and to control for the effects of life experience with faces, WS participants were individually matched to typically developing individuals on the basis of their age and gender. This control group consisted of 17 children and adolescents aged 7 to 19 years ($M = 13.1$; $SD = 1.3$). They were recruited via local schools and day-care centres and they all attended normal classes corresponding to their age level.

All participants were native French speakers, had normal or corrected-to-normal vision and audition, and had no overt physical handicap. Parental informed consent was obtained for all subjects and the local ethics committee approved the experimental procedure.

What Did We Use?

This study focused on the ability to categorize facial emotions. This ability was assessed using a visual task including three types of faces, believed to vary in terms of social relevance: photographs of human faces, human cartoon faces and non-human cartoon faces (see figure 4). Each face was displayed in three different emotional expressions: happiness, sadness and anger. Stimuli comprised 18 black and white pictures of faces (9 female, 9 male). Photographs of human faces were taken from the AR Face Database (Martinez and Benavente, 1998). Human and non-human cartoon faces were inspired from foreign cartoon movies[5] to assure that all subjects were presented with the stimuli for the first time. In order to control for overall familiarization with cartoon faces, exposure to virtual faces (presented on TV programs, comics books, video games, etc.) was assessed for each participant through a parental questionnaire. All faces were cropped at the neckline and presented full face. Pictures subtended approximately $14° \times 11°$ of the visual angle when viewed at 60 cm. Stimuli were displayed using Microsoft Power Point Presentation software in a 14 inch computer screen.

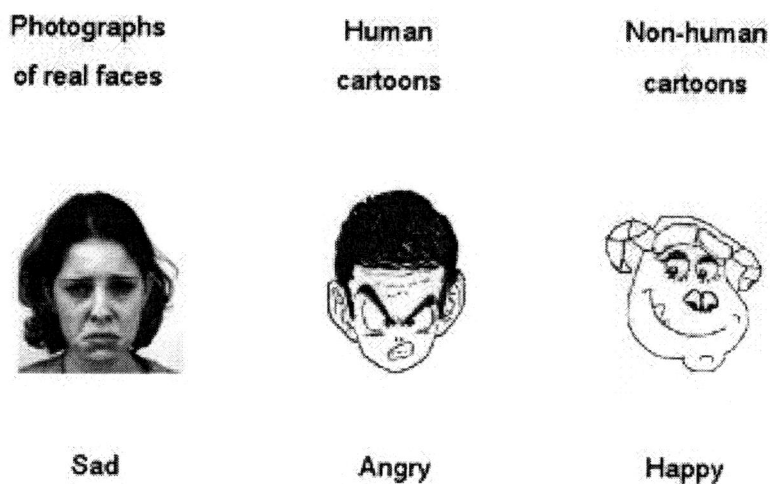

Figure 4. Example of stimuli used in the emotion categorization task. Participants were presented with three types of faces - photographs of real faces, human cartoon faces and non-human cartoon faces – and were asked to judge if faces expressed sadness, anger or happiness.

What Did We Do?

Participants were seated in a quiet room and placed at a distance of 60 cm in front of a computer screen. They were told that faces were going to be presented on the center of the screen and were asked to comment if the presented faces were happy, sad or angry. No information was provided concerning the nature of the faces. The testing session began with

---

[5] der kleine Eisbar, Wickie und die Starken Manner, Samurai Deeper Kyo, Monster and Company, Tabaluga, Sakura

9 practice trials in order to ensure that instructions were understood. During this training session participants were presented with one example of each condition: photographs of real faces (happy / sad / angry), human cartoon faces (happy / sad / angry), and non-human cartoon faces (happy / sad / angry). Following this, all participants were presented with 3 blocks of 18 trials, each containing 6 photographs of real faces, 6 faces of human cartoons and 6 faces of non-human cartoons. The order of block presentation was randomized across subjects. Stimuli remained displayed on the screen until the subject responded. The participants' task was a 3 forced-choice task, as they were explicitly asked to judge if the face was happy, sad or angry. Verbal responses were recorded by the experimenter and scored one if correct or zero if incorrect.

The number of errors produced by each subject in each condition was analysed using ANOVAs[6] (analyses of variance), and Tukey tests for post-hoc comparisons. In order to determine the influence of age and IQ on WS group's performances, correlation analyses were computed using Pearson's r test.

What Did We Find?

Results revealed that although the performance of the WS group was lower overall than those of controls (see figure 5), these group differences were not significant across all conditions. In other words, participants with WS only differed from normal controls (CTR) when they were to categorize emotions in non-human faces (WS = 3.2 vs. CTR = 0.76, p = 0.02). By contrast, when emotions were displayed in photographs of real faces (WS = 1.1; CTR = 0.4) or in human cartoon faces (WS = 2.5; CTR = 1.4) no significant differences were found between groups (all ps > 0.57). Moreover, results revealed that the ability to categorize emotions was not dependent on the face type for controls (all ps > 0.16). Participants included in this group performed as accurately when faces were non-human as well as when they were human. By contrast, no such symmetry was found in the WS performance pattern. Instead, WS individuals were found to produce more errors when categorizing emotions on non-human cartoon faces (3.2) than on human cartoon faces (2.5, p = 0.01) and on photographs of real faces (1.2, p < 0.001).

Finally, results of correlation analysis revealed that neither chronological age (CA) nor IQ exerted an influence on the WS group's performance (all p > 0.05).

---

[6] Results reported in this section were based on a three-way analysis of variance (ANOVA) including Group (WS vs. controls) as between-subject factor and Face (Human Photographs vs. Human Cartoons vs. Non-Human Cartoons) as within-subject factors. Tukey tests were used for post-hoc comparisons.

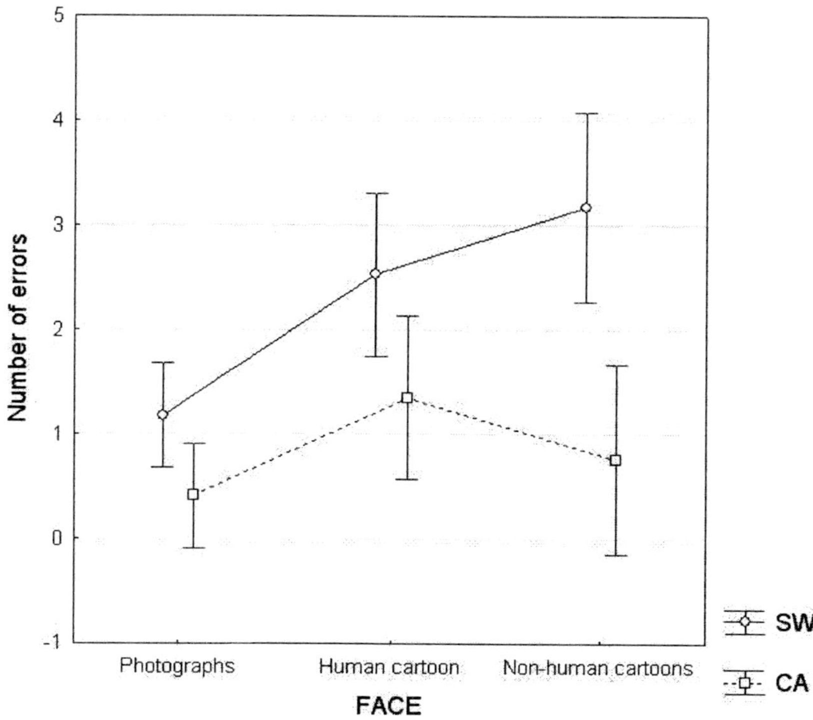

Figure 5. Response patterns (number of errors) observed for each group (WS and Choronological age-matched control (CA)) in each condition (photographs of real faces, human cartoon faces, and non-human cartoon faces).

Discussion

This study aimed at determining the impact of a face's *social status* on emotion processing abilities of individuals with WS when compared to typically developing individuals. When considering overall performance in the facial-emotion categorization task we found that participants with WS performed as accurately as controls for all types of faces except for one. When presented with non-human cartoon faces, WS group's performances were significantly inferior to those of typically developing individuals without MR (see figure 5). This suggests that individuals with WS do have difficulties in recognizing emotions in faces. However, it is important to underline that these difficulties were not found across all experimental conditions, but rather were selective to faces that did not presented human traits. In fact, no group difference was found when participants were asked to categorize emotions in photographs of real faces and human cartoon faces. Strikingly, despite limited intellectual functioning (mean IQ = 57), WS participants were able to perform at similar levels as typically developing individuals of the same (chronological) age with higher IQ. This indicates that WS individuals can decode emotions expressed in faces sharing human features at a higher level than that expected from their intellectual level. These findings thus contradict previous studies arguing for specific impairments in facial-emotion decoding in WS (Gagliardi et al., 2003; Plesa-Skwerer et al., 2006). Most importantly for the purpose of this paper, these results challenge the notion of symmetry in MR by suggesting that individuals with MR can, nevertheless, present spared abilities in specific domains.

Although impairments in social skills have been found in people with MR (e.g., Rojahn, Rabold, and Schneider, 1995), the idea that these impairments affect the whole social sphere has been questioned. Studies show intact abilities for perceiving human bodily movements in contrast with specific impairments in other information-processing capacities in individuals with MR (Moore, Hobson, and Anderson, 1995). The findings of the present study also suggest uneven social-perceptual capacities in individuals with MR, with emotion processing being spared for human faces but impaired for non-human faces, in comparison to typically developing individuals. Curiously, this pattern of performance was found to be independent from IQ levels. Correlational analysis revealed that IQ scores did not account for the WS group's performance in any of the three experimental conditions (all ps > .05). It is evidence that, despite MR, emotion recognition in WS was unaffected by impairments in general cognitive functioning. Also, this supports the idea that spared domain-specific capacities for facial-emotion processing may be found in people with MR. Yet, what determines intactness in some domains and impairments in others? More precisely, what are the reasons underlying normal performances in emotion processing for human but not for non-human faces in WS? In the next paragraphs we will attempt to provide some explanations for this striking dissociation.

First, one may argue that participants with WS have more difficulties in decoding emotions in non-human than in human faces because these stimuli differ in complexity. It is true that the stimuli used in the present study varied in terms of complexity, mainly because real faces present more features and texture variations than cartoons (see figure 4). Nonetheless, performance differences in WS group were found not only between photographs and cartoons (both human and non-human), but also within cartoon conditions (human vs. non-human cartoons). In addition, such difference was not found in typically developing participants that performed as accurately when cartoon faces were non-human as when they were human (see figure 5). Thus, it seems unlikely that a complexity bias underlies the unusual pattern of performance found in WS group.

Second, it can be hypothesized that the well-known visuo-spatial impairments described in WS have an increased impact on the processing of non-human faces. Again, it is true that the task used in the present study was presented through the visual modality. Still, it is important to note that, in contrast to same/different face-processing tasks, this task was not particularly demanding in visual perceptual analysis. Rather, participants were asked to categorize facial emotions on a 3 forced-choice task ("Is he/she happy, sad or angry?"). Since both human and non-human cartoon faces contained identifiable local facial features there is no reason to believe that emotion categorization in non-human faces required more spatial processes than in human faces. Also, if visuo-spatial deficits were to account for WS group's performances, then it should manifest by difficulties not only in human but also in non-human face processing. Within this context, it is also important to point out that the early hypothesis of a general impairment across all areas of visual-cognition in WS (Bellugi et al., 1988) has been recently challenged by studies showing domain-specific rather than generalized deficits. For instance, results of Farran and Jarrold (2003) and of Rondan, Mancini, Livet and Deruelle (2003) suggest that individuals with WS have visuo-constructive deficits but relatively spared visuo-perceptive abilities. As described above, in the present study participants were presented with a visuo-perceptual (not constructive) task. Taken together these arguments seem strong enough to exclude visual-spatial deficits as being responsible for the WS group's performance pattern.

As a third possible interpretation of performance differences as a function of the face type in WS, is the use of different perceptual strategies to process human and non-human faces. It is widely accepted nowadays that typically developing individuals use configural strategies to process faces (e.g., Bukach et al., 2006). Yet, this robust and well-known mechanism is not infallible. This mechanism breaks down as soon as faces loose their usual configuration, as is the case when faces are presented inverted. What if this was also the case for faces presented without human traits? Recent findings of Santos and colleagues (submitted) helps answer this question. In order to determine whether face-processing abilities in WS rely more on social than perceptual mechanisms the authors presented the same stimuli as used in the present study (photographs of real faces, human cartoon faces and non-human cartoon faces) in two different orientations: upright and inverted (see figure 6). Interestingly, results showed a significant performance decrease under disrupted (inverted) presentations in both WS and control groups. Most importantly for our purpose, this so-called face-inversion effect was found not only for human but also for non-human faces. These findings allow us thus to exclude the use of different perceptual strategies when processing human and non-human faces as a possible explanation for the discrepancy found between human and non-human face processing in WS.

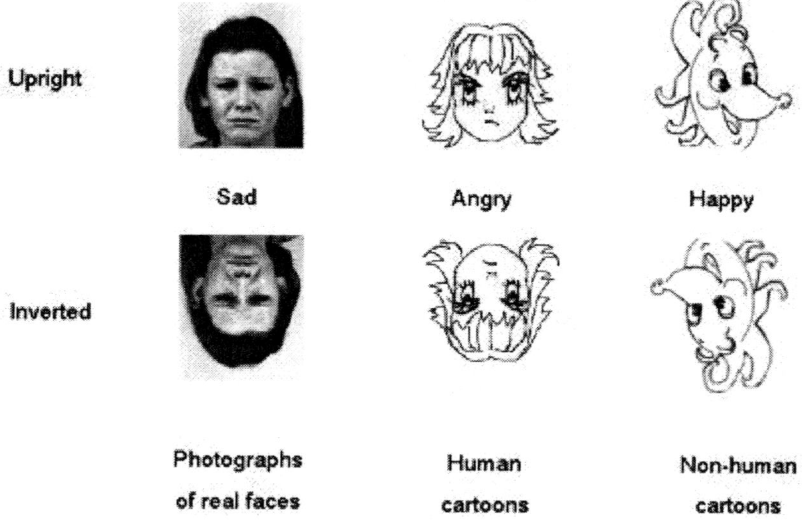

Figure 6. Example of stimuli used by Santos et al. (submitted) in the facial-emotion recognition task. Participants were presented with three types of faces – photographs of real faces, human cartoon faces and non-human cartoon faces – and were asked to judge if faces expressed sadness, anger or happiness. All faces were displayed upright and inverted.

At this stage, it is worth to stress the fact that the results we are discussing here come from an emotion-categorization task. Thus, it seems fair to turn the focus of this discussion from perceptual to more social-cognitive mechanisms.

The human face and particularly facial expressions are powerful sources of social information. From an early age, humans pay increased attention to faces compared to other objects (Morton and Johnson, 1991). This specific interest for faces is believed to result in later expertise in face processing. In line with this idea, one should expect emotions expressed in real faces to be better decoded than that expressed in cartoon faces[7]. This was exactly the pattern found in both groups included in this study (i.e., participants had more difficulties to categorize emotions under cartoon than real photographs), suggesting that expertise may to some extent account for overall performance patterns. While expertise seems to be a reliable argument to explain performance differences between photographs and cartoon conditions, it fails to explain one particular dissociation: that found between human and non-human cartoon conditions in WS. In this study, the level of exposure to virtual faces (presented on TV programs, comics books, video games, etc.) of each participant was assessed through parental questionnaire. Interestingly, no differences were found between exposure to human and non-human cartoons. There is thus no reason to believe that individuals with WS have acquired greater expertise for human than non-human cartoon faces, as both are cartoon faces. It seems thus necessary to look for alternative approaches in addressing the reasons behind this dissociation.

Based on the theoretical framework of adult neuropsychology, our findings of a double dissociation within-syndrome and within-domain could be interpreted in terms of impaired *versus* intact cognitive modules. In this case, we could consider the uneven performance pattern found in the WS group as the result of a dissociation between two independently functioning modules of emotion recognition, one responsible for processing human faces (spared) and another responsible for processing non-human faces (impaired). Within this framework, WS was seen for a long time as a promising model to bolster innate modularity claims, i.e., to demonstrate the existence of innate and independently functioning modules, some of which being intact (e.g., language and face processing) and others impaired (e.g., visuo-spatial cognition). Taking the example of language, many researchers claimed that these abilities were preserved and functionally independent of other cognitive systems in WS (Pinker, 1991; Rossen, Jones, Wang, and Klima, 1995). Relative to other syndromes with MR (e.g., Down syndrome), language performance of individuals with WS is certainly impressive. However, many empirical studies providing evidence for language late onset (Singer Harris, Bellugi, Bates, Jones, and Rosen, 1997) and for atypicalities in several areas of language in WS (e.g., lexicon: Jarrold, Hartley, Phillips, and Baddeley, 2000; pragmatics: Laws and Bishop, 2004) challenged the notion of clear-cut intactness of language skills in this population. According to Karmiloff-Smith (e.g., 1998, 2006), given the dynamics of brain development, cognitive profiles of neurodevelopmental disorders are better interpreted in terms of atypical developmental trajectories rather than using a modular view of cognition (see also, Vazanta, 2005). As a pioneer against the use of adult neuropsychological models

---

[7] Even if children spend long periods of time watching TV or reading comics, their exposure with real faces undoubtedly exceeds the one with cartoon faces.

for explaining genetic developmental disorders, she claims that "it is time that the myths of static, intact modules be dethroned in favour of studying the complex dynamics of developmental trajectories" (Karmiloff-Smith et al., pp. 241). In line with this claim, the next paragraphs will attempt to interpret the dissociation between emotion processing in human and non-human faces in WS in light of a developmental approach, rather than as the outcome of a normal system with a non-human faces' processing module missing, and a human faces' processing module intact. Thus, it seems crucial to ask whether the proficiency to decode emotions in human but not in non-human faces in WS was reached throughout a(n) typical or atypical developmental trajectory.

There is general agreement that development involves contributions from genes and environment. While the WS genotype as been well described, only sparse studies have taken into account the influence of the environment throughout development on later behavioural outcomes in this population. In what concerns emotion processing in WS as well as in typical development, it seems very unlikely that a genetic predisposition *per se* accounts for the whole phenotypic outcome. Hence, the impact of environmental factors in the WS genotype may provide key elements to interpret our findings.

The ability to recognize facial emotions is crucial for effective social interaction and for gathering information about the environment. Moreover, this ability is thought to be linked to the ability to regulate one's own emotions and behave in a socially appropriate manner. For instance, infants who can accurately recognize and interpret facial expressions also tend to engage in pro-social behaviours (Walden and Field, 1982). By focusing on the WS social phenotype, one may find some crucial features that to some extent account for face and emotion processing in WS. These are generally included in the concept of hypersociability and comprise increased social motivation, eagerness to please others, drive to greet and interact with strangers and an empathy with the emotions of others (e.g., Bellugi et al., 2000; Jones et al., 2000). Since the earliest developmental stages, overfriendliness and a special interested in people (in particular people's faces), are remarkable features of WS (for a review see Jones et al., 2000). For instance, observational studies show that, even before language acquisition, children with WS present a "friendly and overly positive nature" and use positive emotional expressions (e.g., prolonged eye contact, smiling) to engage with adults including strangers (Jones et al., 2000, pp. 39). Interestingly, Jones and colleagues (2000) suggested that this "strong attraction to social interaction ... may interfere with their (children with WS) focus on cognitively driven tasks" (Jones et al., 2000, pp. 40). Based on this report, one may wonder about the impact of such gregarious social interest on later emotion processing, and in particular on facial-emotion recognition assessed through a cognitive task, as the one used in the present study.

It is also important to consider environmental influences on the production and interpretation of facial expressions of emotion. People behave differently when alone compared to when they are in the presence of others, and this includes the way emotions are expressed. Studies have shown that when playing with adults in comparison to playing alone, an infant increases smiling and is preferentially directed toward the adult, paying less attention to the toy (Jones and Raag, 1989). There is also evidence that as children mature, they learn to modify their emotional expression in socially-appropriate ways. For example, some of neonatal facial responses are modified during the first year of life, possibly as a result of reinforcement within an environmental context (Ekman, Sorenson, and Friesen, 1969). This flexibility of emotional facial display suggests that facial expressions are co-opted for greater use within social and cultural contexts (Rozin, 1998).

Our findings show that, compared to people without MR, WS individuals are able to process human faces and to decode the emotions expressed on it. Yet, this ability depends on the presence of human facial traits. This suggests that such traits have an increased relevance for WS individuals. We interpret these findings as a possible consequence of the hallmark feature of people with WS – hypersociability (Jones et al., 2000). In light of the WS social phenotype, one may argue that along development the mix of increased interest in social interaction and in people's faces results in increased social exposure and in greater experience with facial expressions. Hypothetically, this may result, in turn, in a certain *expertise* in facial-emotion recognition, despite low-intellectual functioning. In other words, the early impulse to social interaction in WS may have cascading effects over development, resulting in greater experience with facial features. Human features of faces are certainly important cues in social interaction contexts. Therefore, it can be hypothesized that because throughout development individuals with WS are particularly driven towards social interaction and also remarkably attracted by people's faces, they end up to develop an oversensitivity to the presence (or the absence) of the facial features they are (over)exposed to – putatively the human features of faces. This may thus explain why WS participants reached normal levels when they were to extract social information from human faces, but were impaired as soon as faces lost their human traits.

Turning back to the question of whether this outcome was reached throughout typical or atypical developmental trajectories, our findings do not allow us to provide a straightforward answer. Yet, the (over)sensitivity to human facial traits found in WS is more likely to be the behavioural outcome of an atypical combination of genetic (hypersociability) and environmental factors (increased social exposure) over development, rather than from the innate juxtaposition of impaired and intact functions. Validation of this position may help clarify some contradictory aspects of WS, such as the coexistence of hypersociability and social anxiety. Together with recent similar findings in the domain of language (for a review see, Karmiloff-Smith, Ansari, Campbell, Scerif, and Thomas, in press) the findings of the present study may also contribute to overwhelm the misleading notion of an intact social module in WS. Finally, our findings are promising as they challenge the notion symmetry on developmental disorders with MR and provide support to Karmiloff-Smith's (1998) claims for the need of considering development as the key to understand developmental disorders.

Acknowledgements

We are grateful to all the participants, their parents and the Regional Williams Syndrome Associations. Andreia Santos was supported by a grant from the FCT-MCTES (Portugal, SFRH / BD / 18820 / 2004) to conduct this study. We would also like to thank Professor Annette Karmiloff-Smith for her remarkable theoretical contribution to the understanding of both typical and atypical development.

References

American Association on Mental Retardation. (2002). *Mental retardation: Definition, classification, and systems of supports* (10th Ed.) Washington, DC: Author.

Anderson, M. (1992). Intelligence and development: A cognitive theory. Oxford: Blackwell.

Anderson, M. and Miller, K. L. (1998). Modularity, mental retardation, and speed processing. *Developmental Science, 1,* 239-245.

Bellugi, U., Lichtenberger, L., Jones, W., Lai, Z., and St. George, M. (2000). I. The neurocognitve profile of Williams syndrome: A complex pattern of strengths and weaknesses. *Journal of Cognitive Neuroscience, 12* (Suppl 1), 7-29.

Bellugi, U., Sabo, H., and Vaid, V. (1988). Spatial defects in children with Williams syndrome. In J. Stiles-Davis, M. kritchevsky, and U. Bellugi (Eds.), *Spatial cognition: Brain bases and development* (pp. 273-298). Hillsdale, NJ: Lawrence Erlbaum Associates.

Bellugi, U., Wang, P. P., and Jernigan, T. L. (1994). Williams syndrome: An unusual neurophysiologique profile. In S. Broman, and J. Grafman (Eds.), *Atypical cognitive deficits in developmental disorders: Implications for brain function* (pp. 23-56), Hillsdale, NJ: Lawrence Erlbaum Associates.

Berhmann, M., Thomas, C. and Humphreys, K. (2006). Seeing it differently: visual processing in autism. *Trends in Cognitive Sciences, 10,* 258-264.

Bruce, V., and Young, A. (1986). Understanding face recognition. *British Journal of Psychology, 81,* 361-380.

Bukach, C. M., Gauthier, I., and Tarr, M. J. (2006). Beyond faces and modularity: the power of an expertise framework. *Trends in Cognitive Science, 10,* 159-166.

Deruelle, C., Mancini, J., Livet, M. O., Cassé-Perrot, C. and de Schonen, S. (1999). Configural and local processing of faces in children with Williams syndrome. *Brain and Cognition, 41,* 276-298.

Deruelle, C., Rondan, C., Livet M. O. and Mancini, J. (2003). Exploring face processing in Williams syndrome. *Cognition, Brain, Behavior, 7,* 157-172.

Deruelle, C., Rondan, C., Tardif, C. and Gepner, B. (2004). Spatial frequency and face processing in children with autism. *Journal of Autism and Developmental Disorders, 34,* 199-210.

Donnai, D., and Karmiloff-Smith, A. (2000) Williams syndrome: From genotype through to the cognitive phenotype. *American Journal of Medical Genetics: Seminars in Medical Genetics, 97* (2), 164-171.

Einfield, S., Tonge, B., and Florio, T. (1997). Behavioral and emotional disturbance in individuals with Williams syndrome. *American Journal of Mental Retardation, 102,* 45-53.

Ekman, P., Sorenson, E. R., and Friesen, W. V. (1969). Pan-cultural elements in facial displays of emotions. *Science, 164,* 86-88.

Farah, M. J., Wilson, K. D., Drain, M., and Tanaka, J. N. (1998). What is "special" about face perception? *Psychological Review, 105* (3), 482-498.

Farran, E. K., and Jarrold, C. (2003). Visuospatial cognition in Williams syndrome: reviewing and accounting for the strengths and weaknesses in performance. *Developmental Neuropsychology, 23*, 173-200.

Fodor, J. (1983). *The Modularity of Mind.* Cambridge, MA: MIT Press.

Frangiskakis, J. M., Ewart, A. K., Morris, C. A., Bertrand, J. Robinson, B. F., Klein, B. P., Ensing, G. J., Everett, L. A., Green, E. D., Proscel, C., Gutowski, N. J., Noble, M., Atkinson, D. L., Odelberg, S. J. and Keating, M. T. (1996). Lim-Kinase-1 hemizygosity implicated in impaired visuospatial constructive cognition. *Cell, 86*, 59-69.

Gagliardi, C., Frigerio, E., Burt, D. M., Cazzaniga, I., Perrett, D. I., and Borgatii, R. (2003). Facial expression recognition in Williams Syndrome. *Neuropsychologia, 41*, 733-738.

Galaburda, A. M., Holinger, D. P., Bellugi, U., and Sherman, G. F. (2002). Williams syndrome: neuronal size and neuronal-packing density in primary visual cortex. *Archives of Neurology, 59* (9), 1461-1467.

Grelotti, D. J., Gauthier, I. , and Schultz, R. T. (2002). Social interest and the development of cortical face specialization: what autism teaches us about face processing. *Developmental Psychobiology, 40*, 213-225.

Jarrold, C., Baddeley, A. D., and Hewes, A. K. (1998). Verbal and nonverbal abilities in the Williams syndrome phenotype: evidence for diverging developmental trajectories. *Journal of Child Psychology and Psychiatry, 39*, 511-523.

Jarrold, C., Hartley, S. J., Phillips, C., and Baddeley, A. D. (2000). Word fluency in Williams syndrome: Evidence for unusual semantic organisation? *Cognitive Neuropsychiatry, 5*, 293-319.

Jernigan, T. L., and Bellugi, U. (1990). Anomalous brain morphology on magnetic resonance images in Williams syndrome and Down syndrome. *Archives of Neurology, 47* (5), 529-533.

Johnson, M. H., Dziurawiec, S., Ellis, H., and Morton, J. (1991). Newborns' preferential tracking of face-like stimuli and its subsequent decline. *Cognition, 40* (1-2), 1-19.

Jones, S. S. and Raag, T. (1989). Smile production in older infants: the importance of a social recipient for the facial signal. *Child Development, 60*, 811-818.

Jones, W., Bellugi, U., Lai, Z., Chiles, M., Reilly, J., Lincoln, A., and Adolphs, R. (2000). Hypersociability in Williams syndrome. *Journal of Cognitive Neuroscience, 12*, 30-46.

Jones, W., Hickok, G., and Lai, Z. (1998). Does face processing rely on intact visual spatial abilities? Evidence from Williams syndrome. *Cognitive Neuroscience Society Abstract Program, 80*, 67.

Karmiloff-Smith, A. (1997). Crucial differences between developmental cognitive neuroscience and adult neuropsychology. *Developmental Neuropsychology, 13*, 513-524.

Karmiloff-Smith, A. (1998). Development itself is the key to understanding developmental disorders. *Trends in Cognitive Sciences, 2*, 389-398.

Karmiloff-Smith, A. (2006). A tortuous route from genes to behavior : A neuroconstructivist approach. *Cognitive and Affective Behavioral Neurosciences, 6*, 9-17.

Karmiloff-Smith, A., Ansari, D., Campbell, L., Scerif, G., and Thomas, M. (in press) Theoretical implications of studying cognitive development in genetic disorders: The case of Williams-Beuren syndrome. In C. Morris, H. Lenhoff, and P. Wang (Eds.),

Williams-Beuren syndrome: research and clinical perspectives. Johns Hopkins University Press.

Karmiloff-Smith, A, Brown, J. H., Grice, S., and Paterson, S. (2003). Dethroning the myth: cognitive dissociations and innate modularity in Williams syndrome. *Developmental Neuropsychology, 23*, 227-242.

Karmiloff-Smith, A., Klima, E., Bellugi, U., Grant, J., and Baron-Cohen, S. (1995). Is there a social module? Language, face-processing and theory of mind in Williams syndrome. *Journal of Cognitive Neuroscience, 7*, 196-208.

Karmiloff-Smith, A., Thomas, M., Annaz, D., Humphreys, K., Ewing, S., Brace, N., Duuren, M., Pike, G., Grice, S., and Campbell, R. (2004). Exploring the Williams syndrome face-processing debate: the importance of building developmental trajectories. *Journal of Child Psychology and Psychiatry, 45*, 1258-1274.

Korenberg, J. R., Chen, X. N., Hirota, H., Lai, Z., Bellugi, U., Burian, D., Roe, B., and Matsuoka, R. (2000). IV. Genome structure and cognitive map of Williams syndrome. *Journal of Cognitive Neuroscience, 12* (Suppl 1), 89-107.

Kress, T. and Daum, I. (2003). Developmental prosopagnosia: a review. *Behavioral Neurology, 14* (3-4), 109-121.

Laing, E., Butterworth, G., Ansari, D., Gsodl, M., Longhi, E., Panagiotaki, G., et al. (2002) Atypical development of language and social communication in toddlers with Williams syndrome. *Developmental Science, 5*, 233-246.

Laws, G., and Bishop, D. V. M. (2004). Pragmatic Language Impairment and social deficits in Williams syndrome: a comparison with Down's syndrome and specific language impairment. *International Journal of Language Communication Disorders, 39*, 45-64.

Le Grand, R., Mondloch, C. J., Maurer, D., and Brent, H. P. (2001). Neuroperception. Early visual experience and face processing. *Nature, 410*, 890.

Leder, H., Candrian, G., Huber, O., and Bruce, V. (2001). Configural features in the context of upright and inverted faces. *Perception, 30*, 73-83.

Leslie, A. M., and Keeble, S. (1987). Do six-month-old infants perceive causality? *Cognition, 25*, 265-288.

Mancini, J., Rondan, C., Livet. M. O., Chabrol, B., and Deruelle, C. (2006). How children with Williams syndrome do process faces? *Neuropsychiatrie de l'enfant et de l'adolescence, 54*, 159-164.

Martinez A. M., and Benavente, R. (1998). The AR Face Database. *CVC Technical Report, #24*, June 1998.

Maurer, D., Le Grand, R., and Mondloch, C.J. (2002). The many faces of configural processing. *Trends in Cognitive Sciences, 6*, 255-260.

Mervis, C., and Bertrand, J. (1997). Developmental relations between cognition and language: Evidence from Williams Syndrome. In L. B. Adamson and M. A. Romski (Eds.), *Research on communication and language disorders: Contributions to theories of language development* (pp. 75-106). New York: Brookes.

Mervis, C. B., Robinson, B. F., Rowe, M. L., Becerra, A. M. and Klein-Tasman, B. P. (2004). Relations between language and cognition in Williams syndrome. In S. Bartke and J. Siegmüller (Eds.), *Williams Syndrome across Languages*, (pp. 63–92). Philadelphia, PA: John Benjamins Pub.

Mervis, C. B., Robinson, B., Bertrand, J., Morris, C. A., Klein-Tasman, B., and Armstrong, S. (2000). The Williams syndrome cognitive profile. *Brain and Cognition, 44,* 604-628.

Moore, D. G., Hobson, R. P., and Anderson, M. (1995). Person perception – does it involve IQ-independent perceptual processing? *Intelligence, 20,* 65-86.

Morton, J. and Johnson, M. H. (1991). CONSPEC and CONLERN : a two-process theory of infant face recognition. *Psychological Review, 98,* 164-181.

Pinker, S. (1991). Rules of language. *Science, 253,* 530-535.

Plesa-Skewerer, D., Faja, S., Schofield, C., Verbalis, A., and Tager-Flusberg, H. (2006). Perceiving facial and vocal expressions of emotion in individuals with Williams syndrome. *American Journal of Mental Retardation, 111,* 15-26.

Pober, B. R. and Dykens, E. M. (1996). Williams syndrome: an overview of medical, cognitive, and behavioural features. *Mental Retardation, 5,* 929-943.

Pober, B. R., and Filiano, J. J. (1995). Association of Chiari I malformation and Williams syndrome. *Pediatric Neurology, 12* (1), 84-88.

Premack, D. (1990). The infant's theory of self-propelled objects. *Cognition, 36,* 1-16.

Preus, M. (1984). The Williams syndrome: Objective definition and diagnosis. *Clinical Genetics, 25,* 422-428.

Reiss, A. L., Eckert, M. A., Rose, F. E., Karchemskiy, A., Kesler, S., Chang, M., Reynolds, M. F., Kwon, H., Galaburda, A. (2004). An experiment of nature: brain anatomy parallels cognition and behaviour in Williams Syndrome. *Journal of Neuroscience, 24* (21), 5009-5015.

Rhodes, G., Tan, S., Brake, S. and Taylor, K. (1989). Expertise and configural coding in face recognition. *British Journal of Psychology, 80,* 313-331.

Rojahn, J., Rabold, D. E., and Schneider, F. (1995). Emotion specificity in mental retardation. *American Journal of Mental Retardation, 99,* 477-486.

Rondan, C., Mancini, J., Livet, M. O., and Deruelle, C. (2003). Perceptual and visuo-constructive performance in children with Williams syndrome. *Cognition, Brain, Behavior, 7,* 2, 149-156.

Rose, F. E., Lincoln, A. J., Lai, Z., Ene, M., Searcy, Y. M., and Bellugi, U. (2006). Orientation and Affective Expression Effects on Face Recognition in Williams Syndrome and Autism. *Journal of autism and Developmental Disorders,* DOI 10.1007/s10803-006-0200-4.

Rossen, M., Jones, W., Wang, P. P., and Klima, E. S. (1995). Face processing: remarkable sparing in Williams syndrome. *Genetic Counseling, 6* (Special Issue), 138-140.

Rozin, P. (1998). Evolution and development of brains and cultures: Some basic principles and interactions. In M. S. Gazzaniga and J. S. Altman (Eds.), *Brain and mind : Evolutionary perspectives* (Vol. 5, pp. 111-123). Strasbourg, France : Human Frontier Science Program.

Santos, A., Milne, D., Rosset, D., and Deruelle, C. (2006). Human faces do have something special: Evidence from facial emotion processing in Williams syndrome. Manuscript submitted for publication.

Sasson, N. J. (2006). The development of face processing in autism. *Journal of Autism and Developmental Disorders, 36,* 381-394.

Scheiber, B. (2000). *Fulfilling dreams-Book 1. A handbook for parents of Williams syndrome children*. Clawson, MI: Williams Syndrome Association.

Schmitt, J. E., Eliez, S., Bellugi, U., and Reiss, A. L. (2001). Analysis of cerebral shape in Williams syndrome. *Archives of Neurology, 58* (2), 283-287.

Schmitt, J. E., Eliez, S., Warsofsky, I. S., Bellugi, U., and Reiss, A. L. (2001). Corpus callosum morphology of Williams syndrome: relation to genetics and behaviour. *Developmental Medical Child Neurology, 43* (3), 155-159.

Schmitt, J. E., Watts, K., Eliez, S., Bellugi, U., Galaburda, A. M., and Reiss, A. L. (2002). Increased gyrification in Williams syndrome: evidence using 3D MRI methods. *Developmental Medicine and Child Neurology, 44* (5), 292-295.

Searcy, Y. M., Lincoln, A. J., Rose, F. E., Klima, E. S., Bavar, N., and Korenberg, J. R. (2004). The relationship between age and IQ in adults with Williams syndrome. *American Journal of Mental Retardation, 109* (3), 231-236.

Singer Harris, N. G., Bellugi, U., Bates, E., Jones, W. and Rossen, M. (1997). Contrasting profiles of language development in children with Williams and Down syndromes. *Developmental Neuropsychology, 13*, 345-370.

Tager-Flusberg, H., Plesa-Skwerer, D., Faja, S., and Joseph, R. M. (2003). People with Williams syndrome processes faces holistically. *Cognition, 89*, 11-24.

Tanaka, J. W., and Farah, M. J. (1993). Parts and wholes in face recognition. *Quaterly Journal of Experimental Psychology, 46* (A), 225-245.

Tanaka, J. W., Kay, J. B., Grinnell, E., Stansfield, B., and Szechter, L. (1998). Face recognition in young children: When the whole is greater than the sum of its parts. *Visual Cognition, 5*, 79-496.

Thompson, P. M., Lee, A. D., Dutton, R. A., Geaga, J. A., Hayashi, K. M., Eckert, M. A., et al., (2005). Abnormal cortical complexity and thickness profiles mapped in Williams syndrome. *Journal of Neuroscience, 25* (16), 4146-4158.

Tomaiuolo, F., Di Paola, M., Caravale, B., Vicari, S., Petrides, M., and Caltagirone, C. (2002). Morphology and morphometry of the corpus callosum in Williams syndrome: a TI-weighted MRI study. *Neuroreport, 13* (17), 2281-2284.

Udwin, O., and Yule, W. (1991). A cognitive and behavioural phenotype in Williams syndrome. *Journal of Clinical and Experimental Neuropsychology, 13*, 232-244.

Udwin, O., Yule, W., and Martin, N. (1987). Cognitive abilities and behavioural characteristics of children with idiopathic infantile hypercalcaemia. *Journal of Child Psychology and Psychiatry and Allied Disciplines, 28* (2), 297-309.

van der Lely, H. K. J. (1997). Language and cognitive development in a grammatical SLI boy: Modularity and innateness. *Journal of Neurolinguistics, 10*, 75-107.

VanLieshout, C., DeMeyer, R., Curfs, L., and Fryns, J. (1998). Family contexts, parental behavior, and personality profiles of children and adolescents with Prader-Willi, Fragile-X, or Williams syndrome. *Journal of Child Psychology and Psychiatry and Allied Disciplines, 39*, 699-710.

Vazanta, D. (2005). Language cannot be reduced to biology: perspectives from neuro-developmental disorders affecting language learning. *Journal of Bioscience, 30* (1), 129-137.

Walden, T. A., and Field, T. M. (1982). Discrimination of facial expressions by preschool children. *Child Development, 53*, 1312-1319.

Wang, P. P., Doherty, S., Rourke, S. B. and Bellugi, U. (1995). Unique profile of visuo-perceptual skills in a genetic syndrome. *Brain and Cognition, 29*, 54-65.

Wechsler, D. (1996). *Manual for intelligence scale for children* (3rd ed.). New York: The Psychological Corporation.

Wechsler, D. (1997). *Wechsler Adult Intelligence Scale* (3rd ed.). New York: The Psychological Corporation.

Williams, J. C. P., Barret-Boyes, B. G., and Lowe, J. B. (1961). Supravalvular aortic stenosis. *Circulation, 24*, 1311-1318.

Yin, R. K. (1969). Looking at upside-down faces. *Journal of Experimental psychology, 81*, 141-145.

Zigler, E. (1971). The retarded child as a whole person. In H. E. Adams, and W. K. Boardman (Eds.), *Advances in experimental child psychology* (pp. 47-121). Oxford: Pergamon.

In: Mental Retardation Research Advances
Editor: Elizabeth B. Heinz, pp. 175-183

ISBN: 978-1-60021-658-9
© 2007 Nova Science Publishers, Inc.

Chapter IX

Access to Childhood and Adolescent Mental Health Services for Young People with Mental Retardation

***Renato Donfrancesco**[*1] **and Dario Calderoni**[2]*
[1]"La Scarpetta" Hospital – Child Neuropsychiatry Department – Roma (Italy)
[2] National Health System, TSMREE ASL RMB-Child and Adolescent
NeuroPsychiatry Department B District-Rome

Introduction

Mental Retardation (MR) is an intellectual disability originating before the age of 18 that result in significant limitations in intellectual functioning and conceptual, social and practical adaptive skills. The prevalence of Mental Retardation is determined entirely by where we wish to place our cut-off point on the leftward tail of the IQ distribution. If the cut-off point is placed at -2SD from the mean (corresponding to a Wechsler IQ of 70), 2.5% of the children are identified as intellectually retarded (Rutter et al., 1970). However if prevalence rate is based on those children receiving service for mental retardation and/or special school placement, a prevalence rate of 1.3% is obtained (Rutter et al., 1970). In a series of Canadian and European studies reviewed by Scott (1994), based on regional service registers, prevalence was typically less than 1%. Scott concludes that the lower rate is due to the fact that less than one-half of children and adolescents with mild mental retardation are identified as needing services. In adulthood this proportion drops to less than 25%. Many persons with a mild mental retardation have the possibility to perform a manual job and could become a non-specialized worker. So in a social context in which people gives little importance to the academic success, a mild intellectual disability could not be a major problem and a mild MR person could result socially accepted. Therefore DSM-IV-TR and ICD-10 classifications

[*] Authors' Address: Renato Donfrancesco; c/o Ospedale La Scarpetta; Piazza Castellani 23; 00153 – ROMA (Italy); e-mail: oggiposta@yahoo.it; fax: ++390677306011 ; tel.: ++390677306045 mobile : ++393397740368

suggest examining the total functioning of the subject in the social and personal autonomy areas, also using a standardized scale for adaptive skills as the Vineland Scale. This does not necessarily means that those individuals with mild mental retardation who are not identified are functioning in society without difficulty. This matter is not difficult to understand: people with mental retardation is excluded from mainstream society and remain almost invisible in communities, workplaces and in family life. As a result, the health MR people is significantly poorer than that of the general population and little has been done to address the social exclusion of this group. So one of the main social problems for MR people is to advocate strategies in order to promote and deliver the most appropriate care to children and young people with intellectual disability. A review of Ouellette-Kuntz et al. (2005) outlines as the results of several studies indicate that persons with MR in Canada fare worse than the general population on many key health indicators with inadequate access to essential health and other basic services. Krahn et al. (2006) summarizing the literature from 1999 to 2005, describe in U.S. a cascade of disparities in terms of the determinants of health (genetic, social circumstances, environment, individual behaviours health care access), types of health conditions (associated, comorbid, secondary) and in quality health care services. In U.S. the results from a national survey indicate that over a fifth of the children with mental retardation have problems obtaining needed care from speciality doctors and the most common problem includes getting referrals and finding providers with appropriate training (Krauss et al., 2003). Glied et al. (1997) using data from a community survey of children and their parents in U.S., found major gaps in mental health insurance coverage. The low rate of the access to mental health services of the MR people has a wide diffusion. In Sweden where the public health services have a great diffusion and organization, Gustavson et al. (2005), in a unselected series of 82 adults with intellectual disabilities, found that 50% of the subjects have not a previous diagnosis of Mental Retardation and only few had access to a psychiatrist. This kind of gap is a point of vulnerability for MR people because a high percentage of people with an intellectual disability have emotional and behavioural needs (Kerker et al., 2004) and many studies have concluded that mental and emotional disorders are present to a greater degree in mentally retarded than in no retarded people (Borthwick-Duffy, 1994; Bregman, 1991,Lin et al., 2005). This is true also for children. In Rutter's Isle of Wight study (Rutter et al., 1970), 30.4% of the children with an IQ less than 70 were found to have a psychiatric disorder on the parent questionnaire, and 41.8% on the teacher questionnaire. Comparables rates for no retarded persons in the general population were 7.7% and 9.5% respectively. Jacobson (1982), among 30,000 persons receiving developmental disability service in New York State, estimated that 47.7% of the retarded persons displayed some type of problem behaviour. Anxiety and disruptive disorders could be the more frequent psychiatric impairment in MR people. Recently Dekker and Koot (2003) assessed the prevalence, comorbidity and impact of DSM-IV disorders in 7-to 20-year-olds with intellectual disability. The sample of 474 children and adolescents was recruited from Dutch schools for the intellectually disabled. Results showed that a total of 21.9% of the children met the DSM-IV symptom criteria for anxiety disorder, 4.4% for mood disorder, and 25.1% for disruptive disorder. Also in adulthood a significant proportion continue to have problems in a variety of emotional and adaptative domains (Edgerton, 1984, Scott,1994). The low rate of access to mental health service by children and adolescent with an intellectual disability has some serious consequences. McCarthy and Boyd (2002) have studied longitudinally 80 young people from childhood and adolescence to adulthood for the presence of psychiatric and behaviour disorder. Evaluation questionnaires were used during the follow-up study to assess service use from adolescence. The great majority of subjects (64%) with persistent challenging behaviour from childhood into adult life and those with an established childhood psychiatric disorder received no specialist mental health care. Therefore the gap in the utilization of mental health care from MR people becomes a failure in term of quality of life and social costs, so many agencies perform an effort to study a new approach to the problem (Harrison and Berry, 2006). A first question is: why the parents of the disabled children elude the community services for mental health? Liptak et al. (2006) try to answer to this question. One hundred twenty-one families of children with special needs were recruited in a mailed survey. They answered to the Multidimensional Assessment of Parental Satisfation for Children with Special Needs. Families of children with developmental disabilities demonstrate dissatisfaction with several aspects of health care that can serve as areas for intervention by their health care providers. Parents had the lowest ratings for the primary care physicians' ability to put them in touch with other parents, understanding of the impact of the child's condition on the family, ability to answer questions about the child's condition and information and guidance for prevention. The problem of the training of the physicians is not a novelty: in the '90 some author have requested specialized services (Day, 1993). A second problem is the lack of homogeneity of the services for disabled people that is common to many countries. Smiley et al. (2002) found a wide range in the type of services provided by each locality in Scotland and only 21% of the services has completed the process of resettlement. Moreover the problem of a low access to health services is not a specific matter of MR people. Many other chronic health impairments don't receive an optimal medical service. Probably a chronic disease with a life-time expression has more binding needs with major economic costs and this could be another general reason for the lack of health care of many MR persons. As a matter of fact a study (Msall et al., 2003) about chronic disease, comprehensive of developmental disabilities, showed a general lack of medical services not only for children with intellectual disabilities but also for children with asthma , diabetes and so on. Msall and collaborators studied functional disability and school activity limitation in 41,300 children school-age children. They found that 20.8% did not have an identified medical impairment because they had not received medical services in the past year. These results justify the efforts of the public administrations toward a best health care of the chronic diseases in children One example is the State Children's Health Insurance Program (SCHIP) expansions on insurance coverage, use of health care services, and access to care for children with chronic health conditions (Davidoff et al., 2005). The analytic study of the results of this program showed an improvement in insurance coverage and in access to care of the children with chronic condition.

It is very difficult to summarize such data because most studies on family and on access to health care in people with intellectual disabilities have been carried out in the UK or in the USA, and are biased by the societal organization, and political and economic climate of those countries. In the USA and the UK, the care and well-being of children, with or without MR, are seen almost exclusively as the individual family responsibility. In other European country, as Sweden and Italy, policy of welfare state has developed many privileges for all parents in order to help them care for their children, and the support for parents of children with disabilities is provided exclusively by the Government and the community. Other cultural differences could be found if other countries are considered as Taiwan or other oriental countries, concerning the social image of the MR people. We can try to overcome these difficulties focussing our attention only on some factors that are the possible obstacle to a best mental health care of persons with intellectual disabilities. Many differences remain between the several countries, firstly political, economical and cultural but with a certain approximation we can observe if the change of a variable is sufficient to improve the care of MR people. A study with a similar aim was carried out by Olsson and Hwang in Sweden (2003). Their question was: Are families in Sweden experiencing the stressor and life situations described in the studies of parents in more individualistic societies? The variables changed if we consider the UK and USA studies are almost two (but could be several): the insurance coverage that are total for MR people in Sweden, and the community organization for health care. Two hundred and twenty-six families with children with MR and 234 control families with children ranging from 0-16 of age answered mail surveys. Results showed that taken together, parents in Sweden describe most of the stressors proposed in the international literature with the exception of financial strain. Therefore a little more agreeable quality of life is documented by this research but the restrictions in social life and in time seem to be the most evident and bothersome stressors for Swedish families. This condition is common worldwide and difficult to change because of the strict binding with the lack of autonomy of the disabled children in general.

The start point of the research described in these pages is this paper of Olsson and Hwang. The aim is the same: a comparison between two different philosophies concerning health care. The observed variable is the access to mental health care of the children and adolescent with mental retardation. Before to describe the methods of the research it is necessary to summarize the factors that literature seem to have stressed as concerning the access of MR people to services:

- The complete or not insurance coverage
- The ease of the access
- The quality of professional service as the specialization of the physicians and of the others health operators in community care (psychologists, social services, rehabilitators), and the organization of the services.

As described above, the health care organization for disabled children in Italy is deeply different from that of UK and USA, depending from another philosophy and culture.

In Italy society has developed a social protection for children with intellectual disabilities and supports their parents. The three variables above mentioned are absent as an obstacle to the mental health care access of the handicapped children in general:

- In Italy government provides a general insurance coverage for all citizen. MR people have free access to all specialized structure for health care. Also language, cognitive and motor rehabilitation are free.

- The access to service of mental health is direct and easy; it is sufficient to ask for an appointment.
- The community health care for handicapped children is well organized. The services are all specialized. The chief is always a physician specialized in Child Neuropsychiatry. This post-graduate training has the duration of 5 years and is an ideal training for the MR persons care because links a psychiatric with a neurological education. Family and children meet a specialized team with integrated competences. social workers, psychologists and rehabilitators directed by the Child Neuropsychiatrist.

It is possible to consider Italy a sort of social laboratory, in which the variables economic costs, easy access and specialization of services are controlled. Of course there are many other differences between health care organization in Italy and in UK or USA. Moreover the differences are also cultural and political so the results of a research about MR people access to mental health care are usefully only by approximation.

Matherials and Methods

Subjects

The subjects are all users of primary mental health care of the Florence Health Department of Florence district (Tuscany), from 0 to 18 years old. The Florence Health Department served a population of 111.777 children and adolescents 0 to 18. All subjects assessed during one year because of a psychiatric disorder, true or only suspected, in the Child Neuropsychiatry Department are enrolled in the study. This Department is the only agency that, in Florence, receives MR people 0-18 years old, so the result of our study reflects all MR subjects that use any kind of service for mental health.

Measures

Inclusion criteria in the MR people group are the results to standardized test with an IQ lower than 70. The scales used for the cognitive assessment are: WISC-R, WPPSI, Leiter International Scale, Brunet-Lezine. All patients are assessed in person.

Results

The number of child and adolescents with Mental Retardation that had access to mental health care service in the Florence District during 1 year was 423, 0.37% of the total population 0-18. This number is largely lower than expected from the international data above mentioned that are 2.5% in the epidemiological study based on IQ (Rutter et al., 1970) and about 1% considering the national register or other sources (see above).

Discussion

Results show a very low number of accesses during 1 year to the mental services of MR people: only 423 (0.37%). This number is lower than the expected one not only if the type of assessment is considered (IQ with standardized test), that is 2.5% in epidemiological data (Rutter et al. 1970), but also if data from other sources are considered (about 1%). The percentage of 0.37% is very near to the percentage of severe mental retardation that is in Italy 0.34% (Benassi et al.,1990). Nevertheless every comparison between these numbers is difficult because the range of age of the study of Benassi et al is 6 to13-year-olds. A partial explanation of the low rate found is, as a matter of fact, the age target of the research, because during the first year of life is more difficult to diagnose a mental retardation. Moreover it is from the fourth year of life that children have major cognitive requests from the ambient because of the entry in the school. Another explanation could be also invoked; data from this study concern access of MR people during 1 year. Certainly there are some MR subjects, probably only mildly retarded, that use health service every 2 or 3 years. On the contrary many prevalence studies about intellectual disabilities utilize as sources of information the public national registers that accumulate data from several years. If the rate of severe mental retardation in Italy as reported from Benassi and coll. is considered this study confirms the hypothesis of Scott (1994), mentioned in the introduction of this chapter: probably one half of the mild retarded persons during childhood or adolescence don't uses mental health care. These data are also confirmed by van Schrojenstein Lantman-deValk et al. (2006). They found a percentage of 55% of MR people (not only mild retarded persons) that didn't use common MR services, on a total prevalence of 0.78% in Limburg (Netherlands). In conclusion the data of this research show that a general insurance coverage for all citizen, free access to all specialized structure for health care, a direct and easy access and the specialization of the services with well-trained physicians are not sufficient to ameliorate the rate of access to mental health service of MR people.

Then, why many mild retarded people doesn't use mental health care? Probably other factors are involved. They could be cultural or psychological factors.

Cutural and Psychological Factors and Access to Mental Health Care of Mental Retarded People

Cultural and psychological factors are strictly united. When the parents of a mental retarded child confronted himself with the failure in their reproductive competences live a psychological problem that is caused by their public image that is also a cultural product. This feature of the janitorial life of parents of intellectual disabled children is well known from many years (Taylor, 1982). It is important to underline the major stress of parents of MR people (2005), but to understand the quality of this stress is more important. The experience with families of handicapped persons during several years of medical profession suggests the importance of the parents' acceptance of the disease of the son. The comparison with their failure is frequently accepted during the adolescence of the handicapped son. During several years many parents live in a sort of dream in which the limitations of the son is misunderstood. When mental retardation is severe it is inevitable to access to services, but when the handicap is mild it could be easier to elude mental health care justifying the limitation of the children in some way (the teachers are not able to teach, the child is lazy, and so on). The literature about access of MR people doesn't stress sufficiently these kinds of problems. Certainly it is important to underline the need of an insurance coverage for the family of handicapped children and adolescents. It is also important to stress the centrality of an adequate and specialized medical support. Davidoff et al. (2005) have reported data that show an improvement of access to services of MR people with a program of major insurance coverage. Nevertheless data from the research presented in this chapter show that a general insurance coverage for all citizen, free access to all specialized structure for health care, a direct and easy access and the specialization of the services with well-trained physicians are not sufficient to ameliorate the rate of access to mental health service of MR people. Other factors are important, probably cultural and psychological ones. These are the target of future intervention and research. The stress intervention for parents of children with intellectual disabilities is not a novelty (Hastings and Beck, 2004) and it is very important. Nevertheless this kind of intervention is possible after the access of the parents to the services. Probably a better involvement of the primary care, especially of the general practitioners and of the paediatricians of the primary care could determine an improvement of the parents' acceptance of the handicap of the children and consequently a better use of mental health service.

References

Benassi G, Guarino M, Cammarata S, Cristoni P, Fantini MP, Ancona A, Manfredini M, D'Alessandro R (1990). An epidemiological study on severe mental retardation among schoolchildren in Bologna, Italy. *Dev. Med. Child Neurol,* Oct, 32 (10): 895-901.

Borthwick-Duffy SA (1994). Epidemiology and prevalence of psychopathology in people with mental retardation. *J. Consult. Clin. Psychol.* 62 (1): 17-27.

Bregman JD (1991). Current developments in the understanding of mental retardation part II: Psychopathology. *J. Am. Acad. Child Adolesc. Psychiatry.* 30: 861-872.

Davidoff A, Kenney G, Dubay L (2005). Effects of the State Children's Health Insurance Program Expansion on children with chronic health conditions. *Pediatrics,* Jul, 116(1): e34-42.

Day KA (1993). Mental health services for people with mental retardation : a framework for the future. *J. Intellect. Disabil. Res.;* Oct 37 Suppl 1:7-16.

Dekker MC, Koot HM (2003). DSM-IV disorders in children with borderline to moderate intellectual disability. I: prevalence and impact. *J. Am. Acad. Child Adolesc. Psychiatry,* Aug, 42 (8):915-922.

Edgerton RB (1984). Lives in process: Mildly Retarded Adults in a large city. Washington, DC: American Association on Mental Deficiency.

Glied S, Hoven CW, Garrett AB, Regier DA (1997). Children's access to mental health care: does insurance matter? *Health Aff.* (Milwood), jan-feb; 16(1): 167-74.

Gustavson KH, Umb-Carlsson O, Sonnander K (2005). A follow-up study of mortalità, health conditions and associated disabilities of people with intellectual disabilities in a Swedish county. *J. Intellect Disabil. Res.*, Dec, 49 (Pt12): 905-914.

Harrison S,Berry L (2006). Valuing people: health visiting and people with learning disabilities. *Community Pract.*, Feb, 79(2):56-59.

Hastings RP, Beck A (2004). Pratictioner review: stress intervention for parents of children with intellectual disabilities. *J. Child Psychol. Psychiatry,* Nov, 45 (8):1338-1349.

Kerker BD,Owens PL, Zigler E, Horwitz SM (2004) Mental health disorders among individuals with mental retardation: challenges to accurate prevalence estimates. *Public Health Rep.* Jul-Aug; 119 (4):409-417.

Krauss MW, Gulley S,Sciegaj M, Wells N (2003). Access to speciality medical care for children with mental retardation, autism and other special health care needs. *Ment. Retard Oct;* 41 (5): 329-39.

Krhan GL, Hammond L, Turner A (2006). A cascade of disparities: health and health care access for people with intellectual disabilities. *Ment. Retard. Dev. Disabil. Res. Rev;* 12 (1):70-82.

Lin JD, Yen CF, Li CW,Wu JL (2005). Health, healthcare utilization and psychiatric disorder in people with intellectual disability in Taiwan. *J. Intellect. Disabil. Res.,* Jan, 49 (Pt1):86-94.

Liptak GS, Orlando M, Yngling JT, Tehurer-Kaufman KL, Malay DP, Tompkins LA, Flynn JR (2006). *Satisfation with primary health care received by families of children with developmental disabilities.*

McCarthy J,Boyd J (2002). Mental health services and young people with intellectual disability: is it time to do better? *J. Intellect. Disabil. Res,* Mar; 46(Pt3):250-256.

Msall Me, Avery RC, Tremont MR, Lima JC, Rogers ML, Hogan DP (2003). Functional disability and school activity limitations in 41,300 school-age children: relationship to medical impairments. *Pediatrics,* Mar, 111 (3):548-553.

Nachshen JS, Minnes P (2005). Empowerment in parents of school-aged children with and without developmental disabilities. *J. Intellect. Disabil. Res.,* Dec, 49(Pt 12): 889-904.

Olsson MB, Hwang PC (2003). Influence of macrostructure of society on the life situation of families with a child with intellectual disability: Sweden as an example. *J. Intellect. Disabil. Res.,* May-Jun; 47 (Pt 4-5):328-341.

Ouellette-Kuntz H, Garcin N, Lewis ME, Minnes P, Martin C, Holden JJ (2005). Addressing health disparities through promoting equity for individuals with intellectual disability. *An. J. Public Health,* Mar-Apr;96 Suppl. 2:S8-22.

Rutter M, Graham P, Yule W (1970). A neuropsychiatric Study in Childhood. London: *Spastics International Medical Publication and Heinemann.*

Scott S.(1994). Mental Retardation. In: Rutter M, Taylor E.,Hersov L. (eds): *Child and Adolescent Psychiatry* (3rd ed). Oxford: Blackwell.

Smiley E, Cooper SA, Miller SM, Robertson P, Simpson N (2002). Specialist health services for people with intellectual disability in Scotland. *J. Intellect. Disabil. Res.,* Nov, 46 (Pt8):585-593.

Taylor DC (1982). Counseling the parents of handicapped children. *Br. Med. J. (Clin. Res. Ed),* April 3, 284 (6321): 1027-1028.

Van Schrojenstein Lantman-deValk HM, Wullink M, van den Akker M, van Heurn-Nijsten EW, Metsemakers JF, Dinant GJ (2006). The prevalence of intellectual disability in Limburg, the Netherlands. *J. Intellect. Disabil. Res.* Jan, 50 (Pt 1):61-68.

In: Mental Retardation Research Advances
Editor: Elizabeth B. Heinz, pp. 185-196

ISBN: 978-1-60021-658-9
© 2007 Nova Science Publishers, Inc.

Chapter X

Information Technology for People with Mental Retardation

Cecilia Li-Tsang[*1] *and Nichael Wong*[2]

[1] Department of Rehabilitation Sciences; The Hong Kong Polytechnic University;
Hung Hom, Kowloon; Hong Kong SAR;
[2] Department of Rehabilitation Sciences;
The Hong Kong Polytechnic University

Abstract

The development of the information and communication technology (ICT) has made a huge revolution of human's lifestyle in the past few decades. A lot of daily chores could be performed by just pressing a few icons on the computer at home such as paying bills, booking of appointments etc. However, people with mental retardation were often deprived of the opportunities to learn ICT skills. This has created a digital divide among people with mental retardation to get into the ICT world. It is believed that through systematic training and special assistive device (e.g. software programme) designed for people with mental retardation, they can get into the ICT world. The digital barrier could thus be removed. Previous studies have been focused on "Identification of barriers for people with mental retardation to the ICT world", "Training of people with mental retardation in learning various ICT skills" and "Enhancement of people with mental retardation to use ICT skills in vocational and leisure perspectives".

In this book chapter, we shall carefully describe how people with mental retardation manage to get into the ICT world through systematic training and societal support.

---

[*] Correspondence address: Dr. Cecilia Li-Tsang, Associate Head, Department of Rehabilitation Sciences, The Hong Kong Polytechnic University, Hunghom, Kowloon, HK. e-mail: rscecili@inet.polyu.edu.hk; Tel: (852) 2766-6715; Fax: (852) 2330-5124

Introduction

In the past century, there has been a lot of rapid development in human mankind, in particular, the advancement of science and technology. One of the main features is the breakthrough of information and communication technology (ICT). Our modern society now relies heavily on computer technology for work, leisure, communication, learning and performing day to day chores. In Hong Kong, more than 90 % of the families are equipped with computer at home. It remains difficult for a person to survive in this modern society without the computing support. A child learns at school using the computer as a media. A university student searches information using the internet system. An adult works on computer to perform his work at an office and searches information through internet. A housewife pays the bills via the internet and a patient books a medical appointment using the internet. Friends chat with each other using e-mail or MSN system. In this modern world of technology, we all adapt a new life pattern, which relies heavily on the information and communication technology (ICT) system.

Information and Communication Technology (ICT)

Information and communication technology (ICT) is a name given to the modern technology related to computer and Internet, which enable people to get any information interested and facilitate communication around the world without the limit of distance. It is considered to be very useful and helpful. Many tasks could be done through ICT no matter for work, for daily activities or for leisure. Meeting with customers, finding a job, writing essay, hiring a maid for household cleansing, booking sport facilities and playing online games can all be settled by using a computer with Internet access. The letter 'e', derived from electronics, is always be added before nouns to mean that the particular thing which can be done by ICT. 'e-shopping', 'e-mail' and 'e-card' are good examples indicated that shopping, sending mails and cards can be fixed through ICT. 'Tele' is also used to serve the similar purpose of the letter 'e', like tele-conference, tele-rehabilitation meaning that conference and rehabilitation held through ICT.

People with Mental Retardation

Mental retardation is defined by the American Association on Mental Retardation (2002) as "a disability characterized by significant limitations both in intellectual functioning and in adaptive behavior as expressed in conceptual, social, and practical adaptive skills". The World Health Organization (1996) has similar description on mental retardation in the ICD-10; "Guide for Mental Retardation". It was characterized by the impairment of skills resulted from the reduced level of intelligence in the childhood. Thus, the IQ level is used as a guide to diagnose if a person with mental retardation. There are four types of mental retardation in general regarding on the severity, including mild, moderate, severe and profound mental retardation. It may be accompanied with other medical conditions and/or psychiatric disorders, like epilepsy, flatfoot or depression.

Digital Divide for People with Mental Retardation

The development of ICT has boomed over the past two decades all round the world, especially in the developed countries. The usage of computer and Internet is particularly high among the developed countries or cities, such as USA, Sweden, Norway, Hong Kong and Singapore. The penetration rate of computer and Internet for all households in Hong Kong was 70.1 % and 64.6 % (The Government of the Hong Kong Special Administration Region [HKSAR], 2005). For the less developed countries, they are lagging behind in the development of ICT and access of Internet compared to the developed one (Cullen, 2001). It is actually a kind of digital divide. According to the definition from the Organisation for Economic Co-operation and Development (2001), "digital divide is a gap between individuals, households, businesses and geographic areas at different socio-economic levels with regard both to their opportunities to access information and communication technologies and to their use of the Internet for a wide variety of activities". People with low education level, people with lower income, people in old age and people with disabilities are commonly to be deprived of the opportunities to access ICT (Culler, 2001). There are four main issues contributed to it, which are physical accessibility of ICT, ICT skills and support availability, attitudes of the public and individual, as well as content on the Internet.

Bridging the Gap for People
with Mental Retardation

The abilities of people with disabilities in using the ICT were brought up for attention ever since September 1982 (Anson, 2001). There was an article introducing a computer program called 'Adaptive-Firmware Card' that was specially designed for people with disabilities. However, most of the researches were concentrated on the physical accessibility to the computer and Internet for people with physical or speech problems (Anson, 2001). People with mental retardation were not addressed regarding their access to computer and Internet. The reason may be of the assumption that using ICT skills may be too complex for people with mental retardation. It might also be due to lack of opportunities, training and support for this minority group (Abbott and Cribb, 2001; Aspinall and Hegarty, 2001). However, previous research indicated that with the advancement of ICT, people with mental retardation could be further advanced in their life survival skills. Through utilization of the self-regulation and self-management strategies offered by ICT, people with mental retardation can learn various daily tasks more effectively (Davis, Stock and Wehmeyer, 2002a). A number of software was invented for people with mental retardation in facilitating their skills in daily living, at work or for leisure. Training on matching skills (Shimizu, Twyman and Yamamoto, 2003), language abilities (Hetzroni and Schanin, 2002), time management (Davis, Stock and Wehmeyer, 2002a) and vocational skills (Furniss, Lancioni, Rocha, et al., 2001) were few examples on it. Software developed by the companies may not be suitable for people with mental retardation to use (Davis, Stock, and Wehmeyer, 2002b). Thus, a specially designed training program for people with mental retardation was developed in facilitating their computer competencies and preparing them for job hunting.

Studies on ICT Training for People with Mental Retardation

The Competency of People with Mental Retardation in Using ICT

One of the studies conducted by Li-Tsang and her colleagues were to investigate the computer competencies of people with mild to severe grade of mental retardation and their caregivers' or parents' view on factors affecting their learning in ICT (Li-Tsang, Yeung, Chan and Hui-Chan, 2005). A self-developed checklist was used to measure their skills of using mouse and keyboard, as well as browsing the Internet with Internet Explore (IE) (see Table 1). There were eight items related to mouse and keyboard operation, and nine items related to the skills of browsing the Internet with IE. One mark would be given in each item for those who could conduct the action correctly; otherwise, zero mark would be given. Thus, the total score of the checklist was 17. It was developed by adopting the task analysis approach and had high inter-rater reliability (intraclass-correlation coefficient $(3,1) = 0.98$).

Three hundred and fifty three adults were recruited in this study with the consent of their caregivers or parents. The number of male and female was 219 and 134 respectively. The mean age of them was 28.77 years, ranged from 16 to 59 years old. There were 193 subjects with mild mental retardation, 143 subjects with moderate mental retardation, and 17 subjects with severe mental retardation. The percentage of subjects with autism was 11.0% (39) among all the subjects (see Table 2). The result showed that 38.8% of them with total 353 subjects were not able to operate mouse and keyboard, 42.8% were not able to browse the Internet using IE. The percentage of people not able to operate the computer at all was 33.1%. The mean scores of mouse and keyboard operation was 2.47 (SD = 2.69), while that of browsing the Internet was 3.00 (SD = 3.36). Hence, the total mean score was 5.47 (SD = 5.77) out of 17. These skills were the basic requirements for using ICT. It was interested to investigate various factors affecting their performance and abilities in mastering these skills.

Table 1. A self-developed assessment checklist (translated from Chinese version)

Categories	Description
Use of mouse and keyboard	Double click
	Use of arrow keys to move the cursor
	Put the cursor to specific position
	Type the word "HAPPY"
	Deleting two words
	Use of spacebar to insert two blank spaces
	Use of ENTER key to insert a blank line
	Dragging (moving an icon on the desktop)
Internet browsing	Opening the IE browser
	Retrieving a bookmark
	Using the scroll bar
	Browsing by single click
	Use of the BACK key
	Typing webpage address in the correct position
	Pressing ENTER key after typing
	Adding a bookmark
	Close the browser

Table 2. Demographic data of the subjects (N = 353)

	Number of subjects	%
Age (years)		
16-29	217	61.5
30-39	81	22.9
40-49	35	9.9
50-59	20	5.7
Sex		
Male	219	62.0
Female	134	38.0
Type of mental retardation		
Mild	193	54.7
Moderate	143	40.5
Severe	17	4.8
Diagnosis		
Mental retardation	314	89.0
Mental retardation and autism	39	11.0

Factors of People with Mental Retardation to Learn ICT Skills

It was found that younger adults performed better than the older adults. The mean of total score of the youngest age group (16-29 years old) was 6.96 (SD = 5.87), and that of the oldest age group was 1.20 (SD = 2.84). A negative relationship was found between the age of the subjects and their total scores on the checklist with r = -0.42 and p < .000. It might be due to the fact that ICT was developed a few decades ago. It was not common until the past ten years. Computer applications were only introduced into the teaching curriculum of schools in Hong Kong in 1990's. People with older age did not receive any formal ICT training at the local schools. Thus, subjects with younger age should have better performance in ICT skills when compared with those subjects with older age. Subjects with mild mental retardation had the highest scores in both mouse and keyboard operation (mean = 3.62 ± 2.72) and Internet browsing (mean = 4.50 ± 3.36), followed by subjects with moderate (mean = 1.20 ± 1.94 and 1.29 ± 2.40 respectively) and severe mental retardation (mean = 0.59 ± 0.24 and 0.35 ± 1.46 respectively). There was a positive correlation between the intellectual function and computer competence with r = 0.51 and p < .000. People with more severe intellectual disabilities were appeared to have the need of more assistance in learning ICT skills. However, people with dual diagnosis of mental retardation and autism were found to have higher scores when compared with people with mental retardation only. The mean differences between the 2 groups were 1.48 for mouse and keyboard operation, 2.19 for Internet browsing, and 3.68 for total score. Availability of systematic ICT training for people with mental retardation was important as mentioned by the caregivers and parents. The total score of subjects with prior training was slightly higher than that of subjects without receiving any training (mean difference = 5.00, t (351) = 8.79, p < .000). They were found to be deprived of any forms of ICT training before, which was reported by their caregivers and parents. Almost 40% of them did not have any training on ICT before. People with disabilities were lack of appropriate training and suitable software in assisting them in learning ICT as reported by the parents involved in Lindstrand's study (2002).

ICT Training for People with Mental Retardation

A computer training program for people with mental retardation was then developed in developing and enhancing their learning in ICT capability (Li-Tsang, Yeung, Choi, Chan and Lam, 2006). The funding was supported by the Lottery Fund and under the governance of the Social Welfare Department (SWD). It covered the skills of mouse and keyboard operation and Internet browsing using IE based on the self-developed checklist. There were two three-hour sessions with one covered the former and one covered the later. Each session had an instructor to conduct the teaching and tutors were assigned to provide assistance or guidance when necessary for the participants. Training program was given to the instructors and tutors prior to their duties for better understanding of the ICT training program and handling techniques for people with mental retardation. Three training software were developed in line with the program to assist the participants in learning the skill of mouse and keyboard operation, like moving and dragging the cursor, double clicking, typing words and use of ENTER and SPACEBAR keys on the keyboard (see Figures 1 – 3). It offered verbal guideline and audio reinforcement to the participants. The checklist used in the previous study was adopted to evaluate the ICT ability of the subject before and after the training program with one-month follow-up assessment.

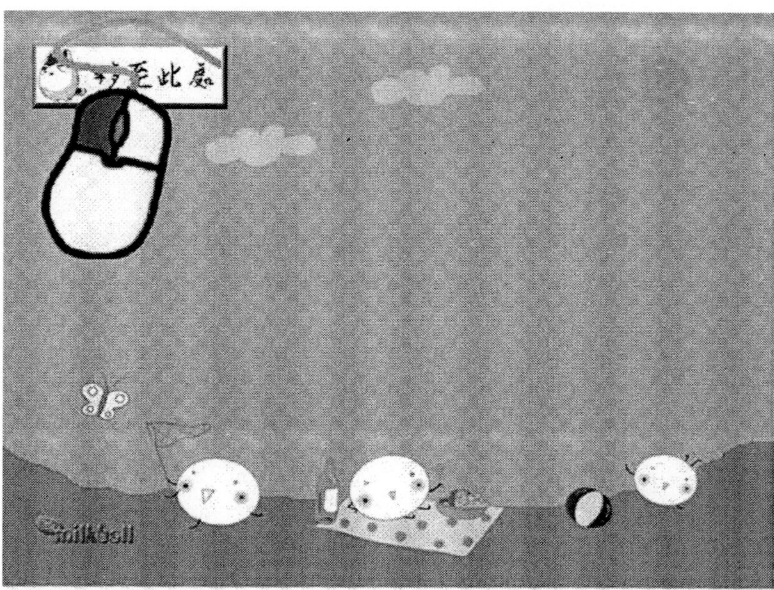

Figure 1. Training software 1.

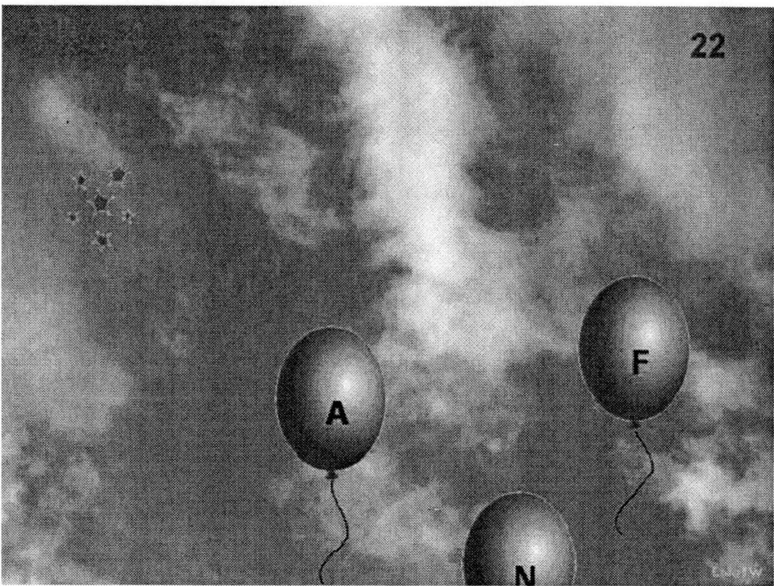

Figure 2. Training software 2.

There were a total of 105 subjects. They were assigned to either experimental group or delayed training group on voluntary basis. There were 76 subjects in the experimental group and 29 in the delayed training group. In the experimental group, the numbers of male and female were 43 (56.6%) and 33 (43.4%) with the mean age of 23.16 ± 10.17 years. In the delayed training group, there were 17 (58.6%) male and 12 (41.4%) female with the mean age of 28.28 ± 9.35 years. The percentage of subjects with mild mental retardation was 82.9 % in the experimental group and 44.8% in the delayed training group. The rest of them were diagnosed with moderate mental retardation, as people with severe or profound mental retardation were excluded in this study.

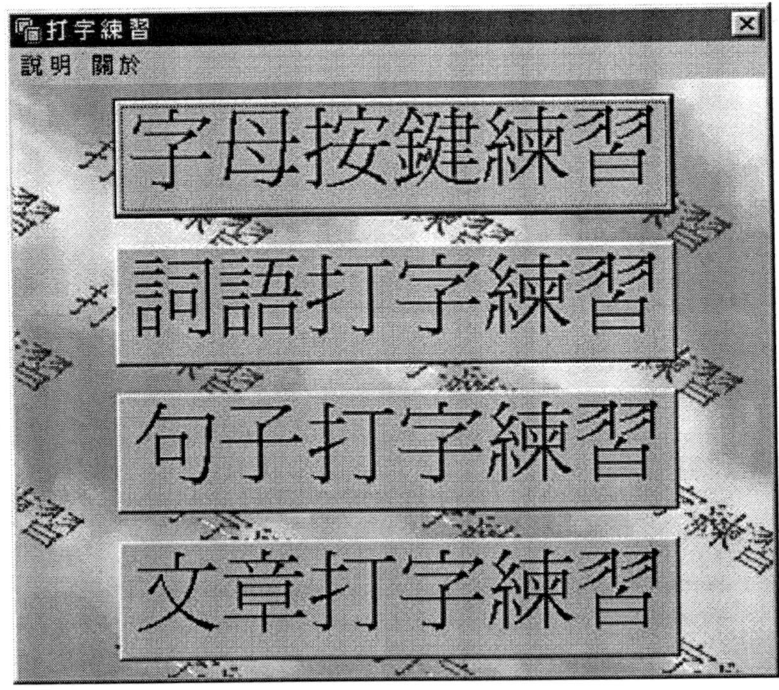

Figure 3. Training software 3.

There were significant improvements in the experimental group (see Table 4) in both skills after the training compared with the delayed training group (see Table 5). The skills learnt were able to be retained by the subjects after the program ended for a month time with $p < .000$ in both main tasks and total score. It suggested that people with mental retardation could also learn ICT skills, provided that appropriate training and assistance were given. The specially designed training program and software were contributed to the success of this training program. Although the mean scores were slightly lower in the one-month follow-up assessment than that after training, there was no significant difference found in the mean scores. It might demonstrate that the subjects could retain the computer skills after one month of follow up. The caregivers and parents reported that it was a precious opportunity to have this kind of training program and software for their children or siblings. They thought that the low tutor to tutee ratio was crucial for the participants to learn more efficiently and effectively.

Table 3. Demographic data of the subjects (N = 105)

		Number of subjects	% / SD
Experimental group	**Sex**		
	Male	43	56.6%
	Female	33	43.4%
	Mean age (years)		
	Male	22.53	SD=10.08
	Female	23.97	SD=10.39
	Type of mental retardation		
	Mild	63	82.9%
	Moderate	13	17.1%
Delayed training group	**Sex**		
	Male	17	58.6%
	Female	12	41.4%
	Mean age (years)		
	Male	23.53	SD=5.19
	Female	35.00	SD=9.95
	Type of mental retardation		
	Mild	13	44.8%
	Moderate	16	55.2%

Table 4. Mean scores of the experimental group before and after training

Main Tasks	Before Training Mean Scores (SD)	After Training Mean Scores (SD)	t	p
Use of mouse and keyboard	1.89 (1.86)	4.09 (2.53)	9.30	.000
Internet browsing	2.42 (2.45)	5.49 (3.18)	11.13	.000
Total score	4.32 (3.94)	9.58 (5.24)	12.21	.000

Table 5. Mean scores of the delayed training group before and after training

Main Tasks	Before Training Mean Scores (SD)	After Training Mean Scores (SD)	t	P
Use of mouse and keyboard	1.41 (2.47)	1.72 (2.64)	1.51	.142
Internet browsing	1.79 (2.81)	1.66 (2.38)	1.00	.326
Total score	3.21 (5.19)	3.41 (5.42)	0.90	.375

Follow up Study on the ICT Training Programme

A six-month follow-up study was carried out after the second study to further investigate the effect of the training program for people with mental retardation (Li-Tsang, Lee, Yeung, Siu and Lam, in press). Fifty-nine subjects were recruited to investigate their abilities in the two skills mentioned above after six months of the end of the training, i.e. mouse and keyboard operation and Internet browsing. There were 36 male and 23 female with the age ranged from 18 to 55. The numbers of subjects with mild, moderate and severe mental retardation were 23, 31 and 5 respectively. Their ICT skills were evaluated by the self-developed checklist in pre-, post-, 6-month follow-up assessment.

There were also significant improvements in the total score over the three assessments using one-way repeated measure ANOVA. The mean score of mouse and keyboard operation was slightly increased from 2.54 ± 2.54 in post-assessment to 2.64 ± 2.63 after six months, while the mean score of Internet browsing skill was decreased in the follow-up assessment from 2.75 ± 3.07 to 2.14 ± 2.84 but still higher than that of the pre-assessment with the value of 1.68 ± 2.79. The total score was also reduced slightly from 5.29 ± 5.35 after training to 4.78 ± 5.20 in 6-month follow-up assessment. However, the mean scores of both skills and the total score were improved after receiving the training program for six months when compared the scores before training. It indicated that the subjects could maintain the skills even after a period of 6 months without formal training.

The success of this program was contributed by the well-organized training protocol, trained instructors and tutors, appropriate training materials (the trainin software) and the low trainer-to-trainee ratio (Li-Tsang, Lee, Yeung, Siu and Lam, in press; Li-Tsang, Yeung, Choi, Chan and Lam, 2006). Feedback from the parents and caregivers, as well as the participants, was positive. They were appreciated with the adequate support from the trainers for the participants, the specially designed training program for people with mental retardation. They thought that the cognitive performance, social interaction skills and behavioral problems of the participants were improved after joining the training. They could better utilize their leisure time through using the computer for playing games, surfing the Internet, etc.

Future Direction

People with mental retardation should be able to master the ICT skills with proper training and support. In addition, when the system becomes more user-friendly in the future, the digital divide for people with mental retardation should be minimized. However, one of the most important factors to facilitate the breaking down of the digital divide may be the social acceptance and acknowledgements. It is often easy to discriminate people with mental retardation away from any technology with the thought of "they might damage the system". This social stigmatization should be minimized.

Conclusion

One of the interesting finding was that people with dual diagnosis of mental retardation and autism performed better in the study. It would be interesting to find out if people with autism could learn more advanced ICT skills. In addition, if they are probably trained and guided, it might be feasible for them to pursue their career in the field of ICT. Thus, their vocational needs may further be fulfilled.

References

Abbott, C. and Cribb, A. (2001). Special schools, inclusion and the World Wide Web – the emerging research agenda. *British Journal of Educational Technology, 32,* 331-42.

American Association on Mental Retardation. (2002). *Definition of mental retardation.* Retrieved 5 Nov 06 from http://www.aamr.org/Policies/faq_mental_retardation.shtml.

Anson, D. (2001). Technology and occupation: The future of computer access. *The American Journal of Occupational Therapy, 55(1),* 106-8.

Aspinall, A. and Hegarty, J. R. (2001). ICT for adults with learning disabilities an organization-wide audit. *British Journal of Educational Technology, 32,* 365-72.

Cullen, R. (2001). Addressing the digital divide. *Online Information Review, 25(5),* 311-20.

Davis, D. K., Stock, S. E. and Wehmeyer, M. L. (2002a). Enhancing independent task performance for individuals with mental retardation through use of a handheld self-directed visual and audio prompting system. *Education and Training in Mental Retardation and Developmental Disabilities, 37(2),* 209-218.

Davis, D. K., Stock, S. E. and Wehmeyer, M. L. (2002b). Enhancing independent time-management skills of individuals with mental retardation using a Palmtop personal computer. *Mental Retardation, 40(5),* 358-65.

Furniss, F., Lancioni, G., Rocha, N., Cunha, B., Seedhouse, P., Morato, P., et al. (2001). Development and evaluation of a palmtop-based job aid for workers with severe developmental disabilities. *British Journal of Educational Technology, 32(3),* 277-287.

Hetzroni, O. E. and Schanin, M. (2002). Emergent literacy in children with severe disabilities using interactive multimedia stories. *Journal of Developmental and Physical Disabilities, 14(2),* 173-190.

Li-Tsang, C. W. P., Lee, M. Y. F., Yeung, S. S. S., Siu, A. M. H. and Lam, C. S. (in press). A six-month follow-up of the effects of an information and communication technology (ICT) training programme on people with intellectual disabilities. *Research in Developmental Disabilities.*

Li-Tsang, C. W. P., Yeung, S. S., Chan, C. C. H. and Hui-Chan, C. W. Y. (2005). Factors affecting people with intellectual disabilities in learning to use computer technology. *International Journal of Rehabilitation Research, 28(2),* 127-33.

Li-Tsang, C. W. P., Yeung, S. S., Choi, J., Chan, C. C. H. and Lam, C. S. (2006). The effect of systematic information and communication technology (ICT) training programme for people with intellectual disabilities. *The British Journal of Developmental Disabilities, 52(1),* 3-18.

Lindstrand, P. (2002). ICT (Information and Communication Technology): A natural part of life for children with disabilities? *Technology and Disabilities, 14,* 75-83.

Shimizu, H., Twyman, J. S. and Yamamoto, J. I. (2003). Computer based sorting-to-matching in identity matching for young children with developmental disabilities. *Research in Developmental Disabilities, 24(3),* 183-194.

The Organisation for Economic Co-operation and Development. (2001). *Understanding the digital divide.* Retrieved 28 Oct 06 from http://www.oecd.org/dataoecd/38/57/1888451.pdf.

The Government of the Hong Kong Special Administration Region. (2005). *Summary of survey results: Household survey on information technology usage and penetration.* Retrieved 31 July 06 from http://www.info.gov.hk/digital21/eng/ statistics/download/ itsurveysummary2005.pdf.

World Health Organization. (1996). *ICD-10 Guide for mental retardation.* Retrieved 31 Oct 06 from http://www.who.int/mental_health/media/en/69.pdf.

Index

A

abortion, 113
academic success, 175
access, 62, 110, 176, 177, 178, 179, 180, 181, 182, 186, 187, 195
accessibility, 187
accounting, 118, 126, 170
accuracy, 29, 155
achievement, 70
acid, 44, 130
ACTH, 89, 93, 94, 101
activation, 5, 6, 30, 31, 42
activity level, 121, 123
adaptability, 122
adaptation, viii, 45, 46, 54, 55, 62, 65, 66, 68, 69, 72, 73, 121
adaptive functioning, 119, 123, 135
ADHD, 115, 132, 133
adjustment, 116, 118, 131, 138
adolescence, 117, 125, 126, 171, 177, 180
adolescent adjustment, 56
adolescents, vii, viii, 1, 4, 7, 8, 9, 10, 13, 15, 17, 18, 19, 20, 21, 22, 24, 26, 29, 31, 35, 36, 37, 38, 39, 40, 41, 42, 43, 44, 60, 65, 70, 74, 101, 115, 120, 125, 130, 142, 145, 160, 173, 175, 179, 181
adulthood, 46, 47, 51, 56, 111, 121, 125, 175
adults, 29, 31, 32, 39, 40, 42, 58, 61, 70, 71, 77, 78, 84, 85, 90, 91, 100, 103, 107, 110, 114, 117, 119, 125, 127, 128, 131, 132, 137, 140, 141, 142, 143, 144, 150, 151, 167, 173, 176, 188, 189, 195
advocacy, 61
aetiology, 93, 94, 110, 112, 115, 117, 118, 137, 138
affective disorder, 114, 116, 125, 130
affective states, 130

age, viii, ix, x, 35, 37, 38, 43, 46, 47, 48, 50, 51, 52, 53, 55, 75, 78, 79, 84, 91, 94, 96, 97, 107, 108, 110, 113, 117, 124, 125, 126, 127, 128, 131, 132, 133, 143, 149, 150, 154, 155, 157, 158, 159, 160, 162, 163, 166, 173, 175, 178, 180, 182, 188, 189, 192, 193, 194
aggression, 110, 111, 115, 120, 123, 125, 128, 129, 130, 142
aging, vii, 35, 36, 71, 86, 127
akathisia, 124, 137
alcohol, 37
alcohol consumption, 37
alertness, 77, 124
alienation, 136
allergy, 124
ALS, 99, 103
alternative, 83, 115, 166
ambivalence, 46, 122
American Psychiatric Association, 138, 142
amino acid, 94, 96
amino acids, 94, 96
amniocentesis, 113
amygdala, 153
amyotrophic lateral sclerosis, 90, 99
anatomy, 172
anger, 111, 161, 165
animal models, 90, 100
animals, 131
animations, 84
anion, 36
anorexia, 125
anorexia nervosa, 125
ANOVA, 162, 194
anoxia, 79
anticholinergic, 124
anticonvulsants, 124

antidepressant, 103
antihypertensive drugs, 124
antioxidant, viii, 35, 36, 37, 38, 39, 40, 41, 42, 43, 44
antipsychotic, 124, 128, 132
antipsychotic drugs, 124, 128
anxiety, 111, 115, 120, 121, 124, 125, 126, 131, 132, 133, 136, 137, 148, 176
anxiety disorder, 131, 176
aortic stenosis, 150, 174
apoptosis, 90, 91, 97, 98, 100
apoptotic mechanisms, 97
appetite, 125, 129
apraxia, 94
argument, 166
Aristotle, 75
arousal, 10
arrest, 90, 100
artery, 93
asphyxia, 89, 90, 92, 93, 98, 101
assessment, viii, x, 32, 36, 37, 38, 41, 105, 108, 109, 111, 112, 118, 120, 121, 123, 127, 128, 129, 134, 135, 136, 137, 143, 145, 160, 179, 180, 189, 190, 192, 194
assets, 57
assignment, 60
assumptions, 108
asthma, 177
ataxia, 94, 98, 102
atherosclerosis, vii, 35, 36
atrophy, 90, 92, 94, 96, 97, 100, 102
attachment, 68, 122
attention, x, 5, 10, 11, 17, 30, 32, 39, 76, 77, 78, 82, 83, 84, 85, 86, 87, 105, 108, 115, 117, 119, 125, 126, 131, 132, 133, 134, 153, 155, 159, 166, 167, 178, 187
attitudes, ix, 46, 54, 65, 122, 187
audition, 160
auditory stimuli, 11
autism, vii, 1, 2, 4, 7, 8, 9, 10, 11, 12, 13, 15, 16, 17, 18, 19, 20, 21, 22, 24, 29, 30, 31, 32, 48, 51, 54, 56, 58, 89, 90, 92, 94, 95, 96, 100, 101, 102, 113, 117, 120, 121, 122, 125, 131, 133, 142, 143, 154, 158, 169, 170, 172, 182, 188, 189, 190, 195
automatisms, 124
autonomy, 178
autopsy, 97
availability, 187
averaging, 18
avoidance, 133

awareness, 78, 129
axons, 97

barriers, xi, 63, 185
basal forebrain, 89, 91, 94, 95, 101
basic services, 176
BBB, 99
BD, 168, 182
behavior, 32, 33, 62, 71, 74, 77, 84, 85, 106, 107, 108, 109, 121, 123, 124, 127, 131, 133, 134, 145, 170, 173, 186
behavioral effects, 135
behavioral problems, 67, 128, 194
beliefs, 49, 65, 68, 136
benzodiazepine, 134
benzodiazepines, 124
bias, 159, 164
binding, 99, 102, 126, 135, 177, 178
biomacromolecules, 41
biomarkers, 42
biopsy, 97
bipolar disorder, 130, 134, 145
bipolar illness, 130
birth, 55, 57, 65, 73, 79, 107, 117, 123
birth weight, 117
births, 113
blocks, 162
blood, 37, 40, 92, 95, 99, 101, 103, 116, 124
blood flow, 116
blood-brain barrier, 99, 103
BMI, 38, 41, 42
body fat, 103
body mass index, 38, 41
bowel, 122
boys, 70, 79, 101, 125, 131, 132
brain, 30, 89, 90, 91, 92, 93, 94, 95, 96, 97, 98, 99, 101, 102, 103, 106, 111, 117, 121, 122, 124, 127, 144, 149, 150, 152, 153, 166, 169, 170, 172
brain damage, 98, 106, 149
brain development, 89, 91, 96, 166
brain functions, 149
brain growth, 94, 96, 97, 98, 99, 102
brain size, 152
branching, 94
breathing, 136
breeding, 106
browser, 189
browsing, 188, 189, 190, 193, 194

B

bulimia, 132
bulimia nervosa, 132
bullying, 122, 138

C

Canada, 176
candidates, 99
carbonyl groups, 37, 40
cardiac surgery, 60
cardiovascular disease, 44
caregivers, 54, 58, 68, 73, 107, 118, 123, 134, 188, 190, 192, 194
caregiving, 54, 62, 66
catalase, viii, 36, 37, 38, 40, 44
catalyst, 61
categorization, 161, 163, 164, 166
causal relationship, 111
causality, 171
cell, vii, 10, 35, 36, 42, 90, 91, 96, 98, 153
cell culture, 98
cell death, 91
cell line, 90
central nervous system, vii, 1, 2, 4, 32, 92, 102
cerebellar development, 96
cerebellum, 10, 11, 91, 96
cerebral palsy, 50, 51, 58, 122, 123
cerebrospinal fluid, 100, 101, 102
certainty, 72
chemotherapy, 98
child development, 65
child well-being, 61, 67
childcare, 73
childhood, vii, 46, 54, 60, 71, 111, 121, 131, 134, 142, 177, 180, 186
cholinergic neurons, 89, 91, 94, 95
chromosomal abnormalities, 128
chromosome, 36, 97, 125, 126, 152, 160
chronic diseases, 89, 90, 92, 98, 177
chronic pain, 128
chunking, vii, 2, 7, 9, 10, 13, 17, 29
cisplatin, 102
classes, 160
classification, 108, 109, 110, 111, 119, 128, 137, 139, 169
classroom, 84, 86
clinical assessment, 120
clinical diagnosis, 152
clinical examination, 95
clinical presentation, 127, 128
clinical symptoms, 96
clinical trials, 90, 100
closure, 95
CNS, 90, 91, 96
coding, 172
coefficient of variation, 18
cognition, xi, 76, 106, 138, 147, 151, 164, 166, 169, 170, 171, 172
cognitive abilities, 83, 120, 126, 128, 129, 135, 160
cognitive deficit, 10, 30, 117, 169
cognitive deficits, 10, 30, 117, 169
cognitive development, 12, 150, 170, 173
cognitive domains, xi, 147, 148, 149
cognitive function, xi, 143, 147, 148, 150, 164
cognitive impairment, 98, 103, 120, 121
cognitive level, 86
cognitive map, 171
cognitive performance, 194
cognitive perspective, 18
cognitive profile, 151, 152, 166, 172
cognitive system, 153, 166
cognitive tasks, 78
cognitive variables, 129
cohesion, 46
communication, xi, 46, 65, 108, 109, 111, 112, 113, 114, 116, 118, 119, 122, 123, 126, 128, 129, 130, 131, 133, 136, 153, 171, 185, 186, 187, 195
communication abilities, 133
communication skills, 123, 126
communication technologies, 187
community, x, 46, 49, 52, 53, 60, 61, 68, 71, 72, 73, 78, 105, 107, 108, 110, 113, 114, 115, 117, 122, 134, 140, 176, 178, 179
community service, 177
community support, 135
comorbidity, 122, 176
compassion, 64
compensation, 63
competence, 60, 61, 135, 190
complete blood count, 124
complex interactions, 135
complexity, 28, 30, 78, 80, 164, 173
compliance, 136
complications, 61, 62, 111, 122, 135
components, vii, 1, 4, 5, 29, 67, 82, 123, 150, 157
comprehension, 86, 121, 127, 137
computer skills, 192
computer technology, 186, 195
computing, 186
concentration, 78, 126

conception, 113
conceptual model, 119
concrete, 123
conduct disorder, 132
conduct problems, 125
confidence, 38, 39, 61, 62, 70
confidence interval, 38, 39
configuration, 155, 157, 159, 165
conflict, 66, 136
conflict resolution, 136
confounding variables, 113
confusion, 119
consciousness, 124
consensus, 54, 108, 119, 137, 149
consent, 80, 92, 135, 136, 188
constraints, 137
construction, 80
control, vii, viii, 2, 7, 9, 10, 11, 13, 15, 16, 17, 18,
    22, 29, 30, 31, 32, 33, 45, 47, 67, 68, 84, 87, 111,
    120, 122, 125, 137, 145, 155, 157, 158, 160, 161,
    163, 165, 178
control group, viii, 2, 7, 9, 13, 15, 45, 47, 67, 68,
    155, 160, 165
conversion, 40
corpus callosum, 152, 153, 173
correlation, 18, 41, 50, 52, 102, 144, 162, 188
correlation analysis, 162
correlation coefficient, 41, 188
correlations, vii, 1, 18, 20, 21, 22, 27, 28, 29, 41
cortex, 10, 94, 95, 96
cortical neurons, 90, 97
costs, 177, 179
counseling, 73, 136
couples, 47
coverage, 176, 178, 180, 181
covering, 49
CSF, 89, 90, 92, 93, 94, 95, 96, 97, 98, 101, 102
cues, 11, 77, 83, 159, 168
cultural differences, 178
culture, 56, 108, 112, 119, 178
curriculum, 190
customers, 186
cycles, viii, 24, 36, 38
cycling, 130

D

daily care, 68
daily living, 106, 122, 187
danger, 80, 85, 86

data collection, 80
death, 97
decoding, 148, 159, 163, 164
defects, 169
defense, 39, 44
deficiency, 85, 87, 107, 113, 150
deficit, x, 87, 105, 115, 117, 119, 125, 134, 142, 149,
    151, 155
definition, 107, 108, 109, 111, 114, 129, 139, 149,
    172, 187
delivery, 65, 73, 103, 107, 136, 139
deltoid, 5
delusions, 112, 119, 120
demand, 82, 134
dementia, 90, 114, 120, 125, 127, 143
demyelination, 91, 97
dendrites, 94, 98
density, 40, 96, 153, 170
Department of Health and Human Services, 145
depression, 46, 57, 66, 67, 111, 115, 117, 121, 127,
    129, 133, 134, 136, 142, 143, 144, 187
depressive symptoms, 145
derivatives, 44
desensitization, 131
desires, 153
detection, 11, 44, 127
developed countries, 113, 187
developing brain, 90
developing countries, 113, 114, 140
developmental delay, 55, 60, 107, 109, 133, 134
developmental disorder, x, 30, 105, 114, 117, 125,
    132, 149, 154, 158, 167, 168, 169, 170, 173
developmental factors, 108
developmental psychopathology, 109
deviation, 18
diabetes, 103, 177
diabetes mellitus, 103
Diagnostic and Statistical Manual of Mental
    Disorders, 109
diagnostic criteria, 114, 119, 130, 132, 160
diathesis-stress model, 129
diet, 37, 41
differential diagnosis, 124
differentiation, 89, 90, 125
diffusion, 176
digital divide, xi, 185, 187, 194, 195, 196
dignity, 108
diodes, 2, 13
disability, viii, 41, 45, 46, 47, 49, 50, 51, 52, 54, 55,
    56, 57, 59, 61, 62, 63, 66, 68, 71, 72, 73, 107,

108, 113, 114, 116, 118, 120, 126, 127, 132, 133, 139, 140, 141, 143, 144, 145, 149, 150, 175, 181, 182, 183, 186

discomfort, 47, 55

discrimination, 85, 151, 159

discrimination learning, 85

discrimination tasks, 151

disease progression, 42

disorder, x, 10, 48, 60, 101, 105, 107, 109, 111, 114, 115, 116, 118, 119, 123, 125, 126, 130, 131, 132, 133, 134, 135, 137, 141, 142, 144, 149, 150, 152, 176, 179, 182

displacement, 5

dissatisfaction, 46, 60, 64, 177

dissociation, xi, 147, 149, 150, 151, 160, 164, 166

distilled water, viii, 36, 38

distortions, 121

distress, 62, 63, 108, 118

distribution, 113, 117, 175

diversity, 108, 143

DNA, 39, 43

DNA repair, 43

doctors, 131, 176

dogs, 79

dopaminergic, 91

dopaminergic neurons, 91

Down syndrome, vii, viii, ix, 1, 2, 4, 5, 6, 7, 8, 9, 10, 13, 18, 29, 30, 31, 32, 35, 36, 37, 38, 39, 40, 41, 42, 43, 44, 47, 48, 50, 51, 54, 56, 59, 60, 61, 62, 63, 64, 65, 66, 67, 68, 69, 70, 71, 72, 73, 74, 82, 92, 101, 113, 114, 122, 125, 126, 127, 140, 144, 154, 166, 170, 173

dream, 180

drug treatment, 127, 129

drugs, 99, 103, 124, 127, 128, 137

dry ice, viii, 36, 38

DSM, 107, 108, 109, 110, 111, 119, 120, 129, 130, 132, 135, 137, 143, 175, 181

DSM-II, 143

DSM-III, 143

DSM-IV, 109, 110, 111, 119, 120, 129, 130, 132, 135, 175, 181

duration, 11, 13, 24, 25, 26, 28, 110, 179

duties, 190

dwarfism, 103

dynamic systems, 22

dysphoria, 56

dysthymia, 129

E

eating, 125, 132

eating disorders, 132

ecology, 56, 71

economic resources, 61

economic status, 113

economics, 114

edema, 102

education, ix, x, 17, 68, 70, 71, 76, 78, 87, 106, 107, 114, 136, 179, 187

Education, 1, 68, 71, 72, 74, 75, 106, 136, 138, 195

educators, 106

EEG, 95, 97, 101, 124

effortful processing, 77, 85

Egypt, 106

elasticity, 69

elastin, 152, 160

elderly, 120, 140, 141

elderly population, 120

electrolyte, 124

eligibility criteria, 63

ELISA, 92, 93

email, 35

emergence, 131, 145, 152

EMG, 4

emotion, xi, 147, 148, 159, 160, 161, 163, 164, 165, 166, 167, 168, 172

emotional disorder, 176

emotional information, 153, 159

emotional well-being, 49

emotionality, 121

emotions, xi, 106, 119, 121, 122, 133, 147, 154, 159, 161, 162, 163, 164, 166, 167, 168, 169

empathy, 148, 152, 167

encephalitis, 79, 95

encephalomyelitis, 98

encephalopathy, 96, 97, 102

encoding, 97, 152, 157

endothelial cells, 102

energy, 59, 62

engagement, 136

environment, 76, 78, 79, 84, 113, 123, 132, 134, 135, 138, 150, 167, 176

environmental context, 126, 168

environmental factors, 113, 115, 117, 129, 135, 167, 168

environmental influences, 152, 167

enzymes, viii, 36, 37, 38, 39, 40, 41, 42, 43, 44

epidemiology, 140

epilepsy, 48, 56, 79, 112, 113, 114, 117, 122, 123, 126, 127, 128, 141, 143, 187
equity, 182
erythrocytes, viii, 36, 37, 38, 43, 44
estimating, 112
ethics, x, 105, 160
ethology, 115
etiology, x, 48, 105, 139
Europe, 112
evolution, 100, 106
exaggeration, 121
exercise, viii, 35, 36, 37, 39, 40, 41, 42, 43, 44, 111
experimental autoimmune encephalomyelitis, 102
experimental condition, 10, 158, 163, 164
expertise, 154, 159, 166, 168, 169
exposure, 161, 166, 168
extensor, 5, 6
externalizing disorders, 125
eyes, 154, 158

F

face recognition, 158, 169, 172, 173
facial expression, 159, 166, 167, 168, 174
facial responses, 167
factor analysis, 143
failure, 77, 83, 86, 94, 109, 177, 180
family, viii, ix, 45, 46, 47, 49, 54, 55, 56, 57, 58, 59, 60, 61, 62, 63, 64, 65, 66, 68, 69, 70, 71, 72, 73, 74, 91, 100, 122, 123, 127, 132, 135, 136, 176, 177, 181
family factors, 62, 132
family functioning, 57, 61, 66, 69
family history, 123
family interactions, 136
family life, 46, 47, 54, 55, 63, 70, 71, 176
family members, viii, 45, 47, 55, 62, 65, 68, 127
family support, 58, 60, 64, 70, 72
family system, 61, 62, 63, 69
family therapy, 136
fatigue, 18, 46, 129
fear, 131, 152
fears, 131, 151
feedback, 10, 18, 24
feelings, 129, 130
females, viii, 2, 9, 45, 52, 55, 113, 126, 131
financial support, 66
flexibility, 168
fluid, 101, 102
fluoxetine, 130

focusing, 64, 84, 123, 129, 154, 167
folate, 124
food, 125, 132
Ford, 22, 32
forebrain, 30, 95, 96
France, 106, 147, 172
free radicals, 98
friends, 46, 63, 65, 70
functional analysis, 134
functional imaging, 116
funding, 63, 190
funds, 66

G

gait, 126
ganglion, 103
gender, 43, 44, 55, 56, 160
gender differences, 56
gene, 36, 91, 95, 97, 126, 150, 152, 160
gene expression, 91
general intelligence, 140, 149
general practitioner, 181
generation, 20, 26, 39, 102
genes, 144, 152, 153, 167, 170
genetic disorders, 111, 115, 133, 170
genetic marker, 152
genetic syndromes, 115, 117, 124
genetic testing, 115, 116
genetics, 102, 115, 173
genotype, 152, 167, 169
gestures, 123
girls, 79, 94, 101, 131, 132
glaucoma, 124
glia, 91
glucose, viii, 36, 37, 38, 40, 41, 42, 43
glutamate, 94, 96, 98, 101, 102
glutathione, viii, 36, 37, 38, 40, 41, 42, 43, 44
glutathione peroxidase, viii, 36, 37, 38, 40, 41, 42, 43, 44
goals, 37, 67, 68, 72, 134
governance, 190
government, 63, 178
Greece, 75, 79
grief, 46, 55, 122, 136
groups, vii, ix, x, 1, 2, 7, 8, 9, 12, 13, 14, 15, 19, 20, 25, 27, 29, 38, 47, 48, 50, 52, 54, 63, 64, 65, 69, 75, 77, 78, 81, 82, 83, 113, 134, 155, 157, 158, 159, 162, 166, 190
growth, 89, 90, 91, 93, 94, 100, 101, 102, 103, 126

growth factor, 90, 94, 100, 101, 102, 103
growth factors, 94, 102
guidance, 177, 190
guidelines, 80, 110, 123
guilt, 120, 122

H

hallucinations, 112, 119, 120, 128
handedness, 24, 32
hands, 7, 17, 18, 21, 22, 24, 25, 29, 31, 32, 33, 126
happiness, 161, 165
harm, 118
hazards, 85
HDL, 40
head injury, 99, 103
head trauma, 79
health, x, 42, 49, 52, 53, 56, 58, 60, 62, 63, 64, 65, 73, 105, 107, 108, 111, 112, 114, 118, 137, 138, 139, 141, 142, 143, 145, 176, 177, 178, 179, 180, 181, 182, 196
health care, 64, 176, 177, 178, 179, 180, 181, 182
health problems, 60, 108, 138, 139, 141
health services, 142, 176, 181, 182
heart rate, viii, 35, 37
hemodialysis, 44
high school, 2, 13
hip, 41, 189
hippocampus, 95
hiring, 186
homogeneity, 177
Hong Kong, 185, 186, 187, 190, 196
hopelessness, 129
hospitals, 64
hostility, 122
House, 71
households, 187
human brain, 32
human rights, 135
hunting, 188
hydrocephalus, 48
hydrogen, 36, 41
hydrogen peroxide, 36, 41
hydroxyl, 36, 41
hyperactivity, x, 87, 105, 115, 117, 119, 125, 126, 128, 142
hypercalcemia, 152
hypoplasia, 10
hypothesis, xi, 47, 137, 147, 158, 159, 160, 164, 180
hypothyroidism, 113

hypoxia, 42, 111

I

ICD, 108, 109, 110, 119, 129, 132, 135, 175, 186, 196
identification, 36, 47, 54, 55, 78, 80, 85, 87, 107, 113, 114, 128, 134, 150
identity, 77, 148, 154, 160, 196
idiopathic, 173
idiosyncratic, 124
images, 170
imaging, 124
imitation, 136
immunization, 113
impairments, 109, 113, 118, 122, 126, 135, 151, 158, 159, 163, 164, 177, 182
implementation, 134
impulsive, 125, 128
in situ, 84, 103, 160
in situ hybridization, 160
in vitro, 36, 37, 90, 100
in vivo, 36, 37, 39, 40, 103
inattention, 5
incentives, 107
incidence, 67, 107, 113, 116, 139, 140
inclusion, 60, 61, 63, 66, 195
income, 187
independence, 108, 138
India, 114
indicators, 44, 120, 129, 176
indices, 42
individual perception, 111
individual rights, x, 105
Individuals with Disabilities Education Act, 107, 138
inertia, 82, 85
infancy, 134
infants, 5, 56, 73, 93, 94, 117, 141, 149, 154, 167, 170, 171
infectious disease, 113
information processing, 7, 9, 18, 24
information technology, 196
informed consent, viii, 35, 38, 135, 137, 160
ingestion, 132
inhibition, 82, 85, 86
initiation, 5
input, 109, 118, 138
insects, 131
insight, 123, 126
insomnia, 137

institutionalisation. 131
instruction, 74, 78, 79
instructors, 190, 194
instruments, 17, 49, 110, 129, 144
insulin, 90, 91, 99, 100, 101, 102, 103
insulin resistance, 99, 103
insurance, 176, 178, 180, 181
integrity, 69
intellect, 106
intellectual disabilities, 46, 57, 65, 67, 72, 84, 87,
    114, 130, 141, 144, 159, 176, 177, 178, 180, 181,
    182, 195
intellectual functioning, 108, 110, 119, 148, 149,
    150, 160, 163, 168, 175, 186
intelligence, vii, x, 105, 106, 107, 115, 128, 132,
    137, 138, 142, 149, 150, 174, 186
intelligence quotient, vii, 149
intensity, viii, 35, 37, 110, 133, 151
intentions, 153
interaction, 19, 20, 26, 61, 63, 106, 122, 136, 138,
    158, 167, 168, 194
interaction effect, 19
interaction effects, 19
interactions, 65, 68, 123, 124, 172
interface, 118
interference, 77, 83, 86
internal time, 23
internalizing, 129
internet, 186
interpersonal skills, 67
interpretation, 155, 159, 165, 167
interrelationships, 154
interval, 2, 4, 5, 7, 10, 11, 12, 13, 18, 19, 20, 21, 22,
    24, 25, 26, 29, 80
intervention, ix, 54, 55, 57, 59, 60, 62, 63, 64, 67,
    68, 70, 71, 72, 73, 74, 107, 109, 116, 128, 134,
    138, 177, 181, 182
intervention strategies, 138
intimacy, 49
inversion, 155, 165
investment, 118
iodine, 113
IQ scores, 150, 160, 164
irritability, 137
ischemic stroke, 42
isolation, 46, 60, 158
Italy, 45, 47, 175, 177, 178, 179, 180, 181

J

Japan, 1
judges, 80
judgment, 132
junior high school, 13, 18

L

lack of opportunities, 187
language, vii, x, 60, 105, 106, 109, 119, 121, 123,
    126, 133, 149, 151, 152, 166, 167, 168, 171, 172,
    173, 178, 187
language acquisition, 167
language development, 133, 151, 171, 173
language impairment, 119, 149, 171
language skills, vii, 121, 123, 166
later life, 127
laughing, 126
LDL, 40
learned helplessness, 87
learning, vii, xi, 30, 32, 59, 60, 61, 62, 63, 64, 71,
    72, 77, 84, 86, 103, 106, 107, 109, 110, 111, 113,
    119, 126, 134, 139, 140, 141, 142, 145, 159, 173,
    182, 185, 186, 188, 190, 195
learning difficulties, 109, 139
learning disabilities, 110, 119, 139, 140, 142, 182,
    195
learning skills, 60
legislation, 60
leisure, xi, 108, 185, 186, 187, 194
leisure time, 194
lending, 115
lens, 2
lesions, 10, 11, 122
life changes, 52
life course, ix, 59, 61
life cycle, 58
life expectancy, 112, 127
life experiences, 131
life satisfaction, 66
life span, 127
lifespan, 60, 70, 71
lifestyle, xi, 185
lifetime, 116, 127
limitation, 177, 181
links, 179
lipid peroxidation, 37, 39, 42, 43
lipids, 39, 41

liquid chromatography, 44
literacy, 195
lithium, 130
liver, 42, 43, 44
location, 77, 86
location information, 86
locus, 97
longevity, 60
longitudinal study, 55, 72

M

Macedonia, 75
magnesium, 43
magnetic resonance, 170
mainstream society, 176
major depression, 123, 129
males, viii, 2, 9, 45, 52, 55, 113, 125, 126
maltreatment, 131
management, x, 69, 73, 105, 107, 112, 113, 115, 119, 121, 122, 124, 128, 131, 132, 134, 135, 136, 142, 144, 187, 195
mania, 115, 121, 130
manic, 130, 145
manic symptoms, 145
manipulation, 32
marital conflict, 61
marriage, 113
masking, x, 105, 121
mastery, 143
matrix, 42
matrix metalloproteinase, 42
meanings, 136
measurement, 49, 93, 107, 124, 129
measures, 49, 54, 57, 111, 120, 135, 150, 154, 156, 160
media, 186, 196
medical care, 182
medication, 110, 111, 123, 124, 137
Mediterranean, 147
memory, 20, 26, 82, 86, 103, 124
men, 47, 111
meningitis, 92
mental age, ix, x, 75, 78, 79, 82, 83, 155, 157, 159
mental disorder, x, 105, 107, 109, 112, 118, 119, 141
mental health, x, 46, 57, 68, 105, 111, 116, 120, 122, 129, 139, 140, 176, 178, 179, 180, 181
mental illness, 71, 106, 107, 108, 109, 112, 113, 114, 115, 116, 117, 123, 127, 137, 138
mental state, 108, 124

mentally retarded adolescents, vii, 1, 9, 10, 13
metabolic disorder, 95, 113
metabolism, viii, 35, 36, 37, 39, 42, 44, 96
metabolites, 42, 96, 98
metaphor, 123
methodological procedures, 37
mice, 91, 102
microcephaly, 91
Microsoft, 161
midbrain, 30
migration, 113, 114
Ministry of Education, 80
minority, 107, 187
mobility, 127
moclobemide, 130
modeling, 131
models, 22, 23, 67, 84, 129, 134, 140, 166
modern society, 186
modules, 149, 166
money, 62, 63
mood, 120, 123, 124, 125, 129, 130, 137, 144, 145, 176
mood disorder, 125, 130, 137, 144, 145, 176
morbidity, 112, 114, 140, 141
morphology, 170, 173
mortality, 113, 114
mothers, viii, 45, 47, 48, 50, 51, 52, 54, 56, 58, 60, 64, 65, 66, 67, 68, 70, 71, 72, 73, 74, 143
motivation, 86, 121, 143, 158, 160, 167
motor behavior, 30, 126, 134
motor control, 7, 11, 17, 30
motor skills, 2, 121
motor task, 17, 24, 31
movement, 4, 5, 7, 9, 10, 13, 17, 18, 24, 29, 30, 31, 32, 63, 119
MRI, 124, 153, 173
multidimensional, 108
multimedia, 195
muscle relaxation, 136
musicians, 26
mutation, 94, 96, 126
mutations, 94, 97, 126
myelin, 97, 98, 102

N

natural environment, 86
negative priming, 87
negative relation, 189
neglect, 131, 143

neonates, 89

nerve, 5, 89, 90, 93, 94, 100, 101, 103

nerve conduction velocity, 5

nerve growth factor, 90, 100, 101, 103

nervous system, 91, 100, 126

Netherlands, 180, 183

network, 70

neural network, 86

neurodegeneration, vii, 35, 36, 96

neurodegenerative diseases, 90, 92, 96, 100

neuroimaging, 95

neuroleptics, 137

neurological condition, 112

neurological disorder, 123

neurologist, 160

neuromotor, 32

neuronal death, 94

neurons, 89, 90, 91, 95, 96, 97, 99, 103

neuropathy, 102

neuropsychological tests, 120

neuropsychology, 124, 166, 170

neuroscience, 170

neurotransmitter, 96

neurotrophic factors, 89, 90, 91, 92, 94, 96, 99

neutrophils, 43

New England, 30

nitrate, 96, 102

NMR, 97

noise, 86

normal children, 31, 47, 122

normal development, 56, 122, 126, 153

North America, 107

Norway, 187

novelty, 177, 181

nuclei, 101

O

obesity, 112, 125

observations, 5, 108, 112, 134

observed behavior, 83

obsessive-compulsive disorder, 131, 134

occipital lobe, 153

occupational therapy, 124

oedema, 96

Oklahoma, 71

old age, 187

older adults, 127, 143, 189

older people, 141

oligodendrocytes, 96, 97, 98

omission, 13

operant conditioning, 136

optical density, 96

optimization, 42

organization, vii, 2, 13, 22, 23, 24, 25, 27, 28, 29, 176, 177, 178, 179, 195

orientation, 124

output, vii, 2, 7, 9, 10, 13, 17, 18, 29

overtraining, 43

oxidation, 39, 40

oxidative damage, viii, 35, 36, 37, 39, 40, 41

oxidative stress, vii, 35, 36, 37, 39, 40, 42, 43, 44

oxygen, 42

P

pacing, 10, 19, 20

panic disorder, 145

parameter, 38, 39

parental care, 113

parenting, 46, 55, 60, 61, 73, 122

parents, viii, ix, 35, 37, 38, 45, 46, 47, 49, 50, 51, 52, 53, 54, 55, 56, 57, 59, 60, 61, 62, 63, 64, 65, 66, 67, 68, 70, 71, 72, 73, 74, 80, 107, 122, 127, 129, 136, 168, 173, 176, 178, 180, 182, 188, 190, 192, 194

parkinsonism, 124

pathogenesis, 89, 90, 92, 94, 100, 101

pathology, 93, 98, 115, 117, 119, 122, 124, 127

pathophysiology, x, 105

pathways, 43, 149

Pearson correlations, 20, 21, 27, 28

peers, 77, 108, 122, 135

perception, 33, 47, 50, 51, 54, 61, 62, 63, 68, 85, 107, 132, 159, 169, 172

perceptions, 49, 55, 60, 62, 64, 65, 68, 70, 119, 121

perceptions of control, 70

perceptual processing, 17, 172

perfusion, 101

perinatal, 111, 113

peripheral nervous system, 92

peripheral neuropathy, 98, 99

peroxidation, 43

peroxide, 36

personal autonomy, 176

personal goals, 46

personal qualities, 70

personality, x, 105, 110, 141, 173

personality disorder, x, 105, 110

personality traits, 141

pessimism, viii, 45, 49, 50, 51, 52, 54, 62
PET, 95
pharmacological treatment, 131
pharmacology, 124
pharmacotherapy, 137
phenomenology, 119, 131, 138
phenotype, 141, 144, 148, 149, 150, 151, 167, 168, 169, 170, 173
phobia, 145
photographs, 154, 160, 161, 162, 163, 164, 165, 166
physical activity, viii, 35, 37, 41, 42, 43, 44
physical aggression, 115
physical exercise, 42
physical health, 66
physical therapy, 124
pica, 132
planning, 7, 66, 114, 116, 118, 121, 135
plasma, 39, 44
plasma proteins, 44
plasticity, 91
polyunsaturated fat, 39
polyunsaturated fatty acids, 39
poor, 82, 89, 92, 93, 94, 113, 121, 122, 126, 127, 152
population, viii, ix, x, 35, 36, 37, 40, 41, 43, 59, 105, 112, 113, 116, 117, 122, 125, 127, 128, 129, 130, 131, 135, 137, 139, 141, 149, 150, 160, 166, 167, 176, 179
Portugal, 168
positive correlation, 20, 190
post-traumatic stress disorder, 131
power, 71, 169
Prader-Willi syndrome, 125
predictive validity, 139
predictors, 43, 56, 58, 121
pregnancy, 123
prematurity, 98, 102
preschool, 143, 174
preschool children, 143, 174
preschoolers, 79
prevention, 102, 134, 138, 140, 177
primary school, 79
primary visual cortex, 153, 170
priming, 77, 86
probability, 31, 134
problem behavior, 63, 127, 134
problem behaviors, 63, 134
problem solving, 59, 67, 83
problem-solving, 87
production, 22, 24, 26, 32, 41, 99, 167, 170

productivity, 49
profession, 180
prognosis, 93, 131
program, viii, 10, 35, 36, 37, 38, 39, 40, 41, 42, 43, 44, 50, 66, 67, 68, 72, 73, 106, 177, 181, 187, 190, 192, 194
programming, 7, 32, 123, 133
proliferation, 94
prophylaxis, 130
protective factors, 70
protein oxidation, viii, 36, 37, 38, 39, 40, 42, 44
proteins, 39, 40, 41, 102
protocol, 38, 194
psychiatric diagnosis, x, 105, 116, 119, 123
psychiatric disorders, 109, 112, 113, 114, 115, 116, 117, 118, 119, 120, 123, 124, 125, 128, 137, 140, 141, 142, 143, 145, 187
psychiatric illness, x, 105, 114, 116, 117, 120, 121, 129
psychiatric morbidity, 117, 137, 141
psychiatric patients, 47
psychiatric side effects, 112
psychiatrist, 120, 142, 176
psychological well-being, 58, 68, 71
psychologist, 80
psychology, ix, x, 67, 76, 86, 174
psychometric properties, 49
psychopathology, 87, 107, 109, 112, 114, 118, 119, 121, 122, 128, 135, 138, 141, 143, 181
psychoses, 114, 144
psychosis, 121, 122, 125, 128, 137
psychosocial functioning, 110
psychotic symptoms, 119
psychotropic drug, 137
psychotropic drugs, 137
puberty, 107
public administration, 177
public health, 176
P-value, 81

Q

quality of life, viii, 45, 46, 47, 49, 50, 52, 54, 55, 56, 70, 112, 127, 133, 140, 177, 178
questionnaires, 120, 177

R

radical formation, 36

rain, 91

range, 49, 78, 79, 80, 112, 114, 122, 124, 125, 131, 133, 134, 136, 137, 150, 152, 177, 180

rating scale, 110, 120, 143

ratings, 177

reaction time, vii, 1, 2, 4, 5, 6, 7, 8, 9, 10, 11, 12, 13, 14, 15, 16, 17, 18, 30, 31, 32, 33, 86

reactivity, 42

reading, 166

reality, 84, 87

reasoning, ix, 75

recall, 18, 19, 24, 154

recalling, 29

receptors, 90, 100

recognition, ix, x, 76, 79, 107, 118, 151, 154, 155, 158, 159, 160, 164, 165, 166, 167, 168, 170, 173

recognition test, 158

recovery, 69, 70, 128

reduction, 40, 67, 121

regression, 50, 94, 97

regulation, 94

rehabilitation, 87, 178, 186

reinforcement, 129, 132, 133, 168, 190

reinforcers, 136

rejection, 122

relationship, ix, 5, 41, 45, 54, 65, 68, 78, 85, 87, 106, 116, 117, 118, 128, 130, 173, 182

relationships, 25, 68, 122, 123, 136, 150, 157

relaxation, 131

relevance, 112, 113, 119, 121, 160, 161, 168

reliability, 49, 119, 188

reproduction, 30

resettlement, 115, 177

resilience, ix, 59, 61, 69, 70, 73

resistance, 40

resources, 60, 61, 62, 63, 68, 70, 77, 82, 134

response time, 31

responsiveness, 10, 44

restructuring, 67

retardation, vii, ix, x, xi, 1, 4, 18, 19, 20, 22, 24, 26, 28, 29, 75, 76, 77, 78, 82, 83, 84, 85, 105, 106, 107, 109, 110, 111, 112, 114, 115, 116, 117, 118, 119, 120, 121, 122, 123, 124, 127, 128, 129, 130, 131, 132, 133, 135, 136, 137, 138, 140, 144, 145, 148, 150, 169, 175, 180, 185, 186, 187, 188, 189, 190, 192, 194, 195

reticular activating system, 10

retinopathy, 98, 102

Rett syndrome, 89, 90, 92, 95, 100, 101, 126, 144

rhythm, 25, 32

risk, ix, 48, 59, 60, 61, 62, 69, 110, 111, 116, 117, 118, 122, 123, 124, 126, 133, 134

risk assessment, 123

risk factors, 69

risperidone, 133

rubella, 79

S

sadness, 161, 165

safety, ix, x, 49, 76, 80, 84, 85, 103, 108, 110, 111

sample, viii, ix, x, 45, 47, 48, 50, 51, 75, 78, 114, 176

satisfaction, 49, 64, 65, 72, 73

Scandinavia, 140, 142

schizophrenia, 107, 114, 116, 119, 125, 128

school, 13, 18, 24, 46, 55, 57, 60, 63, 78, 80, 106, 109, 113, 122, 123, 160, 175, 180, 182, 186, 190, 195

scientific community, 155

sclerosis, 122, 127

scores, 47, 52, 54, 81, 82, 83, 93, 107, 110, 150, 160, 188, 189, 192, 193, 194

search, 76

searches, 186

segregation, 60

seizure, 122, 127, 143

seizures, 127

selective attention, ix, 75, 76, 77, 78, 82, 83, 84, 85, 86

self-efficacy, 67

self-esteem, 46

self-regulation, 187

self-reports, 129

sensitivity, 64, 91, 131, 137, 148, 168

sensory modality, 11, 30

separation, 21

series, 7, 10, 17, 25, 29, 41, 175

serology, 124

serotonin, 95, 101, 130

serum, 40, 42, 43, 89, 92, 94

severe intellectual disabilities, 74, 114, 190

severity, 50, 51, 52, 102, 109, 114, 120, 121, 132, 187

sex, 38, 50, 51, 52, 125

shape, 30, 152, 153, 157, 173

shaping, 65

sharing, 163

shortage, 61

shy, 125

sibling, 70
siblings, 57, 70, 143, 192
side effects, 124, 128, 130, 134, 137
sign, 130, 155
signalling, 99, 102
signs, 97, 108, 109, 121, 125
simulation, 78, 87
Singapore, 187
sites, ix, x, 75, 78, 79, 80, 82, 83, 84, 85, 87, 91, 132
skeletal muscle, 44
skill acquisition, 31
skills, xi, 22, 67, 72, 78, 79, 82, 84, 85, 86, 87, 94,
    106, 108, 109, 110, 117, 120, 121, 123, 127, 132,
    147, 148, 149, 150, 153, 154, 155, 157, 158, 159,
    160, 174, 175, 185, 186, 187, 188, 190, 192, 194,
    195
skills training, 67, 72
skin, 125
skin picking, 125
sleep disturbance, 123, 129
smoking, 37, 43
sociability, 151
social acceptance, 194
social activities, 61
social anxiety, 168
social attributes, 152
social behavior, 56
social behaviour, xi, 147, 148, 152, 153, 159, 167
social change, 134
social class, 113
social context, 42, 175
social costs, 177
social environment, 110, 123
social exclusion, 176
social integration, 41
social isolation, 61, 62
social life, 178
social problems, 176
social services, 55, 107, 178
social situations, 114
social skills, 108, 109, 111, 120, 164
social status, 160, 163
social stigmatization, 194
social support, 55, 56, 58, 67, 71, 73
social withdrawal, 120
social workers, 179
society, 60, 176, 178, 182, 186
socioeconomic status, 63
software, xi, 81, 161, 185, 187, 190, 191, 192, 194
Spain, 35, 60, 64

spatial frequency, 157
special education, 78
specialization, 170, 178, 179, 180, 181
species, 42
specificity, 39, 48, 57, 117, 119, 172
spectrum, x, 48, 101, 105, 111, 114, 119, 144
speculation, vii, 2, 29
speech, x, 60, 94, 105, 111, 124, 126, 127, 136, 187
speed, 7, 11, 12, 28, 80, 169
SPSS, 50, 81
stability, 142
stages, 10, 127, 153, 167
standard deviation, 2, 7, 8, 14, 15, 18, 150
statistics, 114, 196
statutes, 135
stem cells, 44
steroids, 93
stigma, 60
stimulus, ix, x, 4, 5, 7, 13, 30, 75, 76, 77, 82, 83, 86
storage, 2
strain, 178
strategies, x, 24, 27, 36, 47, 55, 105, 134, 136, 138,
    154, 155, 157, 158, 165, 176, 187
streams, 21
strength, 156
stress, vii, viii, ix, 35, 42, 44, 45, 46, 47, 48, 49, 50,
    51, 52, 53, 54, 55, 56, 57, 58, 59, 60, 61, 62, 63,
    65, 66, 67, 68, 69, 70, 71, 72, 73, 74, 118, 121,
    122, 131, 135, 137, 138, 166, 180, 182
stressful events, 70, 73
stressful life events, 128
stressors, 55, 57, 61, 62, 123, 134, 178
students, 2, 8, 13, 24, 56, 87, 138
subgroups, 118, 122
subjectivity, 108
subsidy, 66, 72, 73
suffering, 46, 89, 93, 101, 107
suicidal ideation, 129
supervision, 125, 134
support services, ix, 59, 61, 62, 73
suppression, ix, x, 75, 78, 82, 86
survival, 59, 89, 90, 91, 94, 96, 102, 113, 117, 140,
    187
susceptibility, 77, 96
Sweden, 65, 72, 176, 177, 182, 187
switching, 78
symmetry, xi, 147, 148, 162, 164, 168
sympathetic nervous system, 92
symptom, 111, 130, 176

symptoms, 108, 109, 112, 115, 119, 120, 121, 122,
123, 124, 125, 126, 128, 129, 130, 131, 133, 135,
136, 137, 144
synchronization, 19
syndrome, vii, xi, 1, 2, 3, 4, 5, 7, 10, 13, 31, 32, 37,
42, 43, 44, 50, 51, 57, 60, 61, 62, 63, 64, 65, 66,
67, 70, 71, 72, 73, 74, 89, 90, 92, 93, 96, 97, 100,
101, 102, 103, 111, 112, 113, 114, 115, 117, 118,
119, 125, 126, 140, 141, 143, 144, 147, 166, 169,
170, 171, 172, 173, 174
synthesis, 95, 99, 101
syphilis, 124
systems, 10, 18, 21, 22, 43, 61, 65, 68, 107, 119, 169

T

Taiwan, 140, 178, 182
target behavior, 67, 123
target stimuli, 11, 82
targets, 11, 12
task conditions, ix, x, 76, 80, 81
task demands, 157
task difficulty, 77
task performance, 195
teachers, 65, 136, 181
teaching, 84, 190
technology, xi, 185, 186, 194, 195
temperament, 108, 121
test-retest reliability, 120
thalamus, 97, 153
theory, 10, 32, 61, 63, 73, 85, 87, 144, 152, 169, 171,
172
therapists, 135
therapy, 17, 93, 99, 100, 124, 127, 134, 136
thinking, 121, 127
thiobarbituric acid, 42
threats, 62
thyroid, 124
tic disorder, 122, 132
tics, 127, 132, 133
time, vii, 1, 2, 4, 5, 7, 9, 10, 11, 12, 13, 15, 30, 46,
55, 57, 60, 62, 64, 65, 66, 68, 70, 80, 85, 95, 107,
108, 113, 118, 123, 134, 136, 152, 154, 160, 161,
166, 177, 178, 182, 187, 192, 195
timing, vii, 1, 10, 13, 15, 16, 17, 18, 20, 21, 22, 24,
29, 31, 32, 33
tissue, 42, 101, 133, 134
toddlers, 117, 171
toxic side effect, 130
toxicity, 43

trace elements, 43
tracking, vii, 1, 7, 8, 9, 10, 13, 14, 15, 16, 29, 170
traffic, 78, 79, 82, 84
training, viii, xi, 17, 31, 35, 36, 37, 38, 39, 40, 41,
43, 44, 65, 67, 71, 73, 78, 84, 86, 106, 113, 122,
162, 176, 179, 185, 187, 190, 192, 193, 194, 195
training programs, 41, 84
traits, 163, 165, 168
trajectory, 167
transcription, 31
transformations, 155, 156
transition, 46, 55, 135
transition period, 46
transition to adulthood, 55
transitions, 46
trauma, 69, 93, 111
traumatic brain injury, 101
traumatic experiences, 122
treatment programs, 67
trees, 79
trend, 62, 129
trial, 6, 7, 13, 14, 18, 19, 24, 79, 103
tricyclic antidepressant, 130
tricyclic antidepressants, 130
triglycerides, 40
trisomy, 36, 37, 38, 39, 40, 41, 42
trisomy 21, 36, 37, 38, 39, 40, 41, 42
true/false, 49
tuberous sclerosis, 122
tumor, 42

U

UK, 85, 107, 138, 142, 177, 178, 179
undergraduate, 2, 8, 9, 24
United Kingdom, 107, 113
United States, 60, 106, 112, 127, 140
urinalysis, 124
urine, 95
users, 179

V

validation, 159
validity, 118, 119, 142
values, viii, 36, 38, 39, 40, 69
variability, 5, 17, 31, 114, 119
variable, vii, 1, 2, 4, 9, 10, 13, 16, 19, 20, 26, 28, 55,
114, 119, 178

variables, 38, 50, 52, 78, 84, 134, 144, 178, 179
variance, 50, 162
variation, 10, 19, 20, 26, 27, 55, 113
VEGF, 102
vein, viii, 36, 38
venlafaxine, 130
video games, 161, 166
videotape, 5
vincristine, 102
vision, 106, 128, 160
visual field, ix, 75
visual memory, 86
visual modality, 164
visual perception, 151
visual processing, 169
visual stimuli, ix, x, 76, 151
vitamins, 37
vocabulary, 151
vocalisations, 132
vulnerability, 83, 113, 118, 137, 176

W

waking, 80
Wales, 105, 140
war, 135
warrants, 130
weakness, 151
Wechsler Intelligence Scale, 110, 150
welfare, 177
welfare state, 177
well-being, 49, 57, 58, 65, 67, 177
white matter, 89, 90, 97, 100, 153
withdrawal, 119
women, 42, 47
workers, 195
working memory, 82
World Wide Web, 195
writing, 70, 186

X

X chromosome, 126

Y

young adults, 44, 57
young men, 30, 42, 70